£1.00

WS 141

AF744570

WITHDRAWN
POSTGRADUATE CENTRE
WEXHAM PARK HOSPITAL
SLOUGH, BERKSHIRE
DATE:

SWNHS
C20415095

B. GARREAU

Neuroimaging in child neuropsychiatric disorders

Springer

ISBN 3-540-63634-X Springer-Verlag Berlin Heidelberg New York

LIBRARY OF CONGRESS-IN-PUBLICATION DATA
Neuroimaging and developmental neurophysiology in child psychiatric disorders / Bernard Garreau; [et al.]. 300 p. 19 × 27 cm. Includes bibliographical references and index.
ISBN 2-287-63634-X (hard cover)
1. Pediatric neuropsychiatry. 2. Developmental neurophysiology. 3. Brain-Imaging. I. Garreau, Bernard, 1949. 1. Mental Disorders-in infancy & childhood. 2. Mental Disorders-diagnosis. 3. Magnetic Resonance Imaging. 4. Brain-growth & development. 5. Brain-physiopathology. WS 350 N494 1997] RJ486.5.N48 1997 618.92'89 - dc21 DNLM/DLC for Library of Congress 97-42376 CIP

This work is subject to copyright. All rights are reserved, whether the whole or part of the material is concerned, specifically the rights of translation, reprinting, reuse of illustrations, recitation, broadcasting, reproduction on microfilms or in any other way, and storage in data banks. Duplication of this publication or parts thereof is permitted only under the provisions of the German Copyright Law of September 9, 1965, in its current version, and permission for use must always be obtained from Springer-Verlag. Violations are liable for prosecution under the German Copyright Law.

© Springer-Verlag Berlin Heidelberg 1998
Printed in France

The use of general descriptive names, registered names, trademarks, etc. in this publication does not imply, even in the absence of a specific statement, that such names are exempt from the relevant protective laws and regulations and therefore free for general use.

Product liability: The publishers cannot guarantee the accuracy of any information about dosage and application contained in this book. In every individual case the user must check such information by consulting the relevant literature.

Packaging & Editing: Atelier Brigitte Arnaud, F-75001 Paris.
Design: Michel Ganne.
Printing & Bookbinding: Aubin Imprimeur, F-86240 Ligugé.

SPIN 10511689 90/2918-5 4 3 2 1 0 - Printed on acid-free paper.

Contents

JOHN JAMISON LIBRARY
POSTGRADUATE CENTRE
WEXHAM PARK HOSPITAL
SLOUGH, BERKSHIRE
SL2 4HL

LIST OF CONTRIBUTORS

Jean-Louis Baulieu, MD, PhD
Service de médecine nucléaire in vivo, INSERM U 316, CHU Bretonneau, 2 bd Tonnellé, 37044 Tours Cedex France

Martha Ann Bell, PhD
Department of psychology, Virginia polytechnic institute and state university, Blacksburg, Virginia 24061-0436, USA

Matthew Belmonte, MD
Center for neural science, New York University, 4 Washington Place, Room 809, New York, NY 10003-6621, USA

Nicole Bruneau, PhD
Service universitaire d'explorations fonctionnelles et de neurophysiologie en pédopsychiatrie, INSERM U 316, CHU Bretonneau, 2 bd Tonnellé, 37044 Tours Cedex France

W.I. De Bruin, MD
Department of child psychiatry, Utrecht university hospital, P.O. Box 85500, 3508 GA Utrecht The Netherlands

Jan K. Buitelaar, MD, PhD
Department of child psychiatry, Utrecht university hospital, P.O. Box 85500, 3508 GA Utrecht The Netherlands

Ruth Carper, MD
Department of neurosciences, school of medicine, university of California, San Diego, 9500 Gilman Drive, La Jolla, California 92093-0662 USA

Harry T. Chugani, MD
Division of pediatric neurology/PET center, children's hospital of Michigan, 3901 Beaubien bd, Detroit, MI 48201 USA

Stéphanie Cochin
Service universitaire d'explorations fonctionnelles et de neurophysiologie en pédopsychiatrie INSERM U 316, CHU Bretonneau, 2 bd Tonnellé, 37044 Tours Cedex France

Véronique Delvenne, MD, PhD
Département de psychiatrie, Université libre de Bruxelles, 808 route de Lennik, 1070 Bruxelles Belgium

Claude Dumais-Huber, MSc, DScH
Cell physiology laboratory, Central institute of mental health, J5, 68159 Mannheim Germany

Herbert Van Engeland, MD
Department of child and adolescent psychiatry, university hospital Utrecht, Heidelberglaan 100, P.O. Box 85500, 3508 GA Utrech The Netherlands

Bernard Garreau, MD, PhD
Service universitaire d'explorations fonctionnelles et de neurophysiologie en pédopsychiatrie INSERM U 316, CHU Bretonneau, 2 bd Tonnellé, 37044 Tours Cedex France

Nadine Girard, MD
Université de la Méditérranée, département de radiologie, hôpital nord, 13915 Marseille Cedex 20 France

Marie Gomot
Service universitaire d'explorations fonctionnelles et de neurophysiologie en pédopsychiatrie, INSERM U 316, CHU Bretonneau, 2 bd Tonnellé, 37044 Tours Cedex France

Denis Guilloteau, PhD
Laboratoire de biophysique, faculté de pharmacie, INSERM U 316, 31 avenue Monge, 37200 Tours France

Lisa Jonkman, PhD
Department of analysis and toxicology, section psychofarmacology, university of Utrecht, F.A.F.C. Wentgebouw sorbonnelaan 16, 3508 CA Utrecht, The Netherlands

Chantal Kemner, PhD
Department of child and adolescent psychiatry, university hospital Utrecht, Heidelberglaan 100, P.O. Box 85500, 3508 GA Utrech The Netherlands

Troels W Kjaer, MD
John F Kennedy institute, GI Landevej 7, 2600 Glostrup Denmark

Gilbert F Lelord, MD, PhD
Service universitaire d'explorations fonctionnelles et de neurophysiologie en pédopsychiatrie, INSERM U 316, CHU Bretonneau, 2 bd Tonnellé, 37044 Tours France

Hans C Lou, MD
John F Kennedy institute, GI Landevej 7, 2600 Glostrup Denmark

Joëlle Martineau, PhD
Service universitaire d'explorations fonctionnelles et de neurophysiologie en pédopsychiatrie, INSERM U 316, CHU Bretonneau, 2 bd Tonnellé, 37044 Tours Cedex France

Nancy J Minshew, MD
Departments of psychiatry and neurology, university of Pittsburg, school of medicine, 100 N Bellefield avenue, Bellefield towers, suite 430, Pittsburg, PA 15213 USA

Jay W Pettegrew, MD
Departments of psychiatry and neurology, university of Pittsburg, school of medicine, 100 N Bellefield avenue, Bellefield towers, suite 430, Pittsburg, PA 15213 USA

Charles Raybaud, MD
Université de la Méditérranée, département de radiologie, hôpital nord, 13915 Marseille Cedex 20 France

P.P. Van Rijk, MD, PhD
Department of child psychiatry, Utrecht university hospital, P.O. Box 85500, 3508 GA Utrecht The Netherlands

Mary Robertson, MBCHB, MD, DPM, FRCPsych.
University college London medical school, Middlesex hospital site, Mortimer Street, London WIN 8AA England

Aribert Rothenberger, MD
Kinder-und jugendpsychiatrie, gerg-august universität, Goblerstrabe 23, Göttingen 37073 Germany

Sylvie Roux, PhD
Service universitaire d'explorations fonctionnelles et de neurophysiologie en pédopsychiatrie, INSERM U 316, CHU Bretonneau, 2 bd Tonnellé, 37044 Tours Cedex France

André Syrota, MD, PhD
DSV, DRM, Service hospitalier Frédéric Joliot, CEA, 4, place du Général Leclerc, 91406 Orsay France

M. N. Verbaten, PhD
Department of analysis and toxicology, section psychofarmacology, university of Utrecht, F.A.F.C. Wentgebouw sorbonnelaan 16, 3 CA Utrecht, The Netherlands

Monica Zilbovicius, MD, PhD
INSERM U 316, DRM, DSV, Service hospitalier Frédéric Joliot, CEA, 4, place du Général Leclerc, 91406 Orsay France

Science cannot resolve the
ultimate mystery of nature.
This is because the bottom line is that
we ourselves are part of the mystery
that we are trying to solve.

Max Planck

Introduction

B. GARREAU

Adolescent and child psychiatry is a recent medical speciality which that has been influenced since its birth by a number of psycho analytical ideas. However, in the last fifteen years three broad fields of research have developed, concerning clinical practice, biology and morphological and functional investigations. Clinical research has led to a better definition of abnormalities by proposing criteria for childhood and adolescent mental disorders. Two of these classifications are recognised by the international community: the american psychiatric association's diagnostic statistical manual and the world health organization's international classification of disease. Moreover, the development and use of various methods of assessment has led to considerable advances in early diagnosis. These diagnostic tools have led the clinician to revise his point of view. For instance, childhood autism is now considered as a pervasive developmental disorder. Biological investigations, long oriented towards the definition of biochemical markers, have been enriched by this new clinical approach. Interest has recently shifted to the genetic origin of a number of syndromes in the realm of child psychiatry.

Morphological and functional investigations are at the crossroads of clinical expression and more basic cellular or molecular disorders. These methods have been used to detect concurrent disorders, but also, with other biological studies, to attempt to define markers, as demonstrated by the considerable work devoted to the frontal, temporal or cerebellar hypotheses underlying childhood autism. Their use is currently increasing and the part they play in various fields is likely to grow even more rapidly, particularly pathophysiology and therapeutics, since they are easy to use and yield excellent results.

Such investigations and other biological testes are now orientated towards early development. The central nervous system is constantly changing, from the *in utero* period until a late stage of life, with some phases of substantial, rapid change and others that are more stable. Neuroscience has made considerable progress in the field of cerebral development. Many studies look into the somatic, neurological and behavioural consequences of interference by endogenous or exogenous agents with this developmental processs. In clinical practice this type of interference is usually suspected. In the current state of knowledge, the clinicians' general term "developmental disorder" is apt.

These recent findings are taken into account in this book and a developmental perspective is used as a framework to review the broad trends guiding current research in this field. It is for this reason that the first chapter is devoted to basic aspects of normal development. After presenting the morphological and functional bases of several methods for exploration of the brain, we then concentrate on the results given by the use of these techniques during cerebral maturation. This underlines the importance of age-related morphological and functional modifications. Finally, from this same developmental perspective, we show some examples of brain investigation methods applied to child and adolescent psychiatry.

We do not claim to have carried out an exhaustive review of the literature in this field, but rather to present several studies so as to illustrate the following points:

— obvious ethical rules can be respected while using all morphological and functional exploration methods in paediatrics and particularly in child psychiatry,

— each of these methods has its own clinical applications and limitations. Thus, they are not an end in themselves, but essential tools, their use being determined by the hypothesis we attempt to prove,

— collaboration between child psychiatrists and morphological and functional imaging specialists is necessary and fruitful. Without relegating to the background today's descriptive approach to childhood mental illnesses, which does correspond to clinical reality, child psychiatrists should nevertheless observe and interpret psychiatric symptomatology differently. In the same vein, neurophysiologists or radiologists must keep in mind, while attempting to locate a lesion, that they are exploring a dynamic process with its own temporal pattern. One or more defective elements in this developmental process may cause symptoms, signs or behaviour patterns which defy the laws of normal physiology.

We hope this work will increase awareness among psychiatrists and other clinicians working with children and teenagers and encourage them to co-operate with neuroimaging specialists to improve screening, understanding and treatment of children with mental diseases.

The editing of this book in co-operation with the contributing authors has been a pleasure for me. I also wish to thank:

— Mrs A. Lardeux for illustrating our chapters,

— Mrs L Crespin and M. Barre for their technical assistance,

— Mrs Tovar from Springer-Verlag Éditions in Paris for her friendly support,

My children and my wife for their presence during the creation of this book and for giving me time to do the editorial work.

This book is the result of collaboration between the following organizations:

— Service Hospitalier Frédéric Joliot, DSV-DRM, CEA, Orsay, France, Pr A. Syrota,

— INSERM U 316 Tours, France, Pr L. Pourcelot,

— Université François Rabelais Tours, France, Pr H. Mouray

— CHU Bretonneau Tours, France, Mr M. Moujard,

— Fondation France Télécom, Paris, France, Convention INSERM. Fondation France Télécom 1993.

A child psychiatrist's point of view

G. LELORD (Comité Autisme, France Télécom)

The title of the work by Dr. Bernard Garreau "Neuroimaging in childhood psychiatric disorders" may appear quite ambitious, if not presumptuous. Are not psychiatric childhood disorders both too subtle and too complex to be detected by of the examinations brain? Are these examinations useful in childhood mental disorders? Is not clinical medicine still the only valid discipline in this field? These questions are still posed by many child psychiatrists today.

Dr. Garreau's book clearly shows that research on the safety, validity and reliability of non invasive brain examinations has enabled them to be applied to child psychiatry. Promising results show that different syndromes familiar to clinicians are associated with abnormalities or particularities of electrical, circulatory or secretory activity in the brain.

In this context, autism has been regarded as a painful, emotion-laden "model" of mental disorder in children, who have benefited from these additional examinations early on. It is to be remembered that this syndrome is characterised by a disorder in relations with others (aloneness, withdrawal); difficulties in communicating, with gestures, mimicry, language, bizarre behaviour (impatience, intolerance to change, repeated activities); and disturbances involving perception, motility and emotions. This apparently psychological disorder was long considered to be caused by conscious or unconscious inadequacies or errors of the mother, but decisive examinations have contributed to demonstrating that autism is in fact a disorder of central nervous system function. The history of these examinations has occurred in four steps which were not mutually exclusive.

The first was marked by the study of changing electrical responses of the brain to external stimuli over time (Heuyer et al., 1957). This marked the introduction of functional electroencephalography and showed that the disappearance of the electroencephalogram (EEG) reaction to sound by repetition (habituation) did not occur in autistic teenagers. Inversely, when sound precedes light, the activation normally produced by this signal (anticipation) varies and is even inconstant in these young patients. Study of the EEG has shown that these extremely complex psychological disorders of autistic teenagers are accompanied by more "basic" disorders: the young patient appears not to tire of a simple stimulus that is repeated. He is in difficulty when the stimulus becomes a more complex message.

The second step involved the introduction of functional electroencephalogram averaging techniques (Lelord et al., 1958). They showed that if sound and light are paired several times, sound alone causes an EEG response (evoked potential) in the visual area. This step improved the topographical precision of the EEG and showed that the method could be applied to studying cognitive processes by detecting an "evoked association potential". Work in the following years demonstrated abnormalities in averaged electrical activity in childhood mental pathology. These could involve the "contingent negative variation" of Grey Walter, the "decision wave" (P300) of Samuel Sutton or the "premotor potential" of Kornhüber and Deecke. At the same time, our group noted abnormalities of the "association potential" in childhood autism. The numerous studies of evoked potentials mapping have not been gathered in this book because every three years, since the initial meetings of Dargent and Dongier (1969) and Fessard and Lelord (1972), extensive data were published regularly in the volumes of EPICs (event related potentials international congresses) reporting electrophysiological results in children as well as in adults.

The third step involved studies of cerebral blood flow (Garreau et al., 1994). These studies which our group in Tours through would be of interest arose following a friendly discussion with Pr André Syrota and his team in the Frédéric Joliot Department (SHFJ - CEA - Orsay). In collaboration with Monica Zilbovicius, Bernard Garreau volunteered to conduct pioneering work in childhood autism, thereby turning a research project into reality.

In other pioneering work, Nicole Bruneau (1992) used the Doppler technique developed in the laboratory of Léandre Pourcelot and reported that left hemisphere circulatory reactivity was reduced in the autism syndrome. Bernard Garreau and Monica Zilbovicius (1994) demonstrated decreased circulatory reactivity in the language zone in school-aged children, and (1995) reduced flow-rates in the frontal region of younger patients.

The fourth step occurred as a result of a friendship with Jacques Mallet of Gif-sur-Yvette, and was continued with Jean-Pierre Muh (Herault et al., 1995). This work on childhood autism showed the special features of certain genes involved in the correct function and even development of nerve cells.

The work presented by Bernard Garreau goes beyond the model of autism and addresses a number of childhood psychiatric syndromes. The introduction "Cerebral development and neurophysiological investigations" is remarkable. Its originality resides in the fact that it applies a sort of neuropsychiatric point of view to developmental biology. His comments on nerve cell division and migration, the role of growth factors and the selection of populations of synapses, focus directly on the development of perceptive categorisation and interactive actions. He thinks our knowledge of neuronal genes, in particular the homeogenes controlling development of the antero posterior neural axis, is promising for the understanding of anatomical cerebral and cerebellar abnormalities.

Dr. Garreau goes on to show that the constitution and growth of modules can be expressed at both behavioural and neural levels. The comparison of achievement in the object permanence task and the development of cells in the prefrontal cortex is very striking.

Biochemical and hormonal factors, in particular the development of asymmetry in the brain, are also reviewed, as is the role of the environment and experience. Bernard Garreau concludes with a description of morphological and functional ways of examining the brain which can be applied at different steps in the development of the child and in the course of varied psychopathological events.

Chapter 2, by Jean-Louis Baulieu, is a very clear presentation. The points out the value of the methods discussed in the study of neurotransmitters, receptors and transporters. After the initial work on multiple biochemical examinations performed by Mary Coleman (1976), we studied neurotransmitter derivatives in pervasive childhood developmental disorders with Jean-Pierre Muh. We noted that the levels in certain groups of autistic children were very different from those in control groups. Peripheral levels of homovanillic acid, a dopamine derivative, for example, could be greatly increased. The value is similar to that in very young children, and the decrease related to maturation, particularly marked from seven years of age, does not occur in autistic children. Imaging with markers and radioligands of dopamine, serotonin and endorphins will probably lead to a better understanding of the role of these metabolic features in behavioural disorders of children with biochemical anomalies.

The chapter on the anatomical and physiological bases of the electroencephalogram, by Bernard Garreau was indispensable. First, the cellular bases of the electrical activity of the brain are analysed, then the electrical events of synaptic transmission are described. This leads to a better understanding of the anatomical and physiological bases of the main EEG rhythms. Such an overview is a welcome addition to the literature. The EEG remains a very useful and relatively "simple" method, particularly convenient for use in young children and still remains promising. The relationships between the EEG and states of awareness have been known for a long time, but knowledge of the changes in distribution of cerebral electrical activity as a function of precise tasks enables the mechanism of certain cognitive operations to be better understood. The study of spectral consistency provides new data on the functional relationships of different areas of the cortex. In addition, three-dimensional analysis techniques extend our knowledge of cortical activity and provide information on the functioning of sub-cortical sources. Our child psychiatry group makes extensive use of EEG.

Magnetic resonance imaging (MRI) and cerebral development are very clearly presented by Charles Raybaud and Nadine Girard. This imaging technique has proved, extremely sensitive to changes in brain parenchymal changes and is therefore well suited to depiction of the successive steps in brain maturation. The authors relate the main steps of cerebral development (organogenesis and histogenesis: multiplication, differenciation and migration of neuroblasts; development of the glia; myelination) to the morphological characteristics seen on magnetic resonance images of the foetal brain. Imaging of the infant brain from birth to 18 months is then documented.

MRI affords an exquisite description of morphology in clinical practice at very early stages showing: brain malformations, infections, neuroectodermal syndromes, progressive encephalopathies.etc. But the more frequent clinical problem is assessment of lesions in hypoxic ischaemic encephalopathies of preterm and term neonates. The authors have followed 60 patients for at least two years. They demonstrate the prognostic value of MR data concerning the outcome, both neurological and cognitive, in these patients.

The chapter by Harry T. Chugani, "The ontogeny of cerebral glucose metabolism", is a seminal contribution of great importance. He demonstrates increases in glucose utilisation by 2-3 months in the parietal, temporal and primary visual cortex, in basal ganglia and cerebellar hemispheres, which coincide with the improvement of visuo spatial and sensorimotor integration, the reorganisation of brain stem reflex neonatal behaviour, and increasing cortical EEG activity. There is an increase in glucose consumption in the frontal cortex, particularly the lateral and inferior portions, before the age of six months. Subsequently, around the age of 10 years, glucose metabolism in the cerebral cortex begins to decrease. Chugani links these observations to the different stages of cognitive and emotional development, i.e. visual perception, interactions with the environment, improved performance in the delayed response task and, later on, the acquisition of language skills. He notes that the moment of "autistic regression" in some young patients corresponds to a period of rapid increases in cerebral glucose metabolism.

M.A. Bell presents a valuable review of EEG research, adding her personal original research conducted mainly on infants. She reviews classic EEG development studies from the 1930 s to the 1960 s which remain the cornerstone of the clinical assessment of the examination, showing the ontogeny of the EEG, its gradual increase with age and later the maturational cycles in EEG power and consistency. The EEG is today an indispensable examination in children because of its uncomplicated nature, the case of repeated examinations in longitudinal studies, the possibilities of recording and administering cognitive tasks. Bell demonstrates that the inclusion of cognitive measures in EEG research in infant provides additional information on the neurophysiological processes involved in maturation. She mentiones that several workers have studied EEG maturation cycles using the Piaget stages of cognitive development and places EEG in a special position in research on frontal function and its role in temporal skills, language production and psychomotor processes.

Nicole Bruneau describes a very refined work on the development of a major component of cortical evoked potentials, the N1 wave, throughout childhood. The electric generators of this wave include the temporal auditory cortex, associative regions and frontal areas. In adults, this wave is recorded with maximal amplitude at frontocentral sites, peaking at about 100ms post-stimulation, whereas in children the auditory response displays maximal amplitude at the midtemporal sites, with a positive wave at about 100ms and a large negative wave at approximately 170 ms. Moreover, the modulatory effects of intensity on N1 amplitude are prominent at frontocentral sites in adults and at temporal sites in children.

Before six years of age, an N1 wave of large amplitude is recorded over the frontal area various intermediate aspects between adults and children recordings appear from 7 to 12 years and the very precise data obtained by the author in scalp recordings enable her to discuss the deep generators of these components.

This study is relevant to a number of childhood disorders. Reverse hemisphere dominance was observed in language-impaired children by several workers. Bruneau observed that the amplitude of N1 was significantly lower in autistic than in normal children. Moreover, the intensity effect found at both temporal sites in normal children was not found on the left in autistic children.

Such functional results show how evoked potentials studies are still up-to-date and encourage researchers to make comparisons between the EEG and other imaging techniques such as SPECT and PET in childhood disorders.

Claude Dumais-Huber and Aribert Rothenberger make a thorough and personal contribution to the study of fronto central electric brain activity in normal boys. Their method of electro oculogram (EOG) correction makes it possible to present data on not only the early, but also the late slow negative potentials, which are very difficult to obtain without artefacts in children. they show that EOG correction improves the quality of EEG signals by not only subtracting eye movement-related artefacts, but also enhancing the signal-to-noise ratio. These methods and results are very promising in many childhood psychiatric disorders in which frontal dysfunction is suspected.

In the second part of the book, devoted to pathophysiology, the main childhood neuropsychiatric syndromes are discussed. Tourette's syndrome is characterised by multiple motor tics and one or more vocal tics. Associated behaviour patterns include coprolalia, imitation and attention deficits; obsessive compulsive disorders are also frequent. Mary Robertson reviews several studies conducted with computed tomography (CT) and MRI which draw attention to various cerebral abnormalities (basal ganglia, ventricular size, cavum of the septum lucidum etc.). From recent MRI work, she concludes that this method is reasonably consistent in showing abnormalities of cerebral lateralisation, especially in the caudate nucleus, other basal ganglia structures and normal ventricular asymmetry.

J.K. Buitelaar, W.I. de Bruin and P.P. van Rijk review single photon emission computed tomography (SPECT) studies in this syndrome. Reduced cerebral perfusion has been found in the left putamen, globus pallidus and thalamus, left caudate nucleus, the anterior cingulate areas, and the left dorsolateral frontal area. Studies with a dopamine radioligand (IBZM) revealed decreased binding in the basal ganglia. Using SPECT with technetium (HMPAO), the authors describe an extensive study in children with a combination of Tourette's syndrome and attention deficit disorders: uptake of the radioligand was reduced in three regions on the left side of the brain, the thalamus and frontal and temporal cortex.

Attention deficit disorders are characterised by attention deficit, impulsiveness and temper tantrums. Hans C. Lou and Troels W. Kjaer used SPECT to show a bilateral trend to striatal flow which accompanied increased demands for verbal awareness.

They suggest that a frontal striatal circuit subserving awareness may be impaired by striatal dysfunction in these patients.

In his paper "Electrical brain activity and motor control in Tourette's syndrome and attention deficit disorders", Aribert Rothenberger presents very recent precise electrophysiological data. He carefully studies the negative potentials which precede (premotor or bereitschaft potential, contingent negative variation) and follow (post imperative negative variation) movement. He also uses in adults a technique of transcranial magnetic stimulation which yields information about cortical excitability. He suggests a complete assessment of function of the motor cortex and the fronto cortical system in children with Tourette's syndrome and attention deficit hyperactivity disorders. In tic disorders, the asymmetry in amplitude between left and right primary motor cortex tended to be smaller than in normals and the amplitude of premotor potentials higher over the supplementary motor area. These children also exhibit lower amplitude in some components of the contingent negative variation and post imperative variation. In hyperkinetic children, the amplitude of the premotor potential is reduced over the primary motor cortex and topographical differentiation is weakened along the antero posterior as well as the left-right axes.

Matthew Belmonte and Ruth Carper, members Eric Courchesne's group, describe the panorama of neuroanatomical and neurophysiological aspects of childhood autism. They remind us that this syndrome is a pervasive disorder involving both perceptual processes and interactions with the surrounding world. Precise abnormalities can be observed in autism that are suggestive of temporal dysfunction is: language disorder, decreased tendency to initiate social contact; parietal: lack of attention control, deficits in cross-modal association and frontal: disturbances in executive function and in communication. This diversity suggests malfunction in the reticular formation, brainstem and diencephalic network of the limbic system, basal ganglia and frontal lobe, and of right and left hemispheric balance. The cerebellum, closely connected to the prefrontal cortex, was also studied. It plays a role not only in motility, but also in cognition and language. The authors mention that transmitter systems (dopamine, serotonin, endorphin) involve a large number of these structures and are themselves growth factors whose modification can change cerebral function very early.

Monica Zilbovicius presents a nove promising SPECT study of autistic children. Measurements carried out to date in autistic adults and school-aged children have failed to detect focal anomalies. The author suggests a very simple activation method involving the use of non verbal auditory stimuli. In contrast to controls, autistic children with a dramatic impairment of language acquisition did not activate the posterior associative cortex in the left, language-dominant hemisphere, but did show activation in the right posterior cortex. These findings can be related to both language impairment in autism and to the peculiar spatial abilities shown by some of these children. The results are extended by a longitudinal study in pre school children showing transient frontal hypoperfusion in 2 to 4 year-old autistics. This transient abnormality appears to correspond to cognitive difficulties observed at this age and suggests failure of regulation of neuronal maturation in these children.

The paper by Nancy Minshew and Jay Pettegrew on "Phosphorus magnetic resonance spectroscopy" gives promising data in neuronal events in childhood autism. The authors recall numerous cognitive studies performed in autistic children and conclude that the main deficits involve complex ability in reasoning, memory, language and motor domains, with preservation of simple ability within them. They describe structural abnormalities detected by neuropathological studies as well as cerebral dysfunction revealed by positron and single photon emission tomography.

Their own work uses both very careful neuropsychological investigations and the most recent techniques allowing measures of brain metabolism. They show with phosphorus magnetic resonance spectroscopy remarkable relationships between phospholipid metabolism and clinical deficits. They observe that a positive correlation between falling phosphocreatinine levels and declining test performance is consistent with a hypermetabolic state.

Such findings suggest that brain development in childhood autism is interrupted at a stage of overgrowth and underpruning of neocortex to attain normal connectivity with limbic and cerebellar structures.

The third part of the book is particularly devoted to diagnosis and treatment.

EEG investigations in autistic children were carefully analysed by Stéphanie Cochin and Joëlle Martineau. Several groups have reported spike and spike and wave abnormalities in about 20 % of autistic subjects. Great variations in prevalence (from 4 to more than 30 %) in different studies probably depend on the severity of the syndrome and on the presence of clinical epilepsy. Other workers showed decreased spectral power in the normal alpha band, contrasting with increased delta and sometimes beta rythms. Abnormal orientating reactions and habituation with EEG, electrodermal, respiratory, heart rate recordings were also observed. A very consistent finding is reduced or reversed hemisphere asymetry both at rest and during various cognitive tasks (verbal and nonverbal auditory stimulation, motor imitation etc.). These findings support clinical studies which emphasise abnormal development of hemisphere balance and of normal left hemisphere dominance in autistic children.

A promising investigation is proposed by the authors.Since the initial observations of Schopler, deficiencies in imitative skills have been described in autistic children by many authors, notably in infants by Sauvage's group. Some years ago, we observe that the EEG could reveal imitative reactions over the motor area of individuals looking at a film of an actor performing a movement. Cochin and Martineau have recently performed a study of this "EEG imitation" with much more refined tools (video film alternating fixed or animated grounds, EEG spectral analysis and topographical mapping) in normal adults. They are undertaking a similar study in normal and autistic children.

Véronique Delvenne reports neuroimaging findings in young people with eating disorders. Anorexia nervosa, whose prime symptom is weight loss, accompanied by disturbances in perception of body shape, restlessness and hyperactivity. This syndrome usually commences at puberty, whereas bulimia generally begins around the of 18 years age. Follow-up studies have shown relationships between these two syndromes; bulimia is often associated with strategies for preventing weight gain. The most consistent finding in CT studies is cortical sulcal enlargement, MRI demonstrates a smaller hypophysis and SPECT increased bloodflow in the inferior frontal cortex. Using positron emission tomography (PET) with cognitive tasks in patients with bulimia, Delvenne found increased metabolism in the right frontal cortex and a decrease in the parietal and anterior cingulate cortex. The inconsistency of the results may be explained in part by the influence of nutritional factors and associated pathology.

Joëlle Martineau makes an important contribution concerning pharmacological treatment in autistic children, assessed by what we call the "three marker method". She combines clinical assessment (rating scales), electrophysiological recordings (sound- and light-evoked potential conditioning) and biochemical techniques (monoamine derivatives, particularly homovanillic acid Double-blind and medium- or long-term studies were combined, which compared the effect of vitamin B6 or Mg (catalyst) given separately, and together. She observed higher amplitude and lower variability of conditioned evoked potentials, and decrease of homovanillic acid in B6 + Mg sensitive children. Conditioned evoked responses before treatment were highly variable and homovanillic acid levels were high. She advances several hypotheses to explain the pharmacological activity of vitamin B6 enhancement of dopamine turnover, increased dopamine receptor sensitivity or more complex enzyme deficiencies. This method is a good example of a multi disciplinary contribution, including pharmacology, to brain imaging studies.

Herbert von Engeland and his colleagues, use evoked potentials recordings and show the different sensitivity electroclinical profile between autistic and hyperkinetic children. In the past decade their research group has carried out important series of evoked potential studies in childhood psychiatric patients.

The contribution of Sylvie Roux concerns the multivariate descriptive statistical method in populations of developmentally disordered children, but it gives only a partial look into the work of this engineer in our group. The latter can be described as "reciprocal enrichment obtained by daily co-operation among clinicians, neurophysiologists and computer specialists". As a result of the aspects envisioned by Sylvie Roux, the clinicians and neurophysiologists multiplied their approaches and further defined their assessments. Reciprocal exchanges of information led the engineer to become familiar with the clinical and neurophysiological aspects of autism. The hidden but most novel aspect of this work lies in the resulting exchanges which have given rise to new orientations. The fruitful results of this collaboration are illustrated by three examples.

In an initial study, correspondence analysis identified new major dimensions of behaviour (contact, attention, auditory perception, sensory motility, imitation and verbal communication) in children with developmental disorders. In a second study, relationships were sought between behaviour patterns and certain electrocortical reactivity patterns (intensity of disorders and frontocentral function, attention disturbances and frontocentral reactivity). A third study has further defined bioclinical parameters bearing on autistic behaviour, intellectual impairment and communication disorders. This multidimensional approach involving a clinician and a neurophysiologist has opened new and interesting perspectives for pathophysiological, bioclinical and therapeutic studies.

What are the future perspectives for all this research in neuroimaging and developmental neurophysiology? To and by invoking the example of the intensive studies of pervasive developmental disorders in Tours, we can say that these perspectives are founded on clinical studies, our understanding of cerebral function and molecular biology.

Clinical considerations remind us first that all examinations carried out involve the special Hippocratic relationship between a child, his family and the physician (Sauvage, 1988; Barthélémy et al., 1995). This indispensable and undoubtedly external relationship, however, does not suffice of itself, since it is now recognised that cerebral images are useful to clinical practice. They require renewed observation, interpretation and the definition of the facts observed daily by the clinician. Assessments have thus become necessary, bearing not only on the past history, symptoms and signs, but also on deficient functions (attention, perception, association, imitation, motility, contact and communication), investigated with neurophysiological (Barthélémy et al., 1995) and neuropsychological (Adrien, 1996) methods. This functional analysis is particularly suited to children aged up to 3 years, where the clinician uses not only video techniques, but home movies recorded by many families starting at the child's birth, i.e. before the diagnosis has been made (Sauvage, 1988). This research, combining clinical and imaging data, may have immediate therapeutic implications, providing the opportunity to orientate and define educative psychotherapeutic modalities: exchange and development treatment.

The unifying subject of this book is the study of cerebral function by neuroimaging. The results to be expected in this field from the development of simple psychological and cognitive tests of the young patient performed during the recordings can now be seen. Progress in the use of biochemical markers will also enable us to identify the systems involved during these tests. These cerebral examinations are useful not only for understanding the mechanism of certain deficiencies, but also for evaluating the effects of treatment. For example, it is known that exercise can modify cerebral blood flow. The favourable effect of physical therapy on circulatory insufficiencies (frontal, left hemisphere, etc.) may become better understood.

Molecular biology research look very promising. With Jean-Pierre Muh and his co workers, our group recently demonstrated the characteristics of a gene in autism: Engrailed-2, whose role in the development of the cerebellum is known (Petit et al., 1995). The therapeutic consequences of these recent findings are not immediately evident. Pervasive development disorders are multifactorial syndromes and in most cases not familial diseases in the strict sense. We also know that transmission of vulnerability is very complex. But in our daily lives, we are exposed to substances that modify our genes without our knowledge, i.e. nicotine weakens the action of genes that protect us from cancer. We also know that folic acid can rectify the fragility of a chromosome *in vitro*. It is probable that one day we will learn that remedies used for an entirely different reason (vitamin B6 perhaps) can reinforce or attenuate the effect of a given gene. But for the present, we cannot claim that research on the features of H-Ras or Engrailed genes has immediate consequences.

All this research demands considerable caution, restraint and humanity by those who carry it out. This is indeed the case for Dr. Garreau, an eminent member of our group for 20 years, whose consultations and counsel are greatly appreciated by the children and their families. In the field of cerebral imaging, the object of this work, we are confident in the ability of this neurologist/physiologist and his young co worker, Mrs. Monica Zilbovicius, psychiatrist and biophysicist, as well as Nicole Bruneau, Joëlle Martineau and Sylvie Roux, and in all the authors contributing to this excellent book, to practice and accompany these delicate examinations in. the interest of each child.

References

Heuyer G, Popov C, Lelord G (1957) Étude EEG des réponses aux stimuli simples et combinés des schizophrènes adolescents. IIe Cong Int Psychiat Zurich 4, p 123-134

Lelord G, Calvet J, Fourment A, Scherrer J (1958) Le conditionnement de la réponse évoquée électrocorticale chez l'homme. CR Soc Biol 152: 1097-2000

Fessard A, Lelord G (1972) Averaged evoked responses and their conditioning in normal subjects and psychiatric patients. Int. Colloquium. Tours. INSERM, Paris

⁂

Adrien JL (1996) Autisme du jeune enfant. Développement psychologique et régulation de l'activité. Expansion Scientifique Française, Paris

Barhélémy C, Hameury L, Lelord G (1995) La thérapie d'échange et de développement dans l'autisme de l'enfant. Expansion Scientifique Française, Paris

Bruneau N, Dourneau MC, Garreau B, Pourcelot L, Lelord G (1992) Blood flow responses to auditory stimulations in normal, mentally retarded and autistic children. A transcranial Doppler ultrasonography study in the middle cerebral arteries. Biol Psychiat 32: 691-699

Coleman (1976) The autistic syndromes. North-Holland Publishing Company, New York

Dargent J, Dongier M (1969) Variations contingentes négatives. In: Les congrès et les colloques de l'Université de Liège, Liège

Garreau B, Zilbovicius M, Guerin P, Samson Y, Syrota A, Lelord G (1994) Effects of an auditory stimulation on regional cerebral blood flow in autistic children. Dev Brain Dysfunc 7: 119-128

Herault J, Petit E, Martineau J, Perrot A, Lenoir P, Cherpi C, Barthélémy C, Sauvage D, Mallet J, Muh JP, Lelord G (1994). Autism and genetics: Clinical approach and association study with two markers of H-RAS gene. Am J Med Genet 60: 276-281

Petit E, Herault J, Martineau J, Perrot A, Barthélemy C, Hameury L, Sauvage D, Lelord G (1995) Association study with two markers of a human homeogene in infantile autism. J Med Genet 32: 269-274

Sauvage D (1988) Autisme du nourrisson et du jeune enfant. Masson, Paris

Zilbovicius M, Garreau B, Samson Y, Remy Ph, Barthélémy C, Syrota A, Lelord G (1995) Delayed maturation of the frontal cortex in childhood autism. Am J Psychiat 152: 248-252

A radiologist's point of view

A. SYROTA

In view of various methods' expansion during the last ten years, neuroimaging has come of age in the realm of the neurosciences.This speciality now has its own methods, tools and fields of practice — image processing, animal models, human physiopathology, diagnosis, pharmacology — and even raises unique ethical questions. Psychiatry, and even more so developmental psychiatry, is a field that should necessarily profit from the use of these techniques.

Bernard Garreau's book has the merit of insisting on brain maturation and demonstrating that no matter what morphological or functional neuroimaging method is used, it is important to take into account the main stages of brain development. Using a theoretical model, Bernard Garreau's first chapter outlines the multiple elements involved in development of the central nervous system. It is then possible to imagine the consequences, especially on learning and behavior, of abnormal development of one of these elements, and also to understand the potential insights offered by neuroimaging methods.

Three methods are mainly developped in this book, cerebral electrophysiology (EEG, evoked potentials), single photon emission computed tomography (SPECT) and positon emission tomography (PET). There are various brain investigation methods which way according to the tracer, the detector and the field investigated. They have in common the provision of functional information, i.e. flow, perfusion, metabolism and synaptic mechanisms. The dosimetric data are of particular importance in children. The technical bases of imaging modalities are essential in order to understand the value and limitations of SPECT and PET methods. Thus, Jean Louis Baulieu reviews, not only the physical principles underlying SPECT and PET, but also the anatomical and physiological methods that they imply: mesuring cerebral blood flow and glucose consumption, marking synaptic receptors and transporters. Bernard Garreau adopts the same approach to descibe the anatomical and physiological basis of electrophysiology. Taking another angle, Claude Dumais-Huber and Aribert Rothenberger show the importance of subsidiary factors that ensure the quality of electrophysiological recordings. Their description of the influence of eye movements on recording evoked potentials is a model that can be applied to all functional neuroimaging methods and to their specific examination conditions.

The five following chapters are well justified in this book, addressing several different aspects of brain maturation. Charles Raybaud and Nadine Girard put the accent on the morphological evolution of the central nervous system during life in utero and the first three months after birth. This morphological development must obviously be taken into account in functional neuroimaging studies and in developmental neurophysiology. For example, variations of topography, morphology, latency and amplitude of the components of evoked potentials may be caused by age-linked evolutions of the orientation of their generators. The important role played by developmental factors is also found in the two following studies: Harry T Chugani's description of the stages of metabolic development as shown by measurement of glucose consumption by PET, and Nancy Minshew and Jay W Pettegrew's analysis of brain metabolism by spectroscopic NMR. The variations in function of age are analyzed in electroencephalograms by Martha A Bell and in evoked potentials by Nicole Bruneau and Marie Gomot.

The findings discussed in this section of the book are fundamental. It is astounding to discover such concordant results reported by different authors using different methods. The consequences are of two natures. First, even though this may appear self-evident, studies of children must take into account the main stages of brain development. This means that they must be done on rather narrow comparable age groups. Secondly, this concordance tends to prove the validity of all of these methods.

The second part of Bernard Garreau's book concerns the use of morphological and functional imaging in child and adolescent psychiatry. Far from being an exhaustive overview of all methods used or all diseases under study, this section has the merit of showing the diversity and complementarity of different techniques used to study several important syndromes.

Mary Robertson's chapter presents a review of litterature on tododensimetry and MRI findings in Tourette's syndrome. The apparent contradiction between the results of various studies confirms the important role of the age factor; M. Robertson again justly emphasizes that inclusion of children belonging to a single age grouped is a necessity. On the other hand, chapters by J K Buitelaar, WI de Bruin and P.P. van Rijk and by H.C. Lou and T.W. Kjaer show two complementary physiopathological applications of SPECT in Tourette's disorder and in attention-deficit/hyperactivity disorder. J.K. Buitelaar and colleagues measure regional cerebral blood flow by SPECT using HMPAO among children with Tourette's and attention-deficit disorder as compared with children with attention-deficit disorder alone. H.C. Lou and T.W. Kjaer measure regional cerebral blood flow by SPECT using inhaled xenon among children with attention-deficit disorder alone. These two chapters do not only converge towards comparable findings but both teams go beyond nosographic classifications, suggesting functional definitions of symptomatology. Moreover, they raise the critical question of control groups in child studies. This work is remarkably complemented by Aribert Rothenberger's chapter underlining the contribution of electrophysiological techniques to the study of these disorders. The three chapters underline the complementarity of different methods and their choice according to the aspects under study: anatomical-functional systems in some cases and synchronization of several physiological phenomena in others.

The same approach is used in the next four chapters on childhood autism. A morphological and neurophysiological analysis is provided by M. Belmonte and R. Carper who, using a hypothesis of abnormal cerebellar development in autism, describe the physiological effects of this anomaly on the subsequent development of other systems. Monica Zilbovicius, through measures of regional cerebral blood flow and the influence of auditory stimuli on its modification, and Nancy Minshew and Jay W. Pettegrew, through an analysis of cerebral metabolism using spectroscopic NMR, underline changes observed in abnormalities as the child gets older. These findings insist again on the importance of taking the age factor into account and confirm autism's inclusion among developmental disorders.

Stéphanie Cochin and Joëlle Martineau develop a research in motion perception impairment in autistic children using electrophysiological methods and try to demonstrate changes in cortical rhythms. Spectral analysis and topographical mapping are performed during sequencies of a film. Correlations with clinical assessment are an interesting application of this method. Véronique Delvenne has the same approach using PET in eating disorders in youth people.

The last three chapters address the potential interest of brain imaging, and especially cerebral electrophysiology, in revealing signs of response to treatment or even predicting it. This classical approach is defined by Joëlle Martineau in autism and by H van England, MN Verbaten, L Jonkman and C Kemmer in autistic as hyperkinetic children. Many studies have been published with this aim but their expected practical consequences are not yet evident. Sylvie Roux's chapter is more innovative: she attempts to define biochemical profiles of autistic children, imagining that children with different profiles may respond to different treatments. This approach is certainly an interesting application of the study of neurotransmitters' receptors and transporters. As Bernard Garreau observes in his conclusion, the gap between today's technical possibilities and their actual use in child and adolescent psychiatry seems surprising. Instead of being curtailed by the reasons he evoques: specific ethical issues, psychiatry's clinical complexity, even more present in developmental psychiatry, the rapid evolution of methods, the development of these techniques should be facilitated by this situation. The last few years' progress and the applications that it makes possible should make further investigation among children easier. Development of functional NMR and magnetoencephalography, and coupling morphological and functional methods are promising factors.

It is evident that uncontrolled development of costly facilities is inconceivable. But these units are necessary and even indispensable in order to validate specific techniques and guide their future users' decisions. In recent years, imaging centres have proposed their equipment and know-how to clinicians, inciting them to adjust their hypotheses in order to profit from what these methods had to offer. From now on, the available range of techniques is wide enough to reverse this tendancy. Today, psychiatrists should propose hypotheses and radiologists should guide their choice of a method. This approach requires intensive collaboration between specialists in different fields.

We hope that Bernard Garreau's book will foster this cooperation because it is essential for high quality research and good medical practice.

Part One

Methods and cerebral development

1. Cerebral development and neurophysiological investigations

B. GARREAU

Most childhood psychiatric syndromes appear at a well defined stage of development (Fig. 1) which in part determines their clinical picture. Thus, autism appears very early and affects all adaptive functions: perception, posture-motility, language and communication (Sauvage, 1984). Clinicians justly use the term "pervasive developmental disorders". Schizophrenia appears later and does not affect motor or perception functions and is limited to disorders in consistency of thought (Bleuler, 1911). The first signs of the Gilles de la Tourette syndrome appear only around the age of 7 years and eating disorders such as anorexia bulimia at the onset of adolescence. In addition, symptoms progress with age and childhood psychiatric syndromes are thus intimately linked with the development of the central nervous system in both their genesis and their advancement (Evrard et al., 1992). The causes of these syndromes may be endogenous, e.g. a defect in the expression of development genes, or exogenous such as congenital rubella or certain environmentally-linked disorders. It is clear that these endogenous or exogenous causes affect cerebral development, but the aetiological search in childhood psychiatric syndromes remains problematic. Applying imaging and developmental neurophysiology techniques contributes to this procedure, in addition to the value of these techniques for physiopathological analysis.

Nevertheless, the use of these methods should take into account less the description of the disorder than functional symptomatology and above all the stage of cerebral development.

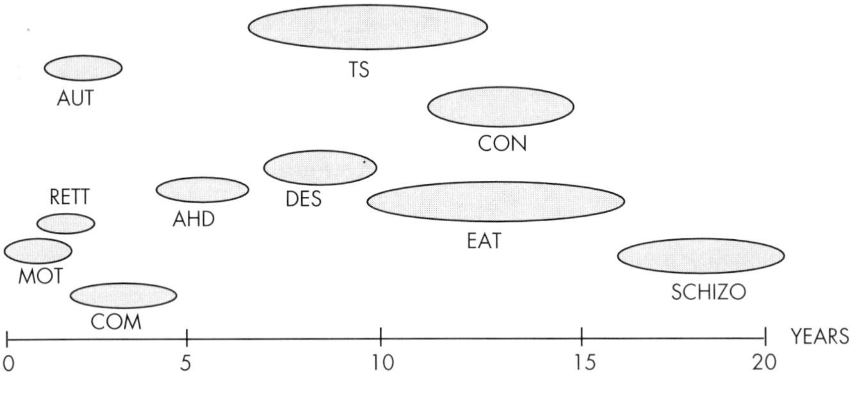

Fig. 1
Stage of development and main pedopsyciatric syndromes
AUT: Autistic disorder;
RETT: Rett syndrome;
MOT: Motor skills disorder;
AHD: Attention and hyperkinetic disorders;
TS: Tourette syndrome;
SCHIZO: Schizophrenic disorder;
COM: Communication disorder;
DES: Disruptive behavior disorder;
CON: Conduct disorder;
EAT: Eating didorders.

In this chapter I look at major current hypotheses the principal steps of cerebral development and finally the major functional levels of the central nervous system. The aim is not an exhaustive presentation of embryogenesis and maturation of the central nervous system, but merely to stress the principal steps of macroscopic, cellular development and synaptic development and to point out the major concepts which today are guidelines for research in this field.

Hypotheses of cerebral development

The development of neurons, synapses and dendrites, neuronal death and synaptic elimination, myeliniation, electrical activity of the brain and glucose consumption all change from the in utero period until adulthood. In parallel, mobility, language, conceptualisation, social interactions and emotions all progress. Since these anatomical, functional, cognitive and behavioural characteristics all change simultaneously, their development must be correlated, in at least overall (Fisher and Rose, 1994). For example, in rhesus monkeys growth and thinning of dendrites and synapses occurs in large cortical regions during cycles which approximately parallel major changes in behaviour patterns (Changeux and Danchin, 1976, Goldman rakic, 1987, Changeux and Dehaene, 1989). In humans, electrical activity in the cortex, a reflection of the operation of neuronal networks and their connections, develops according to patterns closely related to cognitive development and language (Thatcher, 1991).

Theoretical aspects

Behind this overall age-related evolution, the existence of a high degree of synchrony has been shown in the hierarchical development model of Fisher, based on Edelman's theory of the selection of neuronal groups (1987). The basis of Edelman's theory is the hypothesis according to which inputs, already decoded at the subcortical level, undergo parallel processing by a number of networks of cortical neurons. These neuronal networks are genuine modules, each capable of analysing one component of the inputs. In addition, they have their own memory register and co-ordinate their activity and processing to provide an adapted behaviour. Constitution and co-ordination of these anatomico functional modules occurs in three large phases during development (Fig. 2).

At a very early stage of development a cell division phase occurs. During this phase, the activities of many genetically determined factors such as development genes, cell adhesion molecules (CAM) or neuronal growth factors, favour is the selection and growth of definitive neurons and their prolongations, and the programmed death of other nerve cells. At the end of this first phase, synaptic proliferation lead is to the formation of a large number of potential neuronal circuits.

During the second phase, the preceding factors, coupled with experience, lead to the selection of varied populations of synapses, and to the formation of preferential neuronal circuits. These circuits are reproducibly activated by one component of sensory inputs every time this component is present. The constitution of these circuits is shown by the reinforcement of some synapses and by the weakening of others.

The third phase involves the establishment of interactive and co-ordinated anatomico functional modules. Preferential reinforcement and weakening of synaptic networks leads to the formation of modules, i.e., neuronal networks which can analyse a more or less complex component of the inputs. After a certain time and according to a parallel operating mode, interactive neuronal connections are established between different modules which receive independent inputs. The parallel processing of information by individual modules capable of decoding more or less complex components from sensory inputs enables all the modules to provide co-ordinated, simultaneous activity. In addition, experience will enable each of the modules to form its own memory register, whose dynamics will depend on experience.

This principle of the parallel processing of information by co-ordinated, interactive and constituent modules in the course of time, along with development of their own memory register, leads to the phenomenon Edelman calls perceptive categorisation. In order to generate an adapted action, this modular perception and global perception interacts with three structures: the cerebellum, the basal ganglia and the hippocampus.

The cerebellum has direct connections with the cerebral cortex and the spinal cord. It is not indispensable for triggering movement but does play a specific role in its spatial synchronisation and temporal synchronisation (Ivry, 1993). Along with the motor cortex it is the basis for the harmonious production of a gesture. For example, Courchesne et al. (1988) reported hypoplasia of the cerebellar vermis in autistic children; even though the autistic child is in control of fine manipulation considered to involve the pyramidal system, he is clumsy in postural-motor adaptations. The basal ganglia, located at the base of the cerebrum, participate in the planning of motor events and in the choice of types and motor

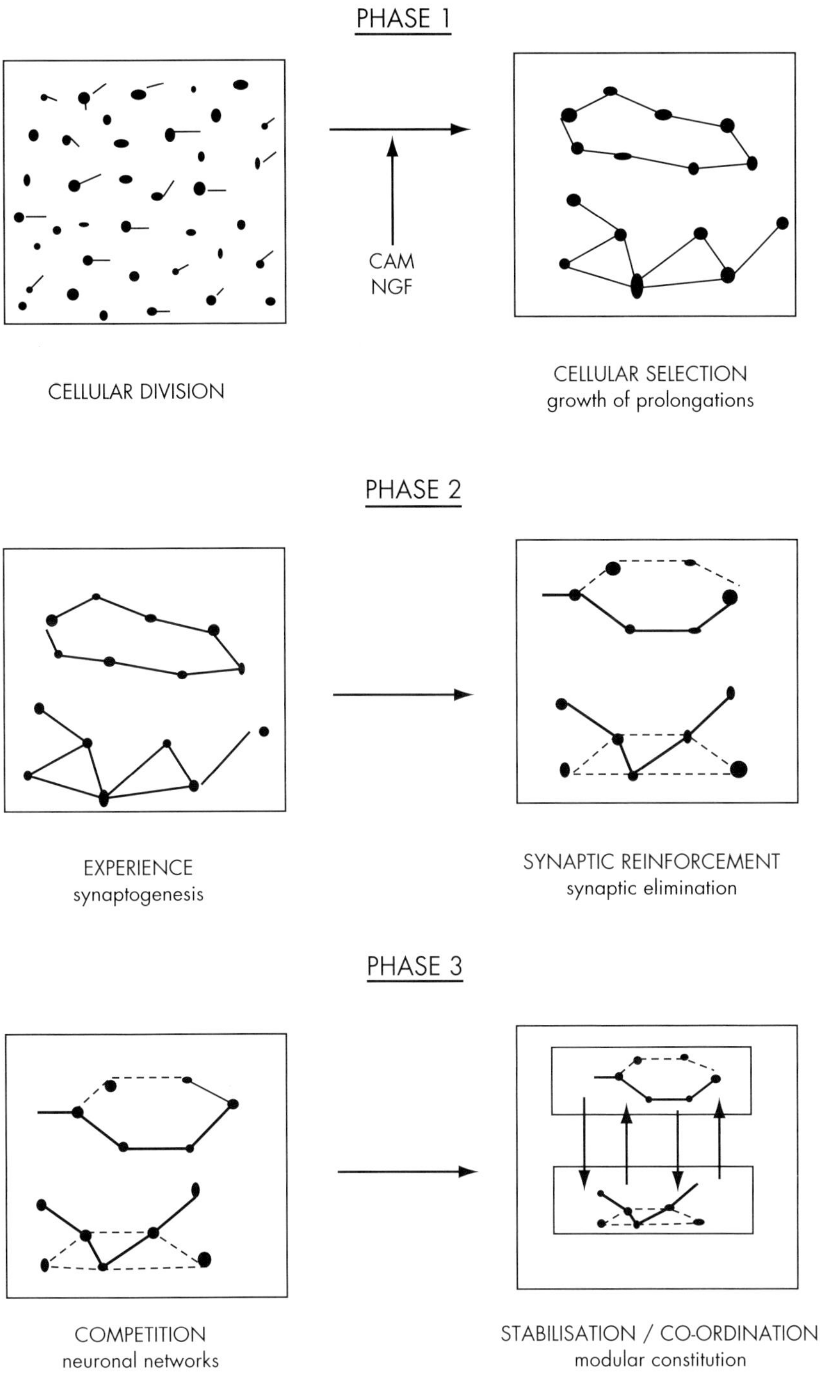

Fig. 2
The theory of neuronal group selection (From Edelman, 1987)

outputs. Thus, not only do the contribute to the regulation of movements via motor programs by coupling overall perceptive responses and motor responses, but they also aid in orienting action along a given plane. The hippocampus lies on the inner side of the temporal lobe. From the entorhinal cortex, it receives connections from all cortical areas. It plays a predominant role in linking short- to long-term memory. Animal studies have confirmed the role of the hippocampus in the transformation of short-term responses for their storage in long-term memory. It helps to order events that have been categorised by the modules and to assure that these events lead to additional synaptic modifications in each module, thereby guaranteeing long-term memory.

Processing information from the body, the environment or even from other neuronal networks by a set of modules will produce a certain type of behaviour that may become very complex (Fisher, 1993). This means that the same network of modules can produce different levels of behavioural complexity as a function of the configuration of their component inputs.

We can illustrate this model by a simple example: place a glass full of water on a table and tell the subject to drink its contents. A large number of components of this perception will be analysed by different modules so as to optimally carry out the action, drinking the contents of the glass, optimally. Thus, the position of the body in space, i.e., with reference to the glass, will be analysed by one module (M1) in the parietal cortex; the shape of the glass by another (M2) in the occipital lobe; its weight by a third (M3); another, in the limbic system, will determine pleasure or displeasure depending on whether the subject is thirsty or not, and whether or not the contents are pleasing (M4); another will analyse the colour of the contents, etc. In addition, each of these modules has its own memory register and so will evaluate the analysis of its current component with its own memory. A coherent, and co-ordinated action will thus occur as a result of a simultaneous, co-ordinated analysis by all the modules, themselves interacting with the cerebellum, basal ganglia, hippocampus and motor cortex (Fig. 3). If no error of appreciation has been detected, this experience will reinforce the memory registers of the different modules participating. If, on the contrary, the contents of the glass are bitter and the subject is expecting water, this experience could modify the M4 memory register, and this may affect a similar experience in the future. The example of the autistic child reflects an overall involvement of this coherency and co-ordination at the highest level. One disorder considered as essential to his condition is inappropriate use of objects.

Constitution and growth modules

The constitution and growth of modules lasts several years. It is not linear, but cyclic. Each growth cycle is composed of a phase of competition between potential neuronal networks, and of a phase of stabilisation and co-ordination among stabilised modules. As we have seen, the competition phase involves reinforcement of potential synapses at the expense of

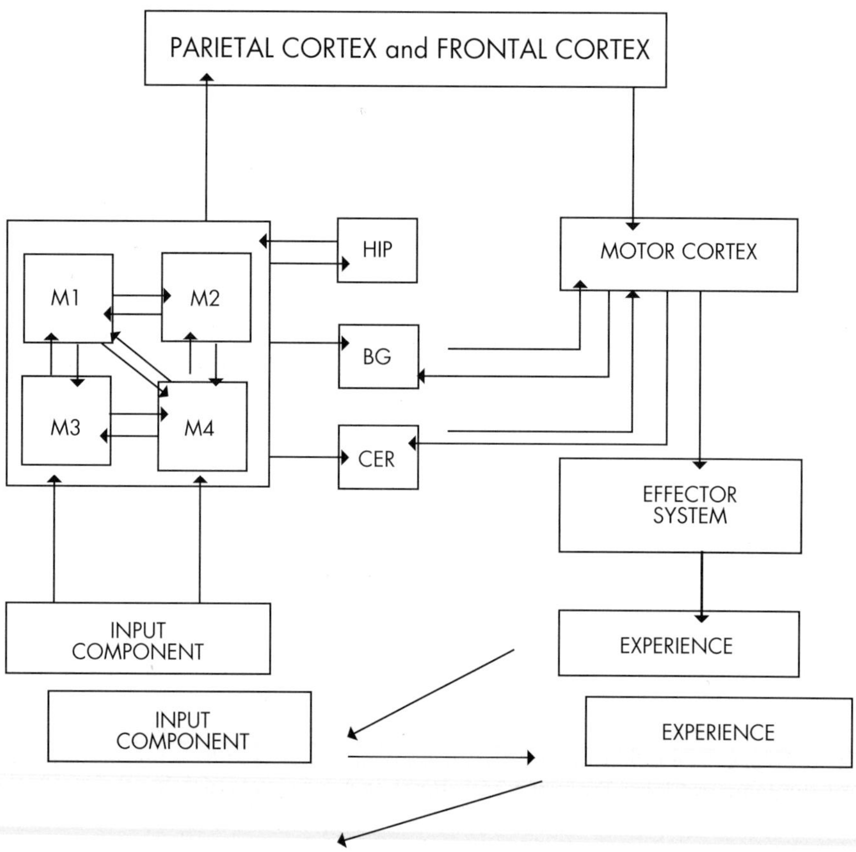

Fig. 3
Example illustrating the theory of neuronal group selection.Each of the modules analyses an input component. A coherent action occurs as a result of a coordinated analysis by all the modules. This coordinated action interacts with the cerebellum (CER), The basal ganglia (BG), the hippocampus (HIP) and the motor cortex. Experience reinforce the memory register of the different modules that may affect a similar experience in the future.

weakening and even disappearance of other synapses The co-ordination phase enables a certain level of functional complexity to be reached. Furthermore, when the stage of competence is reached, it induces the development of other neuronal networks and thus other modules. This competition - stabilisation/co-ordination alternation is also encountered in cell development, be it functional or even behavioural. Neurons, dendrites and their connections multiply (competition phase) and then most die, but the survivors possess powerful functional capacities (stabilisation/co-ordination phase). Another example of this type of cyclic development has been described for the emergence and stabilisation of alpha rhythm power in electroencephalograms (EEG) in the parieto-occipital region between birth and 20 years of age. Matousek and Petersen (1973) showed that, against the background of overall regular growth, alpha power changes in cycles composed of a phase of rapid growth (competition phase) followed by a plateau phase (stabilisation/co-ordination phase). Similar cyclic growth periods have been reported by Chugani and Phelps (1986) and Chugani et al. (1987) for glucose consumption, and by Kitchener et al. (1993) for psychological development. These workers used Piaget's permanence of the object test and showed that success is possible but inconsistent in very young children because their capacity to find a hidden object is unstable while success is constant from 2 years of age.

Thus, several modules composing a modular set will evolve in the course of a cycle composed of competition and stabilisation/co-ordination phases. Their co-ordinated activity enables a certain level of competence to be reached. In addition, their stability and functional maturity also induce development of a second modular set shown by intimate and powerful links with the inducing modular set. This favours acquisition of a new level of competence. The second module will in turn induce development of a third module that reinforces its links with predecessors, and so on (Fig. 4). Fisher and Rose (1994) have shown that development module or modular set could begin only if the inducing module had first reached a stable state. Even though the phase of stabilisation/co-ordination is a plateau in terms of competence, it is apparently very active in terms of the cerebral cortex, in particular for development of cortical connections. Work by Hudspeth and Pribram (1992) and Thatcher (1994), based on examination of consistency of EEG rhythms, has shown the existence of reproducible phenomena at each phase of development. Each phase of stabilisation/co-ordination would be composed of three periods of development of cortical connections, successively involving the left hemisphere, the right hemisphere and then both at the same time. Although this progression is apparently constant in all children, chronology varies from one child to an other. The second phenomenon observed by these workers was the topology of the development of these connections. Each phase of stabilisation/co-ordination stimulates the development of its connections with the right frontal cortex, followed immediately by the occipito-parietal regions and from there a slow development towards the temporal cortex, central zones and the frontal cortex again. (Table I). These results show the precision of cerebral development dynamics. This process represents the principle of the hierarchic and co-ordinated development model.

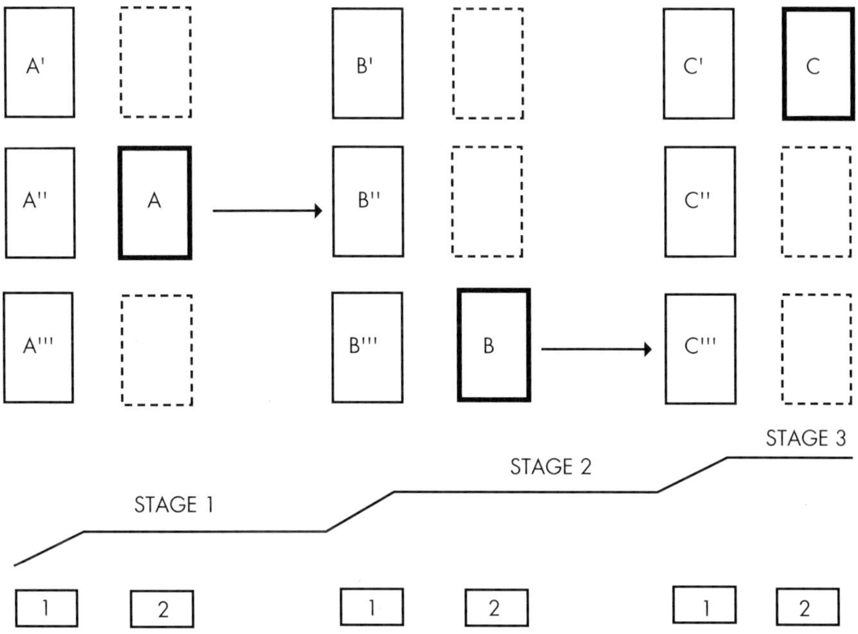

Fig. 4
Constitution and growth of modules.
The constitution and growth of modules is cyclic. After a phase of competition between potential neuronal networks, there is a phase of stabilization and coordination among stabiliazed modules. These stability and functional maturity will induce the development of a second module.

Table 1
Periods of development of cortical connections involving the right and the left hemisphere.

Phase	Age	Latera-lisation
I	1,5	Left
	2,5	
	3	Bilateral
	5	Right
II	6	Left
	8,5	Bilateral
	9	Right
III	11	Left
	13	Bilateral
	14	Right

On the basis of this cerebral development model we can imagine the effects on the future of the child when, due to an endogenous or exogenous factor, induction of a new module and thus of new functions or behaviour does not occur (stagnation or regression) or is suboptimal (behavioural disorder).

Control and specificity

Several modules are activated and co-ordinated in parallel, forming a modular set. In reality, however, several modular sets are active at the same time. Fisher and Rose (1994) believe that co-ordination among several modular sets occurs via the frontal cortex. They believe that one of the principal functions of the frontal cortex is to maintain a piece of data corresponding to the activity of a modular set "on-line" during the time required for the emergence of other information or the occurrence of other activities. This is exactly the same function as that required to co-ordinate two activities, switching them from a state of independence or competition to one of co-occurence and thus of co-ordination. This hypothesis was verified by Goldman-Rakic (1987) in rhesus monkeys, using the permanence of the object test. It was found that columns of cells in the prefrontal cortex enable the solution of the problem to be held "on-line" for a certain period. These cells discharge during the period in which the solution must be retained and resume their basal activity once the problem is resolved. When these columns of cells are destroyed, there is a considerable per cent error in the permanence of the object test.

By recording the EEG during a paradigm of permanence of the object, Bell and Fox (1994) showed that the frontal cortex participates very early in human newborns. During the period of alert preceding that of problem resolution, newborns had intense frontal activity. This was iness concomitant with increased activity of fronto-occipital connections measured with consistency calculation methods, suggesting increased capacities of the frontal cortex to maintain visuo spatial information. The co-ordination of modular sets is thus a basic property of the development of the brain and its behaviour patterns. The different modules are not only competitive, but are co-ordinated via the mediation of the frontal cortex. For example, this co-ordination is lacking in the autistic child, who can be distracted by almost nothing and who also is impatient and quickly loses interest in an object as soon as it is hidden (Adrien, 1996).

As mentioned above, the relative specificity of these modules is reinforced with time, but this specificity is not exclusive. The development of this type of dynamic system requires the permanent interaction of a large number of cerebral modules. The result of this is that participation of these modules may be both general and specific. It is true that the different modules have a specific function and a more general function, resulting from a parallel, non linear evolution and also from considerable zones of overlap. Thus, a given section of brain tissue may participate in the operation of several modules. For example, the module encompassing the areas of Broca and Wernicke, classically described as totally dedicated to language, also participates in non linguistic functions such as the use of the hands (Greenfield, 1991; Lieberman, 1996). This explains the remarkable plasticity of brain tissue, enabling it to supplant defective function following tissue lesion.

Schematically, cerebral development occurs in three phases: the first is principally genetic, while the other two leave considerable room for the experience of the individual in his environment. Before discussing the development of the principal constituents of the central nervous system, I shall examine some general aspects of cerebral growth.

Major steps in development

Before examining the growth processes of central nervous system cell components, I shall describe the major steps in development. The modular system described above gives rise to a complex level of co-ordination after its evolution in major steps that can be identified by both an anatomical-functional study of the brain and a study of cognitive development. This growth process is not linear; the emergence of a new step is marked by successions of rapid growth and plateau phases. This process has been shown by the study of key periods of development and by measurement of variables such as cranial circumference, alpha-rhythm power in the EEG or glucose consumption.

An example of this is the age of eight months in newborns; one of the important stages of development. This age is marked by the appearance of major behavioural and cognitive changes (permanence of the object, distress upon separation, etc.) (Campos et al., 1983; Seibert et al., 1984). It is known that there are also considerable anatomical-functional changes at the same time. Campos et al. (1983) showed that the emergence of autonomous locomotion facilitated the development of a certain degree of dexterity in spatial localisation during this period. There is also a certain degree of convergence concerning alpha rhythm power of the EEG and glucose consumption at the age of eight months.

This panoply of anatomical, functional and behavioural changes at the age of eight months, and at other moments of development, reinforces the hypothesis that cerebral growth and cognitive development are intimately bound. Fisher and Rose (1994) described 12 periods of growth between birth and the age of 21 years, of which seven occur before the age of 2 years: 3-4, 7-8, 10-11, 15-18 weeks, 8, 12 and 20 months, and 4, 7, 11, 15 and 19 years. These growth phases are approximately found by measurements of electroencephalographic variables (Matousek and Petersen, 1973; Dreyfus-Brisac,1979; Emde and Robinson, 1980; Parmelee and Sigman, 1983; Bell and Fox, 1994), glucose consumption (Chugani, 1994) and even cranial circumference, at least during the first year (Fisher, 1987). Finally, it should be noted that most of these phases correspond to phases of synaptogenesis.

Neuronal development

In mammals, the process of cerebral maturation begins in the embryonic stage of gestation, i.e., almost from the beginning of intra uterine life. In humans, it does not end before adolescence and for some cortical structures, not before adulthood.

Maturation of the cortex is a gradual process that for simplicity can be divided into six major periods. 1) Mesodermal signals induce a uniform population of nerve cell precursors from undifferentiated ectoderm (mitotic process). 2) These nerve cells then differentiate and give rise to two cell types: glial cells and neuroblasts. 3) The third period is characterised by migration of neurons from the germinal zone to their final position in the neural plate. 4) At almost the same time, neurons extend their axonal prolongation towards their future target. 5) The axons then develop connections with the target cells, the period of synaptogenesis. 6) Finally, synapses initially formed are modified and will constitute the mature pattern of neuronal connections. The first four steps in humans occur in utero, the fifth extends after birth and the last undoubtedly until adulthood.

Research on the mechanisms involved in the development of the cerebral cortex involves questions shared by all processes of biological development. How does a highly complex structure arise from a group of undifferentiated cells? Current understanding enables two types of factors guiding this major construction project to be distinguished: genetic, so-called intrinsic factors contained by all cells and, increasingly, considerable importance is being given to external, or extrinsic signals. Influence is exerted at several levels, from intercellular interactions up to the environment to which the organism is exposed. These two types of factor play a fundamental role in the early phases of cerebral development.

Every developmental process involves the emergence of an organised structure. In the nervous system, this process gives rise to the proliferation of cells followed by their migration. In the early stages of human development, the nervous system is a neural crest followed by a neural groove and a simple neural tube extending in a caudal direction on the dorsal surface of the embryo. The principal divisions of the brain, resulting from the thickening of the anterior walls of the neural tube, can be seen very early. These local changes in thickness result from the regional modulation of the intensity of cell proliferation inside the neural tube along the central canal or ventricular zone. About 109 cells must be generated in humans to form the mature neocortex of each hemisphere. All cortical cells originate in the ventricular zone and none of them originates from the cortical plate itself (Rakic, 1975). Following cell division, all future neurons migrate to their final position in the cortical plate. A basic aspect of research on brain development is elucidation of the mechanisms that guide these neurons, enabling them to reach their final destination in the brain. In the 1970s, Rakic observed that migrating neurons are guided by other cells in the wall of the neural tube (Rakic, 1972). A neuron thus migrates in a radial direction by a mechanism involving an interaction between it and a transitory population of radial glial cells. These cells lie close to the central canal and have long radial prolongations which reach the outer border of the neural tube. The radial glial cell's guide migrating neurons both mechanically and chemically.

Following their migration, neurons occupy well defined positions in the cortical plate. Autoradiographic studies have shown that the oldest neurons are in the deepest cortical layers (Angevine and Sidman, 1961). Successive waves of neurons then occupy more superficial positions. Recently, McConnell et al. (1988) showed that the final position of a neuron in the cortex is determined very early, at a precise moment in the cell cycle, probably after cell division in the germinal zone. All neurons "born" at the same time will assume the same connections, characteristic of their cortical layer. Caviness (1982) showed that in Reller mutant mice with defective neuronal migration, neurons nevertheless established the connections characteristic of their intended layer, in spite of their abnormal position in the cortex. It thus appears that not only the final position, but also the type of connection developed by the neuron is determined at an early stage in the germinal zone, just before migration (Kennedy et al., 1995).

Once the neuron has reached its final position, and sometimes even before that, it starts extending its axons towards other points of the cortex or towards other subcortical structures. The neuron puts out a prolongation that bears at its extremity a swelling called the "growth cone", described in 1890 by Ramon y Cajal, which grows until it reaches its target neurons. Neuronal connections are established in this way. Growing axons group together to form bundles and can travel considerable distances to their targets. The exact process guiding the axons to their targets is poorly understood. In the 1930s, Weiss (1939) suggested that initial connections were random and that the repeated use of neuronal circuits selected and stabilised the most suitable connections. This theory was partially refuted by the well-known experiments of Sperry (1963) on regeneration after section of the optic nerve. Ganglion axons which compose the optic nerve go towards one or other lateral geniculate body in the optic chiasm, depending on the retinotopic position of the ganglion cells from which they arose. Sperry showed that axons arising from ganglial neurons could recognise their target neuron. In his experiments, the optic nerve of frogs was sectioned and the eyes were rotated 180°. After regeneration of axons from the retina, the behaviour of the frog was the exact opposite of normal. This suggested that in spite of rotation of the retina, ganglial neurons re-established their connections with the same neurons as before the lesion. On the basis of these findings, Sperry formulated the chemoaffinity hypothesis according to which molecules on the surface of target neurons have a chemical code, recognised by specific molecules on the surface of axons (Sperry, 1963). These experiments gave no indication of the nature of this axon-target interaction, but more recent work has shown that the control of growing axons involves a number of glycoproteins produced by glial cells or by neurons. These molecules play an important role in cell adhesion and thereby morphogenesis. Some of the most important glycoproteins, ligands synthesised by glial cells, such as cytotactin (Edelman et al., 1990), laminine (Krotoski et al., 1986), while others are ligands synthesised by neurons, such as astrotactin (Zheng et al., 1996) and N-CAM (Edelman 1983). Immunochemical techniques have enabled Edelman's group to identify molecules cell adhesion molecules responsible for adhesion between cells at different embryonic stages (Edelman, 1983). These molecules apparently impose limits on the movement of migrating neurons or growing axons. The variation in the membrane density of these molecules determines the degree of interneuron adhesion. Thus, in the course of migration CAM density is low (low adhesion) and at the end of migration CAM molecules reappear (high adhesion).

Other chemical substances also contribute to the migration of neurons and to the growth of axons. Three groups play the role of growth factors: factors of decidual or embryonic origin and various neuropeptides. The placenta and decidual membranes synthesise and release a number of substances which can act on the developing brain. Substances produced by decidual cells short-circuit the placental barrier because they are secreted directly into the amniotic fluid with which the neural tube, still open at the initial stages, it is intimate contact. Among these substances there are various prostaglandins (Bryant-Greenwood et al., 1987), prolactin (Sakbun et al., 1987) and the alpha subunit of human chorionic gonadotrophin (HCG). In addition, the placenta and the decidual membranes contain macrophages whose density varies with surrounding conditions and whose production of cytokins in variable quality and quantity could have a great effect on embryonic development.

The principal known growth factors of embryonic origin are the neurotrophins the most important of which are neuronal growth factor (NGF), brain derived neurotrophic factor (BDNF), neurotrophin three (NT 3), insulin and its cousins (IGF 1, IGF 2), basic fibroblast-growth-factors and acid fibroblast growth factors (FGF) and the ciliate neurotrophic factor (CNTF), (Loughlin and Fallon, 1993). The role of these growth factors in the survival of postmigratory neurons and in synaptic plasticity is established. The growth factors participating in the initial stages of development, however, between neural tube formation and neuronal migration, are relatively unknown. It is possible that growth factors arising directly from embryonic tissues play a key role in maturation and differentiation of the primitive brain.

In addition to these neurotrophic factors of decidual or embryonic origin, the role of growth factors has recently been attributed to a number of neuropeptides such as vasoactive intestinal peptide (VIP) (Brenneman et al., 1985, Gressens et al., 1996), calcitonin gene-related peptide (CGRP) (Denis-Donini, 1989), substance P (Narumi and Fujita, 1978) and thyroid release hormone (TRH) (Iwasaki et al., 1989).

Most of these cerebral migration and development phenomena are also dependent on genes called development genes. The value of development genes was shown by embryologists who introduced human genes in the genetic stock of flies: the molecular mechanisms guiding the development of organisms as different as these are in fact practically identical. Regardless of the species, there appears to be a family of homologous or homeotic genes (HOX genes in vertebrates) which control comparable phases of development in all embryos. These genes determine the identity of structures which will develop along the anteroposterior axis of the embryo, in other words, they tell embryonic cells that they are part of the head, thorax or limbs. The proteins coded by these genes have the property of binding to regions that regulate other genes, whose expression they thereby control (McGinnis and Kuziora, 1994). Inactivation of one of these development genes in mice delays the development program of the limbs, such that two phalanges of two digits in each paw do not have time to appear and the limbs are short (Dolle et al., 1993).

These experiments have proved that an early malfunction in embryonic morphogenesis and growth could result from mutation of one of these development genes, responsible for the spatial and temporal development of the different regions of the embryo. The consequences of damage to one of these genes on development of the central nervous system remain to be shown experimentally. Nevertheless, two homeotic genes, "Engrailed" EN-1 and EN-2, are expressed in the murine cerebellum both at the fetal stage and in the adult (Joyner et al., 1988). High resolution morphological imaging, studies of the interface between the genetic anomaly and its functional consequences can be used to study the repercussions of these anomalies and to guide future research in the field of development genes.

Synaptogenesis

Synapse formation starts at the end of the cell division period of immature neuroblasts and remains a dynamic process throughout the existence of the organism, with phases of varying importance. At the end of the cell division phase, neuroblasts form primitive neurites. After neuronal migration, there is rapid growth of axons and dendrites in the direction of their target. We have already seen that intrinsic factors (growth factors, cell adhesion molecules, etc.) guide this growth. Other factors such as calcium and neurotransmitters, in particular biogenic amines, participate during this growth and junction phase. For example, stimulating type Ia serotoninergic receptors on the immature neurons of the frontal cortex slows the rate of growth of neurites and prevents synaptic development (Sikich et al., 1990). The stimulation of D2 receptors on the same neurons, on the other hand, favours neurite growth and synaptogenesis (Todd, 1992).

The number of developed neurites is much greater than the number of synapses in the adult, but the phenomenon of synaptic elimination persists for many years. For example, in region 17 of the human visual cortex, synaptic density is 50-60% higher than that of the baby between 8 and 12 months. The density then decreases progressively, reaching its adult value the age of 12 years. Synaptic density in the frontal cortex is maximal several weeks after birth and then decreases regularly until the age of 16 years (Huttenlocher, 1979; Huttenlocher et al., 1982). This phenomenon of elimination is accompanied by the facilitation of existing synapses, extensively described for the visual system by Hubel et al. (1977), who demonstrated the importance of extrinsic factors, i.e., stimulations of neuronal activity on synaptic development and elimination.

Synaptogenesis thus depends on genetic factors and intrinsic factors during only a short period. Modulation of the number and organisation of synapses by neuronal activity, on the other hand, occurs over a longer period and is undoubtedly the phenomenon most involved in individual differences. Different experience related to the environment affect the synaptic organisation of sensory system, and secondarily motor systems and cognitive development. This automatically leads to a different synaptic organisation, even if the genotype is identical.

Considering the long, slow changes of synaptogenesis and then synaptic elimination and organization, it is obvious that this is an important field for the pathophysiology of infantile development disorders. Toxic agents or infectious agents, nutritional factors, disorders of neurotransmitter metabolism and their effects on neurite growth and synaptic organisation are all plausible hypotheses, as yet unexplored, for a number of development disorders, for which high-resolution anatomical and functional imaging are very valuable tools.

Myelination

Myelin is the lipid produced by Schwann cells in the peripheral nervous system and by oligodendrocytes in the central nervous system. It sheathes most axons and its well known property of an electrical insulator allows rapid nerve conduction. Although demyelination or dysmyelination is evident in some neurological disorders, such as muscular dystrophy, its involvement in the pathogenesis of certain development disorders may be somewhat underestimated. This is shown by the recent hypothesis according to which schizophrenia would be due to a disorder at a certain stage in the myelination of the neurons in hippocampal circuits during adolescence (Benes, 1989).

Myelin in the central nervous system is an extension of the membrane surface of oligodendrocytes. It is composed of two lipid layers alternating with proteins, the most important of which are myelin basic protein (MBP) and proteolipid protein (PLP). During their differentiation into myelin forming cells, oligodendrocytes activate the expression of several genes specific for myelin. These genes code for proteins that play a role in the induction of myelination, the initial deposition of the myelin sheath surrounding the axon and the secondary compaction of myelin. Thus, two principal genes which code for MBP and PLP are on chromosome 18 and the X chromosome in mice. Only in mice it has been shown that mutations of these two genes demonstrate their involvement in myelination.

Myelination is constantly changing during the life of the organism. Even though the first steps of myelination begin in the spinal cord and the caudal part of the brain stem around week 20 of gestation, the process continues into the sixth decade of life (Yakovlev and Le Cours, 1967, Benes 1994). Recently, Hasegawa et al. (1992) used magnetic resonance imaging (MRI) to show changes in myelination in premature and normal babies up to 1 year of age. The first layers of myelin appear in the central nervous system at 25 weeks of gestational age in the globus pallidus, pallidothalamic fibres, posterior part of the internal capsule and ventrolateral nuclei of the thalamus. At 35 weeks, the striatum and pre central_gyri and postcentral gyri myelinate, while this occurs at 37 weeks in the internal capsule and optic radiations.

Myelin is visible macroscopically only after 40 weeks, i.e. at approximately the time of birth, with a chronology of myelination of different structures practically superimposable on that described above. It is nevertheless interesting that at month of age, the principal neuronal structures involved in sensory structures are myelinated and that the major motor systems will be so only at 8 months. During this period, Hasegawa et al. (1992) also reported a temporal shift in protein synthesis PLP being synthesised before MBP.

The subsequent phases of myelination are poorly understood in humans. It is known only that the myelination of the major association systems occurs from the age of 1 year until the end of the second decade, and even the fourth decade in the frontal cortex (Yakovlev and Le Cours, 1967; Benes, 1989)

The study of myelination and its possible involvement in certain developmental anomalies must be considered. Benes (1989) showed that a myelination disorder during adolescence, at a key period in the development of corticolimbic systems, could be linked to the principal symptoms of schizophrenia. In addition, significant in differences myelination between control and mentally retarded children have been shown by MRI (Dietricht et al., 1987). This technique has been considerably improved and it can now be used to study myelination in vivo (Franconi et al., 1994).

Neurotransmission and development

The term neurotransmission covers a vast field which includes the metabolism of neurotransmitters, the study of receptors and, more generally, synaptic function. Even though the development of neurotransmitters in humans remains relatively unexplored, there are several broad notions on neurotransmission. Their clinical, physiological and pharmacological impact is important and imaging techniques are very valuable for studying them.

Schematically, the central nervous system processes information in two basic ways: a rapid, analogue system and a slow, cognitive system. The rapid system is practically mature at birth and the slow system's functional maturation lasts several years. Quantitatively, the rapid system accounts for 95% of neurons and the slow system for 5% (Tassin, 1996).

Even though there undoubtedly exist dozens of neuromediating substances, the rapid system is essentially dependent on an excitatory system whose neuromediator is glutamic acid, an inhibitoty system whose neuromediator is gamma-aminobutyric acid (GABA) and a modulating system whose neuromediators are neuropeptides. This rapid system concerns primarily synapses of the neuronal networks in the cerebral cortex, which is why it is often called the intrinsic system. The slow system is represented by several large systems, of which the most important are those whose neuromediators are acetylcholine, serotonin, noradrenaline and dopamine. The origin of these is subcortical, which is it is called the extrinsic system.

Biochemical analysis of cortical development adds an important functional dimension to morphological and neurophysiological studies. Coyle (1977) established basic themes, including the observation that important projections from caudal brainstem regions are established relatively early in late fetal development. These projections, including the noradrenergic fibres, may be relatively influential early in postnatal life. Another important trend appears to be that a neurotransmitter system's influence is determined by a number of factors, including the differential maturation of uptake systems, synthetic and degrading enzymes, receptor and second messenger systems. A striking discovery is that of a number of instances in which cortical neurotransmitter processes are activated in the early postnatal period. This is particularly interesting in view of the observations that synaptic density in immature primate neocortex is greater than in the adult in several regions. For example, Lidow and Rakic (1992), studied the sheduling of monoaminergic neurotransmitter receptor expression in the prefrontal cortex, primary motor, somatosensory and visual cortex of rhesus monkeys at birth and during the first 60 months of postnatal period. The density of all receptors studied increased rapidly within the first 2 postnatal months to as much as twice that in adult. After the fourth month, density began a decline which subsided around the time of puberty. This course of developmental change was similar in all cortical layers and in all regions examined. However, the magnitude of the transient overproduction and eventual reduction in receptor density varied across the cortical layers and cytoarchitectonic areas in a manner specific to the individual receptor sites. Overall, cortical maturation was associated with the tendency of monoaminergic receptors to concentrate preferentially in the superficial cortical layers. The common developmental course of monoaminergic receptors in different cytoarchitectonic areas reveals an impressive co-ordination in the expression and regulation of these functionally relevant proteins in the cerebral cortex during infancy and adolescence. Recognition that receptor-channel second-messenger mechanisms for important systems of neurotransmission are active in immature cortex opens many possibilities for exploring mechanisms of cortical development and plasticity.

Sexual difference and cerebral development

An influence of sex on the morphological and functional development of the central nervous system has been described in most species, and in particular humans. The mechanisms regulating these differences are based on the hypothesis according to which circulating sex hormones act directly on neuronal organisation. These hormones and their receptors are present at the initial stages of development.

This question of sex-related differences and cerebral development is important in the psychiatry of children and adolescents. Significant differences have been described in terms of the incidence, advancement and severity of development disorders. For example, autism is more frequent in boys but more severe in girls (Rutter and Gapmezy, 1983). Depressive syndromes, on the other hand, are much more frequent in girls.

Considerable work has shown that sex-related morphological and functional differences exist during cerebral development. For example, brain weight increases more rapidly in boys than in girls during the first 5 years (Swaab and Hofman, 1984). Other differences have been reported: the volume of certain nuclei, the size of neurons, synaptic organisation and dendritic organisation and that of neurotransmission systems (De Vries, 1990). These differences involve, in particular, structures such as the hypothalamus, cerebellar amygdala, hippocampus and even some cortical regions (Todd et al., 1989).

A number of functional differences have also been observed, particularly in hemisphere specialisation (Annett, 1980). Thus, boys form a larger proportion of left-handed individuals. During childhood, girls use their verbal competence more than boys, who appear to be more competent in the nonverbal domain (Harris, 1978).

It is thus possible that sex hormones have a direct effect on cerebral development. Up to week 6 in utero, there is no morphological difference between boys and girls. Starting in week 7, testicular development progresses rapidly and is accompanied by the secretion of testosterone (Sitteri and Wilson, 1974). This secretion increases until the third month in utero and again from week 6 post partum (Reyes et al., 1974). One of the metabolites of testosterone is believed to be active on the development of the pituitary and hippocampus (Selmanoff et al., 1977). The ovaries of the female embryo develop starting at week 4 post partum, but their anlagen do not secrete estrogens during embryonic life. Ostrogens required for the development of the female embryo during pregnancy arise primarily from the placenta.

It is thus clear that sex hormones participate actively in the regulation of the different steps of cerebral development, in particular at the stages of neurogenesis, neuronal migration, dendrite growth and neuronal death (Gorski, 1988). The receptors for these sex hormones have been found to lie inside both the cytoplasm and the nucleus (O'Malley and Birnbaumer, 1978).

This first part has enabled us to look at several current concepts of cerebral development,. and thus to note the precision of development dynamics and the extreme diversity of the phenomena occurring. It is not difficult to understand the difficulties in a etiological research on childhood development disorders. It is in this framework that methods of exploring the brain can and should be used.

From the morphological to the functional

Before describing the principles of brain exploration methods, we will briefly discuss the major levels of nervous system functioning.

Functional levels of the cerebral nervous system

The nervous system integrates information it receives from the outside world and from the organism itself, so as to be able to send to effector organs the orders required for the life of the individual and the survival of the species, considering both his evolution and his experience. This is the most highly perfected means of communication, the most elaborate, the most effective and the most rapid that exists among the cells composing the organism.

From a functional point of view, the nervous system may be divided into three parts: a receptive part which receives the information, an effector part and, between the two, an integrating part which carries out information processing and the connection between inputs and outputs. This functional division is encountered anatomically at all levels, especially neurons, and in the entire nervous system itself (Fig. 5).

The neuron is the fundamental anatomical and functional unit of the nervous system. The neuron receives, integrates and transmits information. It is an anatomically specialised cell with highly ramified dendrites which receive and integrate signals. A long axon terminates in endings that send signals to other cells, nerve cells or otherwise. The cell membrane, organelles and constituents of the cytoskeleton are identical to those of other cell types, but adapted to its size and to its specialised local and regional organization. From a function point of view, neurons generate electrical signals and chemical signals. The electrical signals integrate the information produced by the cell and sent along a great distance. This integration occurs by the combination of currents produced by very weak local potentials in dendrites and

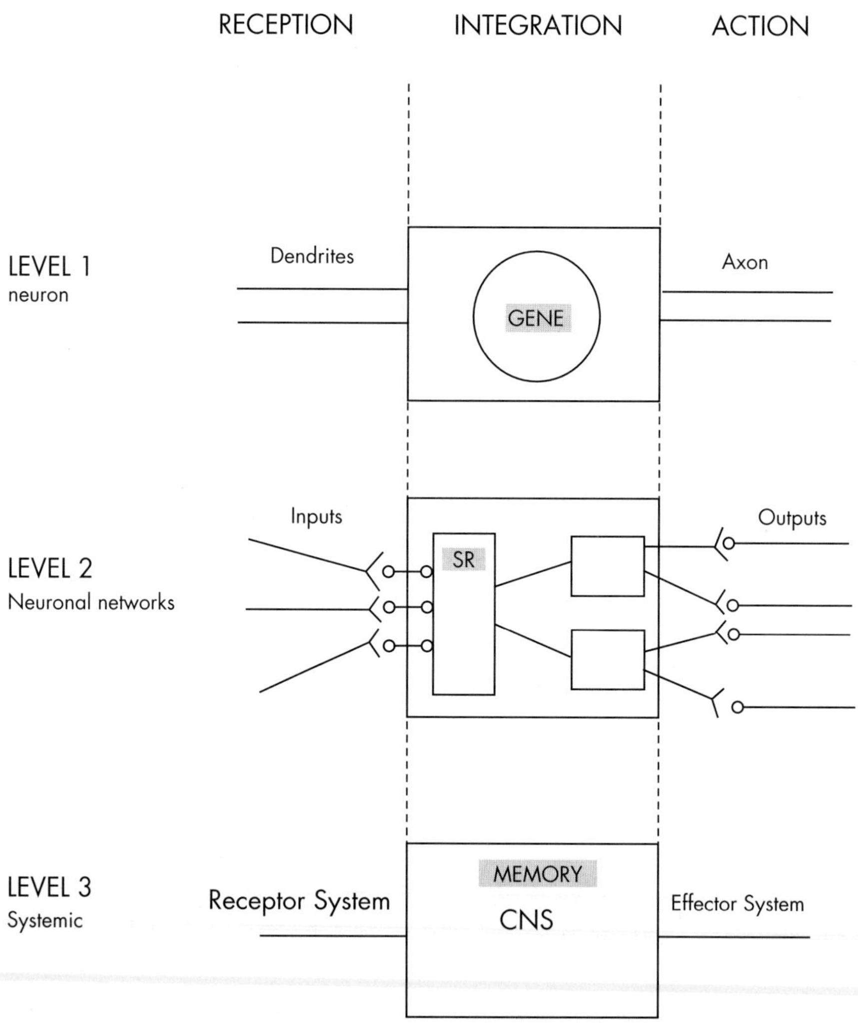

Fig. 5
Functional levels of the central nervous system.

in cell bodies. The resulting action potentials are large, self-maintaining phenomena that rapidly transmit signals along the axon and its termination. These two types of potentials originate in the combination of the activity of specific and regulated ion channels which control the passive movement of ions across the plasma membrane. Neurons communicate among themselves primarily via chemical synapses, where the termination of the axon of one cell contacts the dendrite of another. Arriving action potentials trigger the secretion of synaptic messengers which bind to specific receptors on the postsynaptic membrane.

The interaction between messengers and their receptors causes the emergence of an electrical signal, excitatory or inhibitory, in the postsynaptic cell. Via second messengers, it modifies metabolic pathways, neuronal structure and even gene expression.

Even though the neuron is the basic anatomical-functional structure in the central nervous system, it is included in a network of neurons with anatomical and functional specificity, as described in the first part of this chapter. These neuronal networks have the triple function of reception, integration and action. An example of these neuronal networks is represented by the columns of the cerebral cortex described by Szentagothai (1975) and Rakic (1981). These are highly elaborate three-dimensional structures in which neurons are grouped according to their function and their targets. Each column has receives afferent, receiver fibres, the column or neuron network integrates the inputs and then sends the processed information to another neuronal network, which may or may not be an immediate neighbour.

The third level is the nervous system itself, since the receptor and effector systems have been delegated to the peripheral nervous system. The central nervous system processes and integrates information at its different levels.

Methods for exploring the central nervous system

The temporal resolution or spatial resolution of most methods of cerebral exploration (Fig. 6) is currently at the level of neuronal networks, i.e. modules and modular sets. Three compartments may be the object of morphological and/or functional examination: the neuronal compartments, synaptic compartments and vascular compartments.

Only the neuronal compartment can be subjected to morphological and functional examination. It has been seen that neurons generate and transmit electrical activity in the form of action potentials and this electric activity and the resulting magnetic fields can be recorded.

Synaptic compartment is composed of the axonal termination of the presynaptic neuron, the synaptic slit and the dendritic extremity of the postsynaptic neuron. We have seen that the axonal extremity of the presynaptic neuron releases a chemical neurotransmitting under the influence of the electrical activity of the axon. Binding of the neurotransmitter to a postsynaptic receptor or its reuptake by the presynaptic neuron can be investigated in vivo. In addition, when the neurotransmitter binds to its receptor, this causes a series of energy consuming reactions which can be investigated.

Exploration of the vascular compartment yields an indirect determination of cerebral function. There is dense vascularisation within the neuronal networks. When resting potential is restored after the depolarisation of neurons, energy is consumed. A neuron which has been activated consumes a large quantity of energy-rich substances. Activation of a neuron or group of neurons thus results in a local increase in glucose consumption. The energy indispensable for neuronal function is constantly supplied by the

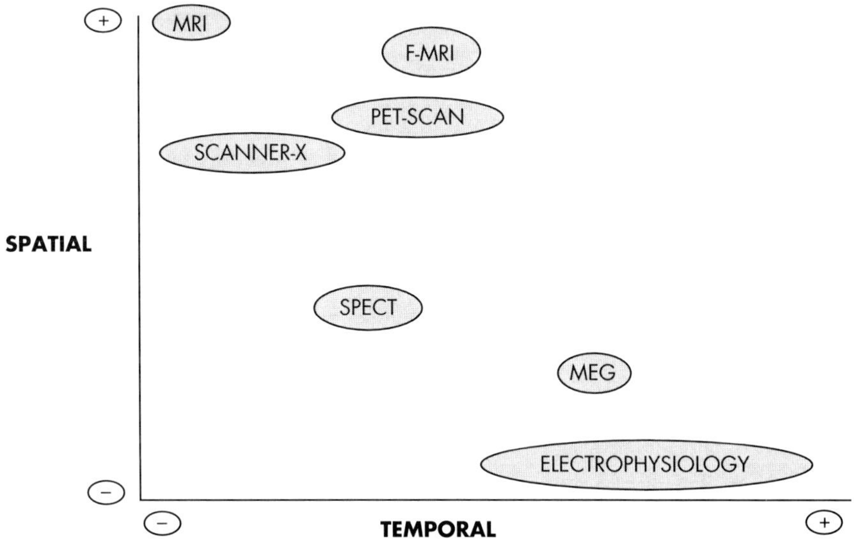

Fig. 6
Main exploration methods for the central nervous system. All of these methods balance between temporal and spatial resolution.

blood. When demand increases, local or regional cerebral blood flow (CBF) increases. Measuring CBF theretone shows the instantaneous activity of the neurons in a given region, in particular when they are stimulated.

Before the main methods of morphological and functional exploration currently available are described several general comments can be made.

Since the beginning of the 1970s, brain imaging and neurophysiology have made considerable progress. Twenty five years ago, methods for examining the brain were limited. Only conventional skull radiographs, angiography and air studies visualised the structures of interest visible and the electroencephalogram gave some indication as to function. In spite of tremendous advances, one method is totally satisfying, morphologically or functionally. We are at the start of a long adventure that should help us understand the development, function and disorders of the nervous system in vivo better.

This book deals with the value of methods for morphological and functional examinations in child psychiatry, but their use in children poses methodological and ethical problems. As we have seen, cerebral development is not a linear phenomenon, but occurs in phases. It is important to bear this in mind and to study defined age groups, limited in comparison with the major developmental phases. The ethical problem is more acute. Only cerebral electrophysiology can be used in children with no known underlying pathology. In the case of all other methods and for obvious ethical reasons, it is impossible to obtain these data, a fact which poses problems of interpretation because of the difficulty in defining criteria of normality.

Regardless of the methods of examination used, they are of value only if accompanied by thorough, objective and rigorous clinical data. A simple descriptive criterion is inadequate, and correlations with functional tests, objective scales for evaluation of behaviour, etc. are not useful, but indispensable.

Finally, in children, the human factor is most important. Whenever an examination if done, we must be prepared for distress and anxiety of child and his parents. This requires: 1) informing the parents: a simple, personalised presentation of every examination is indispensable, explaining the conditions, values and limits of the examination, as well as the expected results; 2) informing the child even if he appears not to understand; in most cases, simply talking to the child is a form of reassurance; 3) preparing the staff who will participate in the examination, explaining the main symptoms of the child and the possible behaviour disorders, parental anxiety, etc.; 4) taking the necessary time, including and waiting to be in optimal conditions before starting and examination.

Following these preliminary comments, I shall briefly describe methods for examing the brain which, for convenience, I have divided into morphological and functional. Figure 6 shows the limits of this type of classification. Subsequent chapters will deal with the anatomical and functional bases of some of them, results as a function of age, and examples of their use.

Morphological methods

The principal methods used to study the structures of the central nervous system are X-ray computed tomography and magnetic resonance imaging.

X-ray computed

This is a technique of axial transverse tomography coupled with computer processing, developed by Hounsfield (Ambrose and Hounsfield, 1973). The process involves sending a beam of X rays which scans the organ to study as fine slices, measuring the absorption of X rays as a function of the election density of the tissues through which it passes. The absorption coefficient is calculated by a computer which rapidly constructs a section of the tissues explored with details whose brightness varies with their election density.

This method was widely used before the advent of MRI. It is of limited interest for examining the central nervous system in child psychiatry. In addition, it has serious limitations as regards study of the brain stem and cerebellum because of X ray absorption by bone. On the other hand, it can be useful for detection and localization of cerebral calcification for correlation with the neuropsychological development.

Magnetic resonance imaging (MRI)

The phenomenon of nuclear magnetic resonance was described by Bloch and Purcell in 1946 and since then has been used for the study of certain molecules. The underlying principle involves determining the frequency that causes the resonance of identical atomic nuclei in a cell, providing they have a magnetic moment. The particles composing atomic nuclei rotate about themselves and so have magnetic moment. If the sum of these magnetic moments is not null, the nucleus itself has a magnetic field.

When placed in an intense magnetic field, nuclei with a magnetic moment become aligned with the field, in the same or the opposite direction. When the nuclei are made to resonate, they are shifted from one population to another. This manoeuvre requires a given energy that will be supplied by exciting the substance with a energy at a suitable radio frequency. For a given magnetic field value, the resonance frequency is specific to a single type of nucleus, for example protons, but also depends on the molecular environment in which the nucleus is situated.

MRI is one application of this principle dating from the 1970s. It involves the combination of the magnetic resonance of protons in the water of the organism, tomography and computerised image processing. The spatial resolution of this method can be very high and this is also true in structures poorly seen on X-ray tomography, such as the cerebellum and brain stem. This method is perfectly suited for the detection of very focal anomalies such as microgyria.

Functional methods

Only cerebral electrophysiology and magnetoencephalography have temporal resolution adequate for distinguishing different data processing events as a function of time. Nevertheless, other methods which that measure the activity of the synaptic or vascular compartments can be considered genuine functional examinations and thus highly valuable.

Cerebral electrophysiology

The electroencephalogram (EEG), described for the first time by Berger (1929), involves recording underlying electrical activity by placing electrodes directly on the scalp. The advantage of this method is that it is enables reliable analysis of cerebral electrical activity over time. It does not general anaesthesia or premedication and is totally safe. Qualitative and quantitative analysis of EEG rhythms, measured in μv^2, affords more detailed analysis.

Repeated sensory stimulation enable the determination of small changes in the normal electric activity of the brain, occurring within about 0.1 s of stimulation. There are referred to as evoked potentials, evoked by auditory, visual, somesthetic, etc., stimulation. Changes caused by a stimulus can be measured over time with high precision.

The advantages of electrophysiology are its safety, low cost and excellent temporal resolution. Its major drawback is poor spatial resolution.

Magnetoencephalogaphy (MEG)

Cohen was one of the first to record magnetoencephalograms. When a neuron is excited across a synapse, ion channels in its membrane open. Since the ionic composition inside and outside the cell is different, opening of these channels causes movement of charged particles in the intra-cellular mediua and extra-cellular mediua. The intensity of the resulting currents is not the same and detectable potential differences are 100 mV inside the cell, but only about 0.1 mV outside it. It is thus the intracellular current that is sufficiently strong to create a magnetic field which can be detected outside the skull. In the EEG,

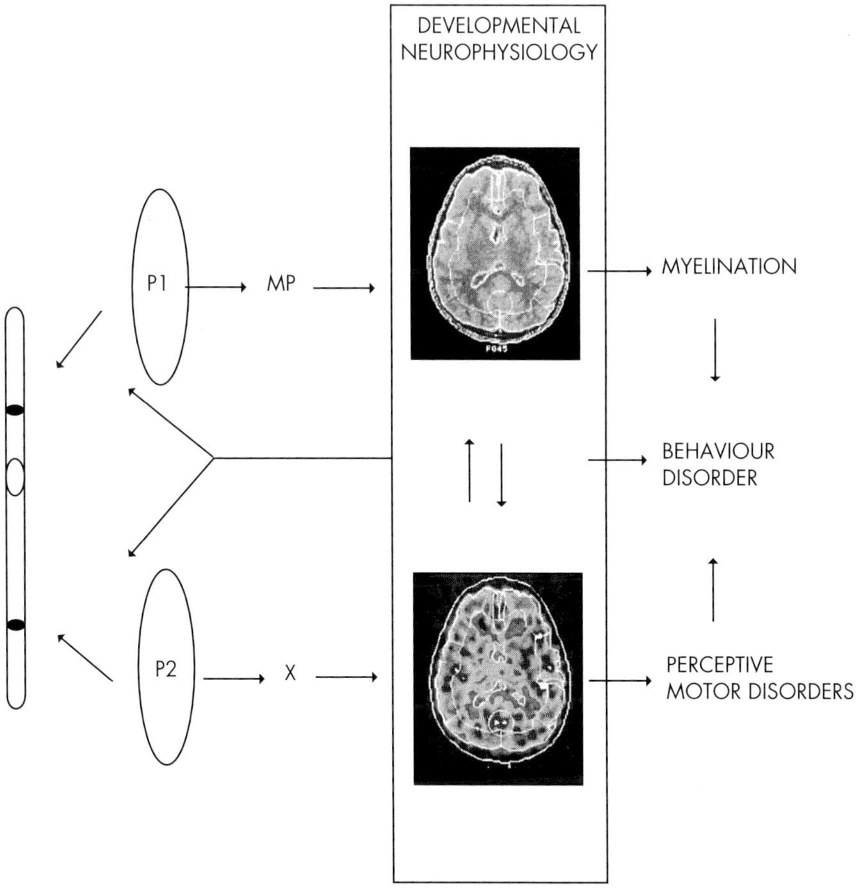

Fig. 7
Morphological and functional explorations are at the croossroads between clinical expression and more basic cell and molecular disorder. *See colour illustrations appendix*

on the contrary, it is differences in extracellular potentials which are measured. In both cases, only the induction created by a population of neurons, whose long axis must be synchronous in order to create a detectable magnetic field or electric field, is detected. This is the case for a cortical macrocolumn when the activity of its neuronal population is synchronised (Nunez, 1990).

Magnetic fields which can be detected by extracranial sensors are created by macrocolumns oriented tangentially to the surface of the scalp, whereas in the case of the EEG, it is the activity of radially-orientated macrocolumns oriented radially. MEG is thus a precise method for studying generators deep inside the cortex while EEG is useful for localising generators on the cortical surface parallel to the scalp. EEG and MEG are thus complementary and should be used together (Cohen et al., 1990).

Positron emission tomography (PET)
Developed around 1975, positron emission tomography uses radioactive elements such as oxygen 15 or carbon 14. When one of these disintegrates inside the organism, it emits a positron which very rapidly encounters an electron in a neighbouring atom. The positron-electron couple annihilates and gives rise to two gamma photons emitted at the same time but in diametrically opposite directions. The two photons pass through the body in a straight line to reach detectors placed in a ring around the patient's head. The event is recorded only if the two photons arrive simultaneously ; if not, they could have come from independent disintegrations, produced at points and times distinct from the event under study. The pair of detectors activated determine the line on which the emission point lay. Several disintegrations from the same site give different lines and so their intersection corresponds to the emitting region. The data recorded are sent to a computer and undergo processing to plot positron emitting regions.

The advantage of this method is its moderaty good spatial resolution, especially when coupled with MRI, and its sensitivity when stimulations are used. In addition, the labelled elements used are atoms which go to form biological molecules and thus have no effect on their physiological properties. Its major disadvantages are its cost and its temporal resolution which is about one minute.

Single photon emission tomography (SPECT)
Single proton emission tomography is a functional imaging technique based on the reconstruction of cross-sectional images, by counting gamma rays emitted by the commonly used nuclear medicine radiotracers such as Tc99m, iodine I123 or xenon Xe133. The practical aspects and performance of this method are relatively diversified and vary with the instruments and tracers used. Its major application in functional examination of the brain is for studying cerebral perfusion. This method has enabled investigators to show that neuropsychological deficits were most often associated with focal, characteristic reduction of blood flow in the brain. It also enables activation studies to be conducted, showing focally increased flow accompaning motor tasks, sensory tasks or cognitive tasks. It can also be applied to the study of neuroreceptors.

The disadvantage of this method is that the gamma-emitting radioisotopes are not constituents of biological molecules. When these molecules are labelled, their spatial configuration and thus their biological properties are modified.

Functional magnetic resonance imaging (F-MRI)
With the development of ultrarapid data acquisition and processing techniques, it has become possible to obtain images in sufficiently short times to follow certain aspects of metabolism: this is F-MRI. The must commonly employed principle depends on the oxygenation of blood; magnetic properties of heamoglobin differ slightly depending on whether or not it is bound to oxygen. Brain activity is thus assessed by obtaining images which show the contrast between regions rich in oxyhamoglobin with the reins, corresponding to a disproportionate increase in cerebral blood flow, and regions with normal flow. As in spectroscopy (see below) the disadvantage of this method is the need for very strong magnetic fields.

Magnetic resonance spectroscopy (MRS)
MRS uses a combination of pulsed radio frequencies and very strong magnetic fields. By analysing magnetic resonance spectra, it is possible to identify certain compounds such as N-acetyl aspartate, GABA, phosphocholine and other phosphorus-containing molecules, and to determine their relative or absolute concentration in a given volume. This method has the advantage of quantifying regional energy metabolism (Andreasen, 1989). Its disadvantage are the use of very strong magnetic fields and low spatial resolution.

Transcranial Doppler Sonography (TCD)
This technique is based on a physical phenomenon described by Doppler in 1843 (Eden, 1992). The Doppler effect is defined as the frequency change undergone by a propagated vibratory phenomenon resulting from relative between the emitter and receptor. When studying blood flow with this technique, ultrasound is used: the difference between the frequency emitted and that received by the probe is proportional to the flow velocity of blood cells. This technique is widely used to study peripheral vessels. Aaslid (1982) reported modifications enabling the technique to be used to examine cerebral arteries,

the principal obstacle to which is passage through the skull. The absorption of ultrasound by the skull was reduced by using frequencies of 2 MHz, lower than those used for the carotid arteries (4 to 8 MHz), and also by placing the probe over natural orifices (transorbital or suboccipital routes) or near zones of thin bone (transtemporal route).

The amplitude of the transcranial Doppler signal is proportional to the flow-velocity of blood but in general the Doppler sonographic examination is not coupled with intracranial imaging. The diameter of cranial blood vessels, and thus the circulation flow-rate, cannot be determined. Even so, in some situations (arterial diameter presumed to be constant, Doppler probe in a fixed orientation, etc.), variations of the mean flow velocity are proportional to DSC variations and the transcranial Doppler is a method of choice for determining brief variations of the DSC, in particular after sensory stimulation (Bruneau et al., 1989).

Conclusion

The nervous system develops from the fetus to the child according to irregular, complex cycles involving genetic factors, soon followed by factors related to the environment and to experience. Methods of morphological and functional examination enable cerebral development and its potential disturbances to be determined. Even if none of these methods taken individually is sufficient, coupled examinations may lead to a better definition of the pathophysiology of certain syndromes and to the search for prognostic and therapeutic features.

References

Aaslid R, Markwalder TM, Nornes H (1982) Non-invasive trancranial Doppler ultrasound recording of flow velocity in basal cerebral arteries. J Neurosurg 57: 769-774

Adrien JL (1996) L'autisme du jeune enfant. Développement psychologique et régulation de l'activité. Expansion Scientifique Française, Paris

Ambrose J, Hounsfield G (1973) Computerized transverse axial tomography. British J Radiol 46: 148-149

Andreasen NC (1989) Nuclear magnetic resonance imaging. In: Andreasen NC (ed) Brain imaging: Applications in psychiatry. American Psychiatric Press, Washington DC, p 67-121

Angevine JB, Siman RL (1961) Autoradiographic study of cell migration during histogenesis of cerebral cortex of mouse. Nature 192: 766-773

Annett M (1980) Sex differences in laterality: meaningfulness versus reliability. Behav Brain Sci 3: 227-228

Bell MA, Fox NA (1994) Brain development over the first year of life: relation between electroencephalographic frequency and coherence and cognitive and affective behaviors. In: Dawson G, Fisher KW (eds) Human behavior and the developing brain. The Guilford Press, New York, p 314-344

Benes FM (1989) Myelination of cortical-hyppocampal relays during late adolescence: anatomical correlates to the onset of schizophrenia. Schizophrenia Bull 15: 585-594

Benes FM (1994) Development of the corticolimbic system. In: Dawson G, Fisher KW (eds) Human behavior and the developing brain. The Guilford Press, New York, p 176-305

Berger H (1929) Uber das Elektrenkephalogramm des Menschen. Arch Psychiat Nervenkr 87: 527-570

Bleuler E (1911) Dementia praecox or the group of schizophrenia. International Universities Press, New York

Brenneman DE, Eiden LE, Siegel RE (1985) Neurotrophic action of VIP on spinal cord cultures. Peptides 6 (suppl 2) 35-39

Bruneau N, Dourneau MC, Garreau B, Pourcelot L, Lelord G (1992) Blood flow response to auditory stimulation in normal, mentally retarded, and autistic children: a preliminary transcraniel Doppler ultrasonographic study of the middle cerebral arteries. Biol Psychiat 32: 691-699Bryant-Greenwood GD, Rees MCP, Turnbull AC (1987) Immunohistochemical of relaxin, prolactin and prostaglandin syntethase in human amnios, chorion and decidua. J Endocrinol 114: 491-496

Campos JJ, Barrett KC, Lamb ME, Goldsmith HH, Stenberg C (1983) Socioemotional development. In: Haith MM, Campos JJ (eds). Infancy and developmental psychobiology. Wiley, New York, p 783-915

Caveness WF (1962) Atlas of electroencephalography in the developing monkey (Macaca mulatta) Addison-Wesley, Reading MA

Caviness VS (1982) Neocortical histogenesis in normal and Reeler mice: a developmental study based upon [3H] thymidine autoradiography. Dev Brain Res 4: 293-299

Changeux JP, Danchin A (1976) Selective stabilisation of developing synapses as a mechanism for the specification of neuronal networks. Nature 264: 705-712

Changeux JP, Dehaene S (1989) Neuronal models of cognitive functions. Cognition 33: 63-109

Chugani HT, Phelps ME (1986) Maturational changes in cerebral function in infants determined by 18 FDG positron emission tomography. Science 231: 840-843

Chugani HT, Phelps ME, Mazziotta JC (1987) Positron emission tomography study of human brain functional development. Ann Neurol 22: 487-497

Chugani HT (1994) Development of regional brain glucose metabolism in relation to behavior and plasticity. In: Dawson G, Fisher KW (eds) Human behavior and the developing brain. The Guilford Press, New York, p 153-173

Cohen D, Cuffin BN, Yunokuchi K, Maniewski R, Purcell C, Cosgrove GR, Ives J, Kennedy JG, Schomer DL (1990) MEG versus EEG localization test using implanted sources in the brain. Ann Neurol 28: 811-817

Courchesne E, Yeung-Courchesne R, Press GA, Hesselnink JR, Jernican TL (1988) Hypoplasia of cerebellar lobules VI and VII in autism. N Engl J Med 318: 1349-1354

Coyle JT (1977) Biochemical aspects of neurotransmission in the developing brain. Int Rev Neurobiol 20: 65-77
Denis-Donini S (1989) Expression of dopaminergic phenotypes in the mouse olfactory bulb induced by the calcium gene-related peptide. Nature 339: 701-703
De Vries GJ (1990) Sex differences in neurotransmitter systems. J Neuroendocrinol 2 1: 1-13
Dietricht RB, Bradley WG, Zaragoza EJ, Otto RJ, Taira RK, Wilson GH, Kangarloo Hooshang AR (1987) Evaluation of early myelination patterns in normal and developmentally delayed infants. Am J Radiol 150: 889-896
Dolle P, Dierich A, Lemeur M, Schimmang T, Schuhbaur B, Chambon P, Duboule D (1993) Disruption of the Hox d-13 gene induces localized heterochromy leading to mice with neotonic limbs. Cell 75 3: 431-441
Dreyfus-Brisac C (1979) Ontogenesis of brain bioelectrical activity and sleep organization in neonates and infants. In: Falkner F, Tanner JM (eds) Human growth: neurobiology and nutrition. Plenum Pess, New York, p 157-182
Edelman GM (1983) Cell adhesion molecules. Science 219: 450-461
Edelman GM (1987) Neural Darwinism: the theory of neuronal group selection. Basic Books, New York
Edelman GM, Cunningham BA, Tiery JP (1990) Morphoregulatory molecules. Wiley, New York
Eden A (1992) The search for Christian Doppler. Springer Verlag, Wien
Emde R, Robinson J (1980) The first two months: recent research in developmental psychobiology and the changing view of the new born. In: Call J, Noshpitz R (eds) Basic handbook of child psychiatry. Academic Press, New York, p 72-105
Evrard P, Miladi N, Bonnier C, Gressens P (1992) Normal and abnormal development of the human brain. In: Rapin I, Segalowitz SJ (eds) Handbook of neuropsychology. Vol 6 Elsevier, Amsterdam, p 11-14
Fisher KW (1987) Relations between brain and cognitive development. Child Dev, 57: 623-632
Fisher KW (1993) Development in context: activity and thinking in specific environments Erlbaum, Hillsdale
Fisher KW, Rose SP (1994) Dynamic development of coordination of components in brain and behavior: a framework for theory and research. In: Dawson G, Fisher KW (eds) Human behavior and the developing brain, The Guilford Press, New York, p 3-66
Franconi F, Sonier CB, Seguin F, Le Pape A, Akoka S (1994) Acquisition of spin echo and stimulated echo by a single sequence application to MRI of diffusion. Magn Reson Imag 12: 605-611
Goldman-Rakic PS (1987) Connectionist theory and the biological basis of cognitive development. Child Dev. 58: 601-622
Gorski RA (1988) Sexual differentiation of the brain: mechanisms and implication for neuroscience. In: Easter SS, Barald KF, Carlson BM (eds) From message to mind. Simauer Associates, Sutherland, MA
Greenfield PM (1991) Language, tools and brain: the ontogeny and phylogeny of hierarchically organized sequential behavior. Behav Brain Sci 14: 531-551
Gressens P, Hill JM, Paindane B, Gozes I, Fridkin M, Brenneman DE (1995) Blochade of vasoactive intestinal peptides function in early mouse embryo induces a severe microcephaly. J Clin Invest In Press
Harris LJ (1978) Sex differences in spatial ability: possible environmental, genetic and neurological factors. In: Kinsbourne M (ed) Asymmetrical functions of the brain. Cambridge University Press, Cambridge, p 405-522
Hasegawa M, Houdou S, Mito T, Takashima S, Asanuma K, Ohno T (1992) Development of myelination in the human fetal and infant cerebrum: a myelin basic protein immunohistochemical study. Brain Dev 14 1-6
Hubel DH, Wiesel TN (1977) Functional architecture of macaque monkey visual cortex. Proc Roy Soc Lon B 193: 1-59
Hudspeth WJ, Pribram KH (1992) Psychophysiological indices of cerebral maturation. Int J Psychophysiol 12: 19-29
Huttenlocher PR (1979) Synaptic density in human frontal cortex: developmental changes and effects of aging. Brain Res 163: 195-205
Huttenlocher PR, De Courten C, Garey LJ, Van Der Loos H (1982) Synaptogenesis in human visual cortex: evidence for synapse elimination during normal development. Neurosci Lett 33: 247-252
Ivry R (1993) Cerebellar involvment in the explicit representation of temporal information. Ann N Y Acad Sci 682 214-230
Iwasaki Y, Kinoshita M, Ikeda K, Takamiya K, Shiojima T (1989) Trophic effect of various neuropeptides on the cultured ventral spinal cord of rat embryo. Neurosci Lett 101: 316-320
Joyner AL, Herrup BA, Auerbach A, Davis CA, Rossant J (1991) Subtle cerebellar phenotype in mice homozygous for a targeted deletion of the En-2 homeobox. Science 251: 1239-1243
Kennedy H, Salin P, Bullier J, Horsburgh G (1994) Topography of developing thalamic and cortical pathways in the visual system of the cat. J Comp Neurol 348: 298-319
Kitchener KS, Lynch CL, Fisher KW, Wood PK, (1993) Developmental range of reflective judgment: The effect of contextual support and practice on developmental stage. Dev Psychol 29: 893-906
Krotoski DM, Domingo C, Bronner-Fraser M (1996) Distribution of a putative cell surface receptor for fibronectin and lamilin in the avian embryo. J Cell Biol 103: 1061-1071
Lemke G (1992) Myelin and myelination. In: Hall ZW (ed) An introduction to molecular neurobiology. Sinauer Associates, Sutherland, p 281-309
Lidov MS, Rakic P (1992) Scheduling of monoaminergic neurotransmitter receptor in the primate neocortex during post natal development. Cerebral Cortex 2 5: 401-416
Lieberman P (1991) Uniquely human: the evolution of speech, thought, and selfless behavior. Harvard University Press, Cambridge
Loughlin SE, Fallon JH (1993) Neurotrophic factors. Academic Press, San Diego
Mac Ginnis W, Kuziora M (1994) Developmental genes. Science, 198: 54-61
Matousek M, Petersen I (1973) Frequency analysis of the EEG in normal children and adolescents. In: Kellaway P, Petersen P (eds) Automation of clinical electroencephalography. Raven Press, New York, p 75-102
Mc Connell SK (1988) Fates of visual cortical neurons in the ferret after isochronic and heterochronic transplantation. J Neurosci 8: 945-974
Narumi S, Fujita T (1978) Stimulatory effects of substance P and nerve growth factor (NGF) on neurite outgrowth

in embryonic chick dorsal root ganglia. Neuropharmacology 17: 74-76
Nunez PL (1990) Localization of basic activity with electroencephalography. In: Sato S (ed) Advances in Neurology Vol 54. Magnetoencephalography. Raven Press, New York, p 39-65
O'Malley BW, Birnbaumer L (1978) Receptor and hormone action. Academic Press, New York
Parmelee AH, Sigman MD (1983) Perinatal brain development and behavior. In: Haith MM, Campos JJ (eds) Handbook of child psychology: infancy and developmental psychobiology. Wiley, New York, p 95-155
Rakic P (1972) Mode of cell migration to the superficial layers of foetal monkey neocortex. J Comp Neurol 145: 61-76
Rakic P (1975) Timing of major ontogenetic events in the visual cortex of the Rhesus monkey. In: Buchwald NA, Brazier M (eds) Brain mechanisms of mental retardation. Academic Press, New York, p 3-40
Rakic P (1981) Development of visual centers in the primate brain depends on binocular competition before birth. Science 214: 928-931
Reyes FI, Boroditsky RS, Winter JSD, Faiman C (1974) Studies on human sexual development: fetal and maternal serum gonadotrophin and sex steroid concentrations. J Clin Endocrinol Metab 38: 612-617
Rutter M, Garmesy N (1983) Developmental psychopathology. In: Hetherington EM (ed) Socialization, personality and social development. Wiley, New York, p 775-911
Sauvage D (1984) Autisme du nourrisson et du jeune enfant. Signes précoces et diagnostic. Masson, Paris
Sakburn V, Koay ES, Bryant-Greenwood GD (1987) Immunocytochemical localization of prolactin and relaxin c-peptide in human decidua and placenta. J Clin Endocrinol Metab 65: 339-343
Seibert JM, Hogan AE, Mundy PL (1984) Mental age and cognitive young handicapped and at risk children. Intelligence 8: 11-29
Selmanoff MK, Brodkin LD, Weiner RI, Sitteri PK (1977) Aromatization and 5 alpha reduction of androgen in discrete hypothalamic and limbic regions of the male and female rat. Endocrinology 101: 841-848
Sikich L, Hickok JM, Todd RD (1990) 5 HT 1A receptors control neurite branching during development. Dev Brain Res 2: 269-274
Sitteri P, Wilson JD (1974) Testosterone formation and metabolism during male social differentiation in the human embryo. J Clin Endocrinol Metab 38: 113-125
Sperry RW (1963) Chemoaffinity in the orderly growth of neural circuits. Proc Nat Acad Sci 50: 703-710
Swaab DF, Hofman MA(1984) Sexual differentiation of the brain: a historical perspective. In: De Vries GJ, De Bruin JPC, Uhgling HBM, Corner MA (eds) Progress in brain research. Vol 61. Elsevier, Amsterdam, p 361-374
Szentagothai (1975) The module concept in cerebral cortex architecture. Brain Res 95: 475-496
Tassin JP (1996) Développement et neurotransmission. Société Française de Neuropédiatrie, Tours 22-24 Janvier
Thatcher RW, Walker RA, Giudice S (1987) Human cerebral hemispheres develop at different rates and ages. Science 236: 1110-1113
Thatcher RW (1991) Maturation of the human frontal lobes: physiological evidence for staging. Dev Neuropsychol 7: 397-419
Thatcher RW (1994) Cyclic cortical reorganization: origins of human cognitive development. In: Dawson G, Fisher KW (eds) Human behavior and the developing brain. The Guilford Press, New York, p 232-266
Todd RD, Swarzenski B, Giovanardi Rossi P, Visconti P (1989) Structural and functional development of the human brain. In: Cicchetti D, Cohen DJ (eds) Developmental psychopathology vol 1, theory and method. Wiley and son, New York, p 161-194
Weiss P (1939) Principles of development. Holt, New York
Yacovlev PI, Lecours AR (1967) The myelogenetic cycles of regional maturation of the brain. In: Minkowsky A (ed) Regional development of the brain in early life. Blackwell, Oxford p 3-70
Zheng C, Heintz N, Hatten ME (1996) CNS gene encoding astrotactin, which supports neuronal migration along glial fibers. Science 272 5260: 418-419

2. Methods: principles, anatomical and physiological bases PET and SPECT

J.-L. BAULIEU, D. GUILLOTEAU

Brain mass represents only 2-3 per cent of body mass; however, its blood flow is 15% of systemic blood flow and its oxygen consumption about 18% of the body's oxygen consumption. These data emphasise the metabolic importance of the brain and reflect the importance and complexity of brain function. The more functional the investigation, the more relevant the information.

Anatomical and functional bases

Blood supply to the brain

The blood supply to the brain is via two arterial systems, one anterior through the carotid arteries and the other posterior through the vertebral arteries. These two systems anastomose in the circle of Willis and in the capillo arteriolar meningo cortical network. Brain perfusion is two directions: centripetal, from the cortex to the white matter and ventricles, and centrifugal, from the brain stem to the thalamus and basal ganglia. These two networks do not anastomose. The vascular systems correspond neither to lobar segmentation nor to functional areas.

The wall of the blood vessels to the brain is composed of three layers: the collagenous adventitia, the smooth muscule media and the intima, formed by tight endothelial cells. This particular organisation of the internal coat is found only in the capillaires of the brain and not in those of other organs. This continuous endothelial wall forms the blood brain barrier. The intercellular junctions are impermeable and cells are unable to perform pinocytosis. The capillary wall is encompassed by cellular processes of the astrocytes which are called "foot processes". Exchange between the plasma and "foot processes" or the interstitium is limited to two mechanisms: passive diffusion of non polar liposoluble substances and active transfer by specific transporters. The first mechanism involves gases (O_2, CO_2, Xe) and the highly lipophilic molecules such as the complexes used as brain perfusion tracers. The second mechanism involves a limited number of proteins transporters which transport electrolytes, glucose and aminoacids (Fig. 1).

Perfusion, metabolism and function

Classically it is accepted that the coupling between neuronal function on the one hand and metabolism and function on the other is mediated by pCO_2, pO_2 and pH. Neuronal activity results in an increase in cellular oxydative metabolism and as a consequence local accumulation of CO_2. The pCO_2 plays an important role in regulating flow, because CO_2 is a potent vasodilator. The same effect occurs after administration of acetazolamide, an inhibitor of carbonic

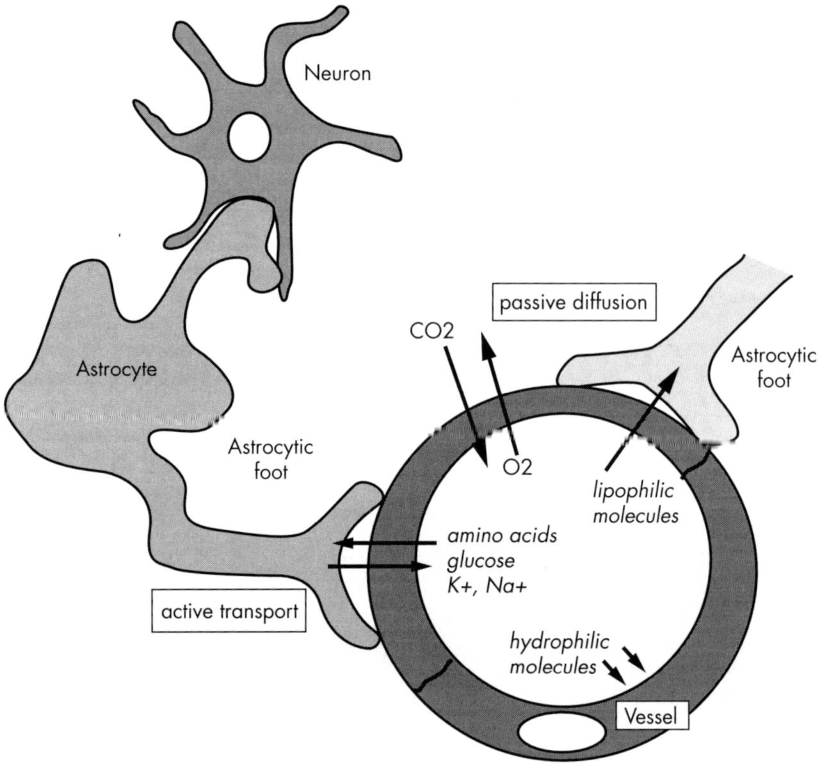

Fig. 1
Blood brain barrier: structure and transferts

anhydrase; pCO_2 seems to be important in the long term regulation of brain flow.

It has recently been shown that other structures and other agents play a role in the short term coupling of neuronal activity and both local metabolism and local perfusion: in particular, the glia and nitric oxide (NO).

Role of the glia

Recent works on the bee retina as a model of the brain and on primary culture of astrocytes showed that (Pellerin and Magistretti, 1994; Takahashi et al., 1995): glucose and fluorodeoxyglucose uptake occurs mainly in the astrocytic cells, neuronal glutamate release is a signal to the astrocyte, which responds by increasing glucose uptake, astrocyte glucose uptake is mediated by the glucose transporter which is coupled to the sodium transporter, and there is a saturable lactate transporter in the neuron.

These findings the hypothesis that lactate, which does not cross the blood brain barrier, could be the energy substrate of the activated neuron. Neuronal activation and metabolic production of energy could be coupled according to the following sequence: synaptic glutamate release; glial response of glucose uptake and glycolytic lactate production; and neuronal lactate uptake and incorporation into the Krebs cycle after conversion into pyruvate by lactate dehydrogenase.

A diagram of the metabolic events during neuronal activation can therefore be drawn, emphasing the role of the glia (Fig. 2).

Role of nitric oxide

The hypothesis of spatio temporal coupling between neuronal function and local perfusion is the basis of brain activation studies using brain blood flow measurement or imaging as the methods for monitoring brain activity. Regulation of local blood flow or perfusion by local neuronal activity has been established (Ladecola, 1993). However the exact molecular mechanism is not yet understood.

Major interest has recently developed concerning nitric oxide (NO) a ubiquitous molecular mediator involved in many physiologic processes, mainly relaxation of vessel smooth muscle fibres of the vessels (Moncada and Higgs, 1993). NO is a highly reactive, diffusible molecule and has a half life of only a few seconds; it is difficult to detect and measure (Archer, 1993). An indirect approach is to use agents which modify the enzymatic activity of NO synthase. This enzyme allows NO production by the reaction L.arginine - L. citrulline + NO.

Two series of experiments have shown the role of NO in perfusion-activity coupling. Firstly, cyclic GMP increase in the rat cerebellum induced by NMDA (N-methyl-D-aspartate) glutamate receptor activation is increased by L.arginine and blocked by NO synthase inhibitors (Moncada et al., 1989;

Garthwaite, 1991): this show that NO plays a role in the cellular response to activation of glutamate receptors. Secondly, the local increase in blood flow induced by NMDA is antagonised by NO synthase inhibitors (Faraci and Breese, 1993). NO might therefore mediate adaptation of perfusion during neuronal activity, as shown in figure 3. However, it is probable that other vasoactive substances also play a role which is not understood to date.

The synapse

The chemical transmission of the neuronal signal consists of the release of a presynaptic fibre neurotransmitter which binds to a specific postsynaptic receptor. The neurotransmitter present in the synaptic cleft is rapidly inactivated either by reuptake into the presynaptic fibre, involving a molecular transporter, or by enzymatic degradation, e.g. by acetyl cholinesterase.

The neurotransmitter substances are small molecules (monoamines, aminoacids, peptides). The neuronal brain network can be divided into different systems (cholinergic, dopaminergic, serotoninergic, adrenergic, GABAergic, peptidergic etc) on the basis of chemical neurotransmission.

Close specificity exists between the neurotransmitter and the receptor or transporter. However, it is possible to bind some analogues, for example, neuroleptic drugs bind to the dopamine transporter. The use of gamma-emitting analogues as radioligands is the basis of the scintigraphic approach to neurotransmission. This is an in vivo functional investigation of the nervous system. It provides pathophysiological and diagnostic information. It is also useful for guiding treatment and follow-up, because the receptors and the transporter are the targets of many drugs active on the brain. The criteria for a suitable radioligand are: passage through the blood brain barrier; specific, stable binding to receptors or transporters; absence of toxicity, and absence of pharmacological activity at the dose used.

The following receptors can be investigated by scintigraphic procedures: dopaminergic, cholinergic, serotoninergic and benzodiazepine receptors. The dopamine transporter can also be explored. It is therefore necessary to consider further the physiological and neurochemical properties of these different systems.

Dopaminergic system

The dopamine system consists of different neuronal pathways arising from brain stem nuclei. The axons reach different brain structures in which dopaminergic receptors can be found.

There are three ascending pathways: the nigro striatal, which controls motility; the meso limbic which plays a role in instinctive and affective behaviour; and the meso cortical which plays a role in arousal, attention, cognition and memory.

There are two descending pathways: the tubero infundibular pathways which regulates growth hormone and prolactin secretion, and the incerto hypothalamic which plays a role in hunger, thirst and blood pressure regulation.

Disturbances of this system occur in many disease conditions, namely movement and psychiatric disorders.

Receptors

The dopaminergic receptors bind dopamine and other agonists or antagonists. According to the binding properties and the molecular mechanism of their action, different dopaminergic receptor subtypes have been identified, which correspond to genetically controled molecular structures.

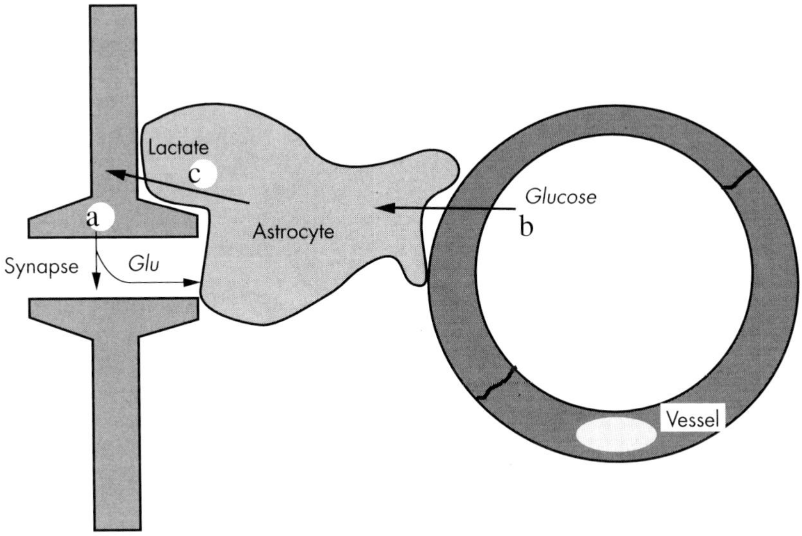

Fig. 2
Neuronal activation and metabolism
a Neuronal activation, glutamate release and uptake by astrocyte
b Glucose transport from the blood into the glia cell, glycolysis, lactate production
c Lactate transport from the glia cell to the neuron

D1 and D2 subtypes differ according to their molecular mechanism of action: the D1 receptor activates adenylcyclase whereas the D2 receptor has no effect on it (Kebabian and Calne, 1979; Seenan, 1981). The dopaminergic receptor is a glycopeptide of 400 amino acids with seven hydrophobic transmembrane domains, one extra cellular N terminal position bearing the glycosyl moiety, one intracytoplasmic C terminal position and, in some subtypes, a protein G binding site located on the third intracytoplasmic loop. This loop is short in the D1 and long in the D2 receptors (Schwartz et al., 1992). The receptor subtypes have the same transmembrane chain and it is accepted that dopamine binds to the receptor by the phenolic groups and two serine residues of the fifth transmembrane loop (Zhou et al., 1990; Hutchins, 1994). The D3 receptor was cloned in 1992 by Sokoloff et al.(1992); it has a higher affinity than the D2 receptor for dopamine and is found mainly in the limbic region (Strange, 1993; Meador-Woodruff et al., 1994). The D4 receptor was cloned in 1991 (Van Tol et al., 1991); it is also found mainly in the limbic region and has a high affinity for clozapine, an atypical neuroleptic without extrapyramidal side effects.

The D5 receptor was cloned in 1991 (Sunahara et al., 1991). D5 receptor mRNA is mainly found in the hippocampus and the thalamus whereas D1 receptor mRNA is mainly expressed in the striatum, the acumbens nucleus and the olfactory tubercle (Ogawa, 1995).

D2 receptors are easy to explore because of suitable available radioligands and high striatal concentration (about 15 picomoles/cc) (Wagner et al., 1984).

Transporter

The neuronal dopamine transporter is a 800 kDa protein, which is specific to the fibres described. It plays an essential role in inactivating the neurotransmitter released into the synaptic cleft. It is blocked by cocaine and some derivatives.

Serotoninergic system

Receptors

The serotoninergic systems are formed by descending and ascending pathways from the median raphe nuclei to the locus coeruleus, spinal cord, hypothalamus, striatum, hippocampus and the anterior cortex. They are involved in sleep, aggressive behaviour and pain.

A great variety of receptor types exists. Seven types or subtypes have been identified according to their affinity for different ligands, localisation and physiological role: 5 HT1A, 5 HT1B, 5 HT1c, 5HT1D, 5 HT2, 5 HT3, 5 HT1p. The best understood are the 5HT2 receptors which are found in the brain and at the periphery in smooth muscle fibres (Hartig and Lever, 1990).

To date, only one radiolabelled ligand has been used for human SPECT: iodo ketanserine, a 5HT2 receptor ligand. It has been used to show an increase in receptor sites in the fronto parietal cortex of depressed patients (Bossuyt et al., 1991); Other applications such as investigation of schizophrenia, are under consideration (Busatto, 1996).

Transporter

A specific serotonin transporter exists in the serotoninergic fibres. Its molecular structure is similar to that of the dopamine transporter (Hoffman et al., 1991). The serotonin transporter is the therapeutic target of some antidepressant drugs (Johnson, 1989).

Cholinergic system

Acetylcholine is an important neurotransmitter in both the central and peripheral nervous system. It binds to two receptor types which differ in localisation, pharmacological agonists and molecular mechanism of action .

Nicotinic receptors are present in the peripheral nervous system, in the autonomic system ganglions and at the neuromuscular junction. The nicotinic receptor is a membrane glycoprotein organized in five subunits. It is directly coupled to an ion channel.

Muscarinic receptors are in the central nervous system. They are coupled to the ion channels through a GTP binding protein which has the role of signal tranducer. Muscarinic receptor activation involves an interaction with a G protein. After release into the synapse, acetylcholine is inactivated not by reuptake but by acetylcholine esterase enzymatic degradation.

Glutamatergic system

Glutamate and aspartate are excitatory aminoacid neurotransmitters. They are involved in many mental and neurosensory functions, including cognition, memory, movement and sensation. They act on synaptic connection plasticity during development. In many diseases, excess glutamatergic system activation results in neuronal lesion and death (Lipton and Rosenberg, 1994). The disease processes are characterised by an excess of neuronal calcium ion influx through the ion channels, triggered by the glutamate receptors.

Receptors

The excitatory aminoacid receptors belong to two types according to the molecular mechanism of action, ionotropic receptors which are directly coupled to the ion channel in the cell membrane, and metabotropic receptors which are coupled to a G protein and to a second intracellular messager. The ionotropic receptors are subdivided into different types according to their selective antagonists: NMDA, AMPA (amino-3-hydroxy-5-methyl-4-isoxazole propionate) and kainate.

Transporter

Release of excitatory amino acids into the synapse and the extracellular fluid is followed by re uptake into the neurons and astrocytes. This re uptake is not only an inactivation process but also a link in the coupling chain between neuronal activation, perfusion and metabolism (Fig. 2 and Fig. 3). These transporters, which have a high affinity for their ligands, were recently cloned (Kanai and Hediger, 1992).

Benzodiazepine receptors

Benzodiazepines represent a chemical class of substances with anxiolytic, anticonvulsive and sedative pharmacological effects. Benzodiazepines radiolabeled with tritium (e.g. ^{3}H diazepam) or with carbon 11 (e.g. ^{11}C flunitrazepam) have been used to characterise binding sites as receptor sites. These receptors are unusual because they do not have any known endogenous ligand. Benzodiazepine receptors are classified into two types according to their localisation and central and peripheral receptors

The central receptors are found exclusively in the central nervous system on the neuron membrane. They are coupled to aminobutyric acid receptors (GABA) receptors and to chloride channels within a macromolecular complex (Olsen, 1982). GABA is the main inhibitory transmitter in the central nervous system. The GABA receptors are in the cerebral cortex and cerebellum. Benzodiazepine receptor ligands are agonists, as are benzodiazepines such as diazepam, chlorazepam, flunitrozepam, or belong to other chemical classes as pyrido-dihydro-pyrrolopyrazinc (zopiclone) with sedative effects. Some ligands are reverse agonists, as are β carbolines which have convulsant effects and generate panic attacks. Other ligands such as flumazenil or RO-15 1788 are agonists, which block the effects of the agonists.

Peripheral benzodiazepine receptor sites have been characterised in the kidneys, liver and lungs. They also exist in the steroid hormone secretory glands, activated monocytes and glial cells of the nervous system. Unlike central receptors, the peripheral receptors are on the mitochondrial membranes. Search for the endogenous ligand suggests that porphyrins might be receptor ligands (Verma et al., 1987). The porphyrin type seems to be variable from one tissue to another, however protoporphyrin IX seems to be the main substance (Snyder et al., 1990). The chemical relationships between porphyrins and haemoglobin on the one hand and porphyrins and cytochromes on the other, and also their cellular and subcellular localisation, suggest that the peripheral benzodiazepine receptors could play a role in oxidative reduction processes, steroid hormone synthesis and chemotaxis.

Methodological principles

There are various scintigraphic brain investigation methods which way according to the tracer, the detector and the field investigated. They have in common the provision of functional information, i.e. flow, perfusion, metabolism and synaptic mechanisms.

The dosimetric data are of particular importance in children. The technical bases of imaging modalities are essential in order to understand the value and limitations of PET and SPECT methods.

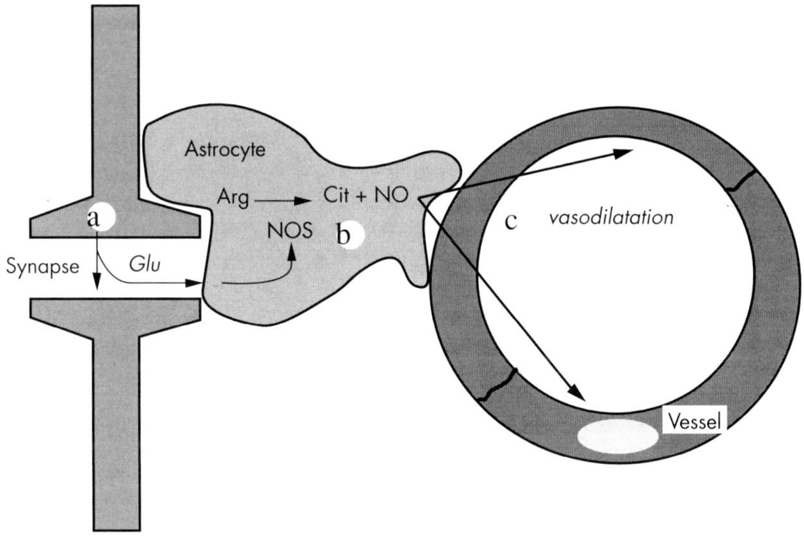

Fig. 3
Neuronal activation and perfusion (hypothesis)
a Neuronal activation, glutamate release and uptake by astrocyte
b Stimulation of NO synthase (NOS) and NO production
c NO diffusion and microvessel smooth-muscle relaxaxion

Investigations

Flow, perfusion

Cerebral blood flow is a physiological parameter which is expressed in milliliters per minute per gram of tissue; perfusion is a more qualitative concept which is not measurable and which depends on capillary flow, exchange area and membrane permeability.

The measurement of cerebral blood flow is most often based on a diffusible tracer tissue clearance study, for example $H_2^{15}O$ or ^{133}Xe. Oxygen 15 is positon emitter with a short half life (125 seconds). It is injected as $C^{15}O_2$ and $H_2^{15}O$ is produced in the lung by carbonic anhydrase. The classical method necessitates study of blood kinetics by arterial sampling and is relatively invasive (Ter-Pogossian et al., 1969). Alternative methods have been suggested to avoid arterial sampling, e.g. external detection of vascular activity (Nelson et al., 1993), ignoring arterial activity when measuring variation in local flow during activation testing (Volkow et al., 1991). The advantages of oxygen 15 are low radiation dose and the possibility of repeated injections in different neuropsychological conditions. The drawback is the need for a PET facility.

Xenon is an inert, diffusible, liposoluble gas. Isotope 133 is a β emitter (mean energy 110 kev) and a γ emitter (81 kev) with a 5.31 day half life. It is most often administered by inhalation through a closed circuit system. Detection is not optimal because its low energy leads to depth attenuation. In the past external probes were used and SPECT machines are more often used today. SPECT machines must have high sensitivity and be able to perform a tomographic acquisition every 10 seconds. Some, such as Tomomatic* (Medimatic, the Netherlands) and Ceraspect* (Digital Scintigraphic Inc., USA) are dedicated to brain imaging. It is anticipated in the near future that conventional three-headed gamma cameras will be able to measure brain flow using xenon (Devous et al., 1993). The algorithms for calculating the absolute blood flow use the scintigraphic data collected during the initial wash-in during 2 - 3 minutes' inhalation and the 4 - 5 minutes' wash-out phase after inhalation ceases (Celsis et al., 1981). The xenon method provides the gold standard brain blood flow measurement. Use of this method in children is limited by the relatively high radiation dose.

The so called "brain perfusion" tracers deliver a lower radiation dose. They have the following common properties: passage through the lung; crossing the blood brain barrier which requires high lipophilicity, neutral electric charge, molecular weight between 350 and 500 daltons and a low affinity for plasma proteins; first pass brain extraction; cerebral retention due to a chemical change which decreases lipophilicity; and rapid clearance from the blood and surrounding tissues.

The important properties are first pass extraction and complete retention. Given these two properties, these tracers give information on brain perfusion at the time of injection (not at the time of imaging). Imaging can be performed later, over as long a time as necessary. The first brain perfusion tracer was iodo amphetamine radiolabelled with iodine 123 (Holman et al., 1984). The advantages of iodo amphetamine are one hundred per cent brain extraction, good correlation between early uptake and flow out a wide range of values (Moretti et al., 1987) and good response to the acetazolamide-induced vasodilatation (Khul et al., 1982). Its drawbacks are high, variable uptake and release in the lung, with consequent degradation product redistribution and relatively high radiation dose, especially to the retina. Moreover the cost of iodine 123 is high and availability is limited. For these reasons alternative tracers, 99m technetium radiolabelled lipophilic complexes, have emerged since 1985: the first was hexamethylpropylene-amine-oxime (HMPAO Ceretec*, Amersham UK) and the second the ethyl- cysteinate-dimer (ECD Neurolite*, Dupont Pharma France). Brain uptake is rapid (1 - 2 minutes) and represents about 3.5 - 4% of the injected HMPAO activity or about 5 - 6% of the ECD dose. The mechanism of HMPAO retention has not been completely clarified: it seems to be a consequence of the conversion of lipophilic complexes into secondary complexes: hydrophilic complexes, by demethylation to a lower pH in the brain than in the blood (Nakamura et al., 1989), and secondary complexes bound to glutathione (Suess et al., 1992). ECD retention is the consequence of a specific intracellular transformation of the diester by esterases into anionic mono- and diacid complexes which cannot cross back through the cell membrane (Kung, 1990). Due to these properties, the topographical distribution of radioactivity reflects regional brain perfusion in the healthy subject (Leveille et al., 1989). However, in disease, the changes in permeability and metabolism may alter uptake and retention in a way as yet unknown. ECD offers several advantages over to HMPAO: better in vitro stability (6 hours for ECD, 30 minutes for HMPAO), higher brain uptake and higher contrast between brain and other tissues and between normal and hypoperfused regions of the brain. However, the relative diagnostic performance of these tracers in disease remains to be assessed.

Metabolism

The parameters which can be studied are oxygen and glucose metabolism rates. These fundamental studies are carried out only using PET. Measurement of local oxygen metabolism rate is based on continuous inhalation of $^{15}O_2$ followed by $C^{15}O_2$. A classical and particularly elegant method for the calculation of the O_2 tissue extraction coefficient was developed by

Subramanyam et al. (1978), who established that the oxygen extraction coefficient could be calculated by dividing the equilibrium images obtained with $^{15}O_2$ and $C^{15}O_2$ pixel by pixel. This calculation necessitates mesuring arterial concentration of $^{15}O_2$ and $H_2{}^{15}O$ during $^{15}O_2$ inhalation and of $^{15}O_2$ during $C^{15}O_2$ inhalation. It is therefore necessary to obtain two arterial samples which makes performing this method more difficult in children; an indwelling cannula can, of course, be used.

Measurement of local glucose metabolic rate is based on the method of Sokoloff et al. (Sokoloff et al., 1977) using 2-fluoro-2 deoxyglucose radiolabelled with fluorine 18 (FDG). FDG is a substrate for the transmembrane glucose transporter and for hexokinase. This enzyme transforms FDG into phosphorylated FDG, which is not metabolised further. FDG kinetic can therefore be described by a three compartment model. Integrating the data obtained by venous sampling and dynamic brain PET recording into such a model, it is possible to calculate regional brain glucose metabolic rate (Phelps et al., 1979).

Neurotransmission

Many systems: cholinergic, monoaminergic (dopamine, epinephrine, serotonin), GABAergic systems (benzodiazepines), peptidergic (somatostatin, opioïd substances) involving different neurotransmitters can be investigated by PET or SPECT. Table 1 shows that a large number of radioligands have been used for PET and for SPECT (Wagner et al., 1984), SPECT ligands has been radiolabelled with iodine 123. This isotope is relatively expensive, not immediately available and delivers a radiation dose which is not negligible. In the next few years its replacement by 99m technetium will probably decrease the cost and the radiation dose. 99m technetium radioligands will be of most interest for nuclear imaging in children (Meegalla et al., 1995; Madras et al., 1996)

Dosimetry

For ethical reasons, it is not possible to determine directly the radiation dose received by children submitted to scintigraphic investigation. The dose is extrapolated from that measured in adults (table 2) (Ter-Pogossian, 1981; Mejia et al., 1991; Atkins et al., 1991; Soundy et al., 1990; Verhoeff et al., 1993;Kung et al., 1989; Kuikka et al., 1994). It is important to keep in mind that doses received by the child are proportionately higher than those received by the adult.

Table 1
PET and SPECT radioligands for investigation of brain neurotransmission

			equivalent dose (mSv)			
tracer	reference	activity (Mbq adult)	brain	target organ	ovaries	testes
^{15}O-oxygen (inhalation)	(Ter Pogossian, 1981)	7000		tracheal mucosa 38		
^{18}F-deoxyglucose	(Mejia et al., 1991)	185	5.4	bladder wall 22		2.8
^{133}Xe-xenon (inhalation)	(Atkins et al., 1991)	300		lung 0.9	0.1	0.1
^{99m}Tc-HMPAO	(Soundy et al., 1990)	500		bladder wall 27	3.8	1.1
^{123}I-iomazenil	(Verhoeff et al., 1993)	185	28	brain 28	3.1	8.1
^{123}I-IBZM	(Kung et al., 1989)	185	basal ganglia 74	basal ganglia 74		
^{123}I-ßCIT	(Kuikka et al., 1994)	185	1.7	basal ganglia 50	2	1.1

Figure 4 shows the activities recommanded by the Paediatric Task Group of the European Association of Nuclear Medicine (PTGEA, 1990).

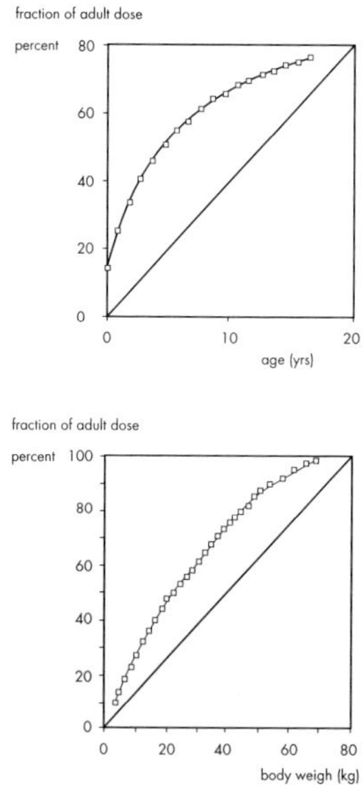

Fig. 4
Usual activities administered to children.

Detectors

Without going into excessive detail, it is useful to describe some aspects of signal detection and scintigraphic imaging: emission tomography principles; the differences between PET and SPECT; brain dedicated camera definitions and descriptions; and problems of quantification and image fusion.

Emission tomography principles

Emission tomography is based on the detection of radiation emitted by the body, the organ or the lesion under study. It is thus basically different from transmission tomography (X-ray CT) which consists of detection of radiation from an external source through the body. The radiation source is a gamma emitting radioisotope, which is passing in the body usually after intravenous injection. The radioisotope is in the elementary state or coupled to a molecule which acts as a vector. There are several consequences of this. The radiation dose to the body depends only on the activity delivered and the pharmacokinetics. It is not dependent on the duration of imaging nor on the number images or the area they

Table 2
Adult dosimetry of radiotracers used for brain PET and SPECT
The EDE (effective dose equivalent) is an equivalent of the dose to the body weighted by the dose to the critical organs (bone marrow, gonads, etc.).

		PET	SPECT
Dopamine	Receptors D1	^{11}C-SCH23390 (Ravet et al., 1987; Farde et al., 1987)	^{123}I-TISCH (Billings et al., 1991)
Dopamine	Receptors D2	^{76}Br-lisuride (Maziere et al., 1986)	^{123}I-iodolisuride (Loc'h et al., 1991)
		^{11}C-methyhlspiperone (Wagner et al., 1984)	2' iodospiperone (Iwasaki et al., 1995)
		^{11}C raclopride (Farde et al., 1986)	^{123}I-iodobenzamide (Kung et al., 1989; Baulieu et al., 1992)
			^{123}I-IBF (Ichise et al., 1986; Laruelle et al., 1994)
	Transporter	^{11}C-nomifensine (Aquilonius et al., 1987)	^{123}I-ßCIT (Innis et al., 1993)
		^{11}C-ßCIT (Farde et al., 1994)	
Serotin	Receptors	^{11}C methyl-bromo LSD (Hartig and Lever, 1990)	^{123}I-ketanserin (Bossuyt et al., 1991)
Serotin	Transporter	^{11}C(+)McN5652 (Szabo et al., 1995)	^{123}I-ßCIT (Brucke et al., 1993)
			^{123}I-nitroquipazine (Jagust et al., 1995)
Benzodiazepine	Receptors	^{11}C-flumazenil (Shinoto et al., 1986)	^{123}I-iomazenil (Schubiger et al., 1994)

cover. The radiation is altered by attenuation and diffusion before being detected. This alteration distorts both resolution and quantification. The data and images are closely related to the physico chemical, biochemical and pharmacological properties of the radioactive isotope vector. The information gained is basically functional and metabolic, i.e., blood flow, perfusion, specific receptor binding, specific molecular transport.

Tomographic imaging consists of the reconstruction of slices in different orientations (transverse, sagittal, coronal) from the planar projections obtained at different angles during rotation through 180° or 360°. The reconstruction algorithms are similar to those used in transmission imaging and usually involve a filtered back projection. Back projection, filtering, display and filing are performed by a data processing system which plays an important role and is coupled to the detector.

Differences between PET and SPECT

PET and SPECT differ according to the radiation detected: in PET, the radioisotopes emit positron (positive electron). After travelling a few millimeters the positron combines with an ordinary electron in an annihilation reaction and gives rise to two 511 keV gamma rays (mass-energy equivalence) in exactly opposite directions (motion quantity nil). These can be detected by two detectors facing each other, thus performing electronic collimation. The detection yield is high and the scintigraphic signal reflects the total radioactivity present in the field of detection without significant attenuation. PET is limited by the short half life of the radioelements (^{15}O 2min, ^{13}N 10min, ^{11}C 20min, ^{18}F 112min) and of the cost of the cyclotron required to produce them and of PET cameras.

In SPECT, the photons are emitted as single units in any direction from the source. A physical collimation is necessary, in the form of a lead shield pierced by parallel, convergent or divergent channels (parallel convergent or divergent collimator) or by a single hole (pinhole collimator) which select the direction of the photons to be detected. The collimator considerably reduces the number of photons which reach the scintillation crystal. These photons have relatively low energy (140 kev in the case of 99m-technetium) and undergo attenuation and diffusion causes of error in quantitative detection. SPECT is limited by low sensitivity and inaccurate quantification. Its advantages compared to PET are availability and low cost.

Brain dedicated camera

A solution to the limitations of PET and SPECT could be the use of brain dedicated SPECT cameras. These consist of a battery of detectors or a cylindrical detector close to the skull, increasing both the yield of detection and the spatial resolution. An example is the annular stationary crystal camera (Ceraspect* Digital Scintigraphy Instrument Boston Ma - USA). This is relatively small and devoid of visible moving parts during imaging. These characteristics contribute significantly to reduction of fear in children induced by the imaging examination.

Quantification

Quantification comprises several steps: measurement of radioactivity by external detection, drawing of structure or regions of interest, and calculation of physiological parameters by modelisation. The parameters are blood flow, metabolic substrate consumption, molecular receptor or transporter concentration. Measurement of radioactivity by external detection necessitates taking into account attenuation, diffusion and partial volume effect: these corrections are of greater importance in SPECT and require preliminary studies with appropriate phantoms. Structure and regions of interest often cannot be satisfactorily delineated from the scintigraphic image because of poor spatial resolution. The anatomical structures are best drawn on morphological imaging modalities such as X-ray or MRI. The imaging data therefore have to be transferred, reset and merged.

Physiological parameter calculation uses models which take into account the biological properties of the tracer. For example, brain blood flow can be calculated from xenon 133 wash in and wash out using Fick's principle (Celsis et al., 1981) or neuroreceptor concentration can be calculated from the bound and unbound portions of a specific ligand using a compartmental model or Scatchard's analysis (Abi-Dargham et al., 1994).

In conclusion, a great variety of possibilities is offered by PET and SPECT for functionnal brain imaging of children with psychiatric disorders. Significant progresses is to be expected in diagnosis of psychiatric diseases and in research in cognitive sciences. Relevant data will soon be available in Tourette's syndrome and in hyperkinetic, autistic and anorectic children, as described in the following chapters.

References

Abi-Dargham A, Laruelle M, Seibyl J, Rattner Z, Baldwin M, Zoghbi S, Zea-Ponce Y, Bremner J, Hyde T, Charney D, Hoffer P, Innis R (1994) SPECT measurement of benzodiazepine receptors in human brain with iodine-123-iomazenil: kinetic and equilibrium paradigms. J Nucl Med 35: 228-238

Aquilonius S, Bergström K, Eckernäs S, Hartvig P, Leenders K, Lundqvist H, Längstrom B (1987) In vivo evaluation of striatal dopamine reuptake sites using (11C) nomifensine and positron emission tomography. Acta Neurol Scand 76: 283-287

Archer S (1993) Measurement of nitric oxide in biological models. FASEB J 7: 349-360

Atkins H, Robertson J, Croft B, Tsui B, Susskind H, Ellis J, Loken M, Treves S (1991) Report n°9 Radio xenons in lung imaging In: Loevinger R, Budinger T, Watson E (eds) Mird Primer The Society of Nuclear Medicine, New York, p 70-77

Baulieu JL, Guilloteau D, Chalon S, Markabi S, Gaymard B, Ribeiro Barras MJ, Autret A, Tranquart F, Besnard JC (1992) Scintigraphie des récepteurs cérébraux D2 de la dopamine: résultats préliminaires obtenus avec l'iodobenzamide (123I-IBZM). J Med Nucl Biophys 16: 52-57

Billings J, Kung M, Chumpradi S, Mozley P, Alavi A, Kung H (1991) In vivo characterization of [123I] TISCH; a high affinity and selective imaging agent for the CNS D1 dopamine receptors. J Neurochem 58: 227-238

Bossuyt A, Bossuyt Piron C, Mertens J, Gijsemans M, D'Hænen H (1991) 5HT2 receptor imaging with I-123-ketanserin in depression. J Nucl Med 32: 952

Brucke T, Kornhuber J, Angelberger P, Asenbaum S, Frassine H, Podreka J (1993) SPECT imaging of dopamine and serotonin transporter with 123I ßCIT: binding kinetics in the human brain. J Neural Transm Gen Sect 94 2: 137-146

Busatto G (1996) Radioligands for brain 5-HT2 receptor imaging in vivo: why do we need them? Eur J Nucl Med 23: 867-870

Celsis P, GoldmanT, Henriksen L, Lassen N (1981) A method for calculating regional cerebral blood flow from emission computed tomography of inert gas concentrations. J Comput Assist Tomogr 5: 641-645

Devous M, Gong S, Payne J (1993) Dynamic quantitative Xe-133 RCBF SPECT on the Prism 3-headed tomograph: stimulation and phantom studies. J Nucl Med 34: 91

Faraci F, Breese K (1993) Nitric oxide mediates vasodilatation in response to activation of N-methyl-D-aspartate receptors in brain. Circ Res 72: 476-480

Farde L, Hall H, Ehrin E, Sedvall G (1986) Quantitative analysis of dopamine-D2 receptor binding in the living human brain using positron emission tomography. Science 231: 258-261

Farde L, Halldin C, Stone-Elander S, Sedvall G (1987) PET analysis of human dopamine receptor subtypes using 11C-SCH 23390 and 11C-raclopride. Psychopharmacology 92: 278-284

Farde L, Halldin C, Muller L, Suhara T, Karlsson P, Hall H (1994) PET study of [11C]β-CIT binding to monoamine transporters in the monkey and human brain. Synapse 16: 93-103

Garthwaite J (1991) Glutamate, nitric oxide and cell-cell signalling in the nervous system. Trends Neurosci 14: 60-7

Genna S, Smith A (1988) The development of ASPECT, an annular single crystal brain camera for high efficiency SPECT. IEEE Trans Nuclear Science 35: 654-658

Hartig P, Lever J (1990) Serotonin receptors. In: Frost J, Wagner H (ed) Quantitative lmaging. Neuroreceptors, neurotransmitters and enzymes. Raven Press, New York, p 153-154

Hoffman B, Mezey E, Brownstein J (1991) Cloning of serotonin transporter affected by antidepressants. Science 254: 579-581

Holman B, Lee R, Hill T (1984) A comparison of two cerebral perfusion tracers: 123I-IMP and 123-HIPDM in humans. J Nucl Med 25: 25-30

Hutchins C (1994) Three-dimensional models of the D1 and D2 dopamine receptors. Endocrine Journal [illegible]

Ichise M, Ballinger J, Golan H, Vines D, Luong A, Tsai S, Kung H (1996) Noninvasive quantification of dopamine D2 receptors with Iodine-123-IBF SPECT. J Nucl Med 37: 513-520

Innis R, Seibyl J, Scanley B (1993) Single photon emission computed tomographic imaging demonstrates loss of striatal dopamine transporters in Parkinson's disease. Proc Nat Acad Sci 90 24: 11965-11969

Iwasaki Y, Yonekura Y, Saji H, Nishizawal S, Fukuyama H, Iida Y, Magata Y. (1995) SPECT imaging of dopamine D2 receptors with 2'-iodospiperone. J Nucl Med 38: 1191-1195

Jagust WJ, Eberling JL, Biegon A, Scott E, Taylor SE, Henry F, Vanbrocklin, HF, Jordan S, Hanrahan SM, Roberts JA, Brenham KM, Mathis CA (1996) Iodine-123-5-iodo-6-nitroquipazine: SPECT radiotracer to image the serotonin transporter. J Nucl Med 37: 1207-1214

Johnson A (1989) An overview of the animal pharmacology of paroxetine. Acta Psychiat Scand 80 (suppl 350): 14-20

Kanai Y, Hediger M (1992) Primary structure and functional characterization of a high-affinity glutamate transporter. Nature 360: 467-471

Kebabian L, Calne D (1979) Multiple receptors for dopamine. Nature 277: 93-96

Khul D, Barrio J, Huang S (1982) Quantifying local cerebral blood flow with 123I-IMP tomography. J Nucl Med 23: 196-203

Kuikka J, Bergström K, Ahonen A, Länsimies E (1994) The dosimetry of iodine-123 labelled 2ß-carbomethoxy-3ß-(4-iodophenyl) tropane. Eur J Nucl Med 21: 53-56

Kung H (1990) New technnetium 99m-labelled brain perfusion imaging agents. Semin Nucl Med 20: 150-158

Kung H, Pan S, Kung M, Billings J, Kasliwal R, Reilley J, Alavi A (1989) In vitro and in vivo evaluation of 123I IBZM: a potential CNS D2 dopamine receptor imaging agent. J Nucl Med 30: 88-92

Kung H, Alavi A, Chang W, Kung M, Keyes J, Velchik M, Billings J, Pan S, Noto R, Rausch A, Reilley J (1990) In vivo SPECT imaging of CNS D-2 dopamine receptors: initial studies with iodine-123IBZM in humans. J Nucl Med 31: 573-579

Ladecola C (1993) Regulation of the cerebral microcirculation during neural activity: is nitric oxide the missing link? TINS 16: 206-213

Laruelle M, van Dyck C, Abi-Dargham A, Zea-Ponce Y, Zoghbi S, Charney D, Baldwin R, Hoffer P, Kung H, Innis R (1994) Compartmental modeling of Iodine-123-iodobenzofuran binding to dopamine D2 receptors in healthy subjects. J Nucl Med 35: 743-754

Léveillé J, Demonceau G, De Roo M (1989) Characterization of 99 mTc-ECD for brain perfusion imaging. Part 2: biodistribution and brain imaging in humans. J Nucl Med 30: 1902-1910

Lipton S, Rosenberg P (1994) Excitatory amino acids as a final common pathway for neurologic disorders. N Engl J Med 330: 613-622

Loc'h C, Bourguignon M, Mazière B, Stulzaft O, Ottaviani M, Hantraye Ph, Chabriat H, Raynaud C, Syrota A, Mazière M (1991) 123I-iodolisuride, un nouvel agent pour l'étude des récepteurs dopaminergiques D2 par tomographie d'émission monophotonique (SPECT). J Med Nucl Biophys 15: 420-427

Madras B, Jones A, Mahmood A, Zimmerman R, Garada B, Holman B, Davison A, Blundell P, Meltzer P (1996) Technepine: A high-affinity 99mtechnetium probe to label the dopamine transporter in brain by spect imaging. Synapse 22: 239-246

Mazière B Loc'h C, Stulzaft P, Hantraye M, Ottaviani M, Comar D, Mazière M (1986) 76Br-bromolisuride: a new tool for quantitative in vivo imaging of D2 dopamine receptor. Eur J Pharmacol 127: 239-247

Meador-Woodruff J, Mansour A, Saul J, Watson S Jr (1994) Neuro-anatomical distribution of dopamine receptor messenger RNAs. In: Niznik HB (ed) Dopamine receptors and transporters. Marcel Dekker, New York, p 401-415

Meegalla S, Plössl K, Kung M, Andrew Stevenson D, Liable-sands L, Rheingold A, Kung H (1995) First example of a 99mTc complex as a dopamine transporter imaging agent. J Am Chem Soc 117: 11037-11038

Mejia A, Nakamura T, Masatoshi I, Hatazawa J, Masaki M, Watanuki S (1991) Estimation of absorbed doses in humans due to intravenous administration of fluorine 1 fluorodeoxyglucose in PET studies. J Nucl Med 32: 699-705

Moncada S, Palmer R, Higgs E (1989) Biosynthesis of nitric oxide from L-arginine: a pathway for the regulation of cell function and communication. Biochem Pharmacol 38: 1709-1715

Moncada S, Higgs A (1993) The L-arginine nitric oxide pathway. N Engl J Med 329: 2002-2010

Moretti J, Defer G, Delmon L (1987) Acetazolamide: effet sur la perfusion cérébrale appréciée par la tomoscintigraphie à l'123I-IMP Résultats préliminaires. J Biophys Biomec 11: 69-73

Nakamura K, Tukatani Y, Kubo A (1989) The behavior of 99mTc-HMPAO in blood and brain. Eur J Nucl Med 15: 100-107

Nelson D, Miraldi F, Muzic R, Greg P, Leisure G, Semple W (1993) Noninvasive arterial monitor for quantitative oxygen-15-water blood flow studies. J Nucl Med 34: 1000-1005

Ogawa N (1995) Molecular and chemical neuropharmacology of dopamine receptor subtypes. Acta Med Okayama 49: 1-11

Olsen R (1982) Drug interactions at the GABA receptor-ionophore complex. Am Rev Pharmac Toxic 22: 245-277

Paediatric Task Group of the European Association of Nuclear Medicine (1990) A radiopharmaceutical schedule for imaging in paediatrics. Eur J Nucl Med 17: 127-129

Pellerin L, Magistretti PJ (1994) Glutamate uptake into astrocytes stimulates aerobic glycolysis: a mechanism coupling neuronal activity to glucose utilization. Proc Nat Acad Sci 91: 10625-10629

Phelps M, Huang S, Hoffman E, Selin C, Sokoloff L, Kuhl D (1979) Tomographic measurement of local cerebral glucose metabolic rate in humans with (F-18)2-Fluro-2-deoxy-d-glucose: validation of method. Ann neurol 6: 371-386

Ravert H, Wilson A, Dannals R, Wong D, Wagner H (1987) Radiosynthesis of selective dopamine D-1 receptor antagonist: R(+)-7-chloro-8-hydroxy-3-(11C)Methyl-1-Phenyl-2,3,4,5-Tetrahydro-1-H-3-Benzazepine (11C)SCH 23390). Int J Appl Rad Isot 38: 305-306

Schubiger P, Hasler P, Beer-Wohlfahrt H, Bekier A, Oettl R, Cordes M, Ferstl F, Deisenhammer E, de Roo M, Moser E, Nitzsche E, Podreka J, Riccabona G, Bangerl I, Schober O, Bartenstein P, Van Rijk P, Van Isselt J, Van Royen E, Verhoeff N, Haldemann R, Von Schulthess G (1991) Evaluation of multicentre study with Iomazenil - a benzodiazepine receptor ligand. Nucl Med Commun 12: 569-582

Schwartz J, Giros B, Martes M, Sokoloff P (1992) The dopamine receptor family: molecular biology and pharmacology. Semin Neurol 4: 99-108

Seeman P (1981) Brain dopamine receptors. Pharmacol Rev 32: 229-313

Shinotho H, Yamasaki T, Inoue O, Itoh T, Suzuki K, Hashimoto K, Tateno Y, Ikehira H (1986) Visualization of specific binding sites of benzodiazepine in human brain. J Nucl Med 27: 1593-1599

Snyder S, Mc Enery M, Verma A (1990) Molecular mechanisms of peripheral benzodiazepine receptors Neurochem res 15: 119-123

Sokoloff L, Reivich M, Kennedy C (1977) The (14C) deoxyglucose method for the measurement of local cerebral glucose utilization: theory, procedure and normal values in the conscious and anesthetized albino rat. J Neurochem 28: 897-916

Sokoloff P, Martres M, Giros B, Bouthenet M, Schwartz J (1992) The third dopamine receptor (D3) as a novel target for antipsychotics. Biochem Pharmacol 43: 659-666

Soundy R, Tyrrell D, Pickett R, Stabin M (1990) The radiation dosimetry of 99mTc-exametazime. Nucl Med Commun 11: 791-799

Strange P (1993) New insights into dopamine receptors in the central nervous system. Neurochem Int 22: 223-236

Subramanyam R, Alpert N, Hoop B, Gordon J, Brownell G, Taveras J (1978) A model for regional cerebral oxygen distribution during continuous inhalation of $^{15}O_2$, $C^{15}O$, $C^{15}O_2$. J Nucl Med 19: 48-53

Suess E, Huck S, Reither H (1992) Uptake mechanism of $_{99}$mTc-HMPAO in cell cultures of dissociated postnatal rat cerebellum. J Nucl Med 33: 108-114

Sunahara R, Guan H, O'Dowd B, Seeman P, Laurier L, Georges S, Torchia J, Van Tol H, Niznik H (1991) Cloning of the gene for a human dopamine D5 receptor with higher affinity for dopamine than D1. Nature 350: 614-619

Szabo Z, Kao PF, Scheffel U (1995) Positron emission tomography imaging of serotonin transporters in the human brain using [$_{11}$C](+)McN5652. Synapse 20: 37-43

Takahashi S, Driscoll BF, Law MJ, Sokoloff L (1995) Role of sodium and potassium ions in regulation of glucose metabolism in cultured astroglia. Prod Nat Acad Sci 92: 4616-4620

Ter-Pogossian M (1981) Special characteristics and potential for dynamic function studies with PET. Semin Nucl Med 11: 13-23

Ter-Pogossian M, Eichling J, Davis D (1969) The determination of regional cerebral blood flow by means of water labeled with radioactive oxygen-15. Radiology 93: 31-40

Van Tol H, Bunzow J, Guan H, Sunahara R, Seeman P, Niznik H, Civelli O (1991) Cloning of the gene for a human dopamine D4 receptor with high affinity for the antipsychotic clozapine. Nature 351: 610-614

Verhoeff N, Busemann Sokole E, Hengst D, Stubs J, Van Royen E (1993) Dosimetry of iodine-123 iomazenil in humans. Eur J Nucl Med 20: 580-584

Verma A, Nye J, Snyder, S (1987) Porphyrins are endogenous ligands for the mitochondrial (peripheral type) benzodiazepine receptors. Proc Nat Acad Sci 84: 2256-2260

Volkow N, Mullani N, Gould L, Adler S, Gatley S (1991) Sensitivity of measurements of regional brain activation with oxygen-15-water and PET to time of stimulation and period of image reconstruction. J Nucl Med 32: 58-61

Wagner H, Burns H, Dannals R, Wong D, Längström B, Duelfer T, Frost J, Ravert H, Links J, Rosenbloom S, Lukas S, Kramer A, Kuhar M (1984) Imaging dopamine receptors in the human brain by positron emission tomography. Science 221: 1264-1266

Zhou Q, Grandy D, Thambi L, Kushner J, Van T, Cone R, Pribnow D, Salon J, Bunzow J, Civelli O (1990) Cloning and expression of human and rat DI dopamine receptors. Nature 347: 76-80

3. Anatomical and physiological bases of the main electroencephalographic rhythms

B. GARREAU

The electroencephalogram (EEG), described for the first time by Berger (1929), was for a long time the only method available for functional exploration of the brain and was thus used for diagnostic purposes. At first, few workers considered the anatomical and physiological bases of the main EEG rhythms (Adrian and Matthews, 1934). In the early 1980s, quantitative methods of EEG analysis appeared and were found to be of value in neuropsychiatry, giving rise to a large volume of work on the anatomical and physiological basis of EEG rhythms.

The classical EEG of a normal adult in standard recording conditions is composed of a basal rhythm, the alpha rhythm, and a number of rhythms denoted as slow and fast by reference to the alpha rhythm (Table 1). In this chapter, I discuss the cellular basis of the electrical activity of the brain and then move on to the physiological basis of the principal rhythms.

Cellular bases of the electrical activity of the brain

Most signals from the central nervous system (CNS) are generated by ion permeability changes in the postsynaptic membrane, in particular for sodium, potassium, calcium and chloride (Kandel et al., 1991). This permeability change is caused by the release of transmitting molecules at the extremity of the presynaptic neuron.

Neurons maintain a potential difference of about 70mV across their external membrane. This is called the resting membrane potential and results from an inequal distribution of Na+, K+, Cl- and organic anions across the membrane of cells, which leaves the inside of the nerve cell membrane negative in relation to the outside. This unequal distribution of ions is maintained by the Na+/K+ pump, which establishes the ionic gradients for Na+ and K+ that characterise the nerve cell. By transporting Na+ and not K+ out of the cell, this pump keeps the Na+ concentration ten times as low and the K+ concentration about 50 times as high within the cell as outside. The resting membrane potential results from two properties of the cell: the concentration gradients established by the Na+/K+ pump, and the high permeability of the membrane to K+. At rest, the membrane is normally 50 to 100 times as permeable to K+ as it is to Na+; Potassium diffuses easily through the resting membrane, whereas Na+ does so with much more difficulty. Because of its high concentration inside the cell, K+ tends to be driven out of the cell under the influence of the concentration gradient, but leaves behind a major negative charge on the inside surface of the membrane, which making it about 70mV more negative on the inside, than on the outside.

Nerve fibres use this resting membrane potential to transmit nervous impulses, which in turn are used to send a signal from one part of the nervous system

Rhythm	Frequency (Hz)	Amplitude (uV)	Localisation	Reactivity
Delta	Below 3.5	100		
Theta	4/7.5	50	Frontal	↘ Motor activity
Alpha	8/13	30	Occipital	↘ Light
Mu	8/13	30	Rolandic	↘ Motor activity
Beta	above 13	20	Frontal	↗ Motor activity

Table 1. Characteristics of the main EEG Rhythms.

to another. When the membrane potential of a nerve cell is reduced by 20 mV , an all-or-none action potential is initiated. These action potentials are abrupt changes in membrane potential lasting several tenths of a second. They move along the fibre, generating a signal. Any stimulus that abruptly increases membrane permeability to sodium ions can trigger an action potential in a nerve fibre. The action potential results from a sudden change in membrane permeability to sodium and potassium: permeability to sodium is suddenly multiplied by a factor of 5000, returning immediately to a normal level, while permeability to potassium increases considerably. As a result, the membrane potential instantaneously passes from its negative resting value to a positive value, and then becomes negative again.

The action potential is composed of two distinct phases, membrane depolarisation and repolarisation. The sudden increase in permeability to sodium ions leads to a massive influx in to the cell, causing an inversion of the membrane potential. This abrupt disappearance of the normal negative potential is called depolarisation. The momentary appearance of a positive potential inside the fibre is called potential inversion. Immediately after depolarisation, sodium channels once again become practically impermeable, while potassium channels are wide open . Sodium ions no longer enter the fibre, while there is a massive efflux of potassium because of the transmembrane concentration gradient. Potassium ions are positively charged and so this expulsion of excess positive charge restores the normal negative resting potential: this is repolarisation.

An action potential triggered anywhere on an excitable membrane tends to propagate by successive excitation of adjacent zones on the membrane. Sodium permeability of a nerve fibre excited at a given point on its trajectory is suddenly increased at that point. The depolarised zone is the site of a positive current towards the inside and in the resting membrane there is a positive current towards the outside, forming a circuit. For a reason as yet unknown, the output current through the resting membrane results in increased membrane permeability to sodium, enabling these ions to penetrate the membrane and to initiate the self-sustained increase of sodium permeability. This part in turn depolarises and the nervous impulse travels as successive portions, or volleys. New circuits of local currents then appear, causing increasingly closer depolarisation.

Synaptic transmission

Transmission between nerve cells occurs via a succession of events which can be summarised as follows:

action potentials arrive at the axon end of the presynaptic neuron, neurotransmitters are released into the synaptic space; and a postsynaptic potential is produced.

Neurotransmitters are synthesised by presynaptic neurons and stored in vesicles formed by the Golgi apparatus. When action potentials arrive at the end of the axon of the presynaptic neuron, membrane permeability changes, thereby favouring the release of neurotransmitters from vesicles into the synaptic space. The neurotransmitter diffuses into this space and binds to receptors on the postsynaptic membrane. There is a non-negligible interval between depolarisation of the presynaptic membrane and production of postsynaptic action potentials: this synaptic interval is about 0.5 ms. If it is an excitatory synapse, the reactions caused by neurotransmitter binding to its receptor will cause relative depolarisation, the excitatory postsynaptic potential (EPSP). On the other hand, if it is an inhibitory synapse the production of an inhibitory postsynaptic potential (IPSP) will cause hyperpolarisation. The postsynaptic potential is proportional to the quantity of neurotransmitter released, then bound to receptors. Furthermore, when the postsynaptic potential has reached a certain threshold, action potentials will be produced. After their production, there is an absolute refractory period of several ms, during which no new action potential can be produced.

The action potentials produced by a nerve cell can be recorded with an electrode placed on the outer surface of its membrane. An electrode placed within the axon will record the initial -70 mV resting potential and an electrode placed on the outer surface of the resting cell membrane will record the extracellular space potential, by convention equal to zero. As the wave of membrane depolarisation approaches the electrode, the local currents preceding it will cause an increase in the positive potential of the extracellular space, but when it reaches the electrode there is a sudden and brief increase in the negative potential of the extracellular space, immediately fol-

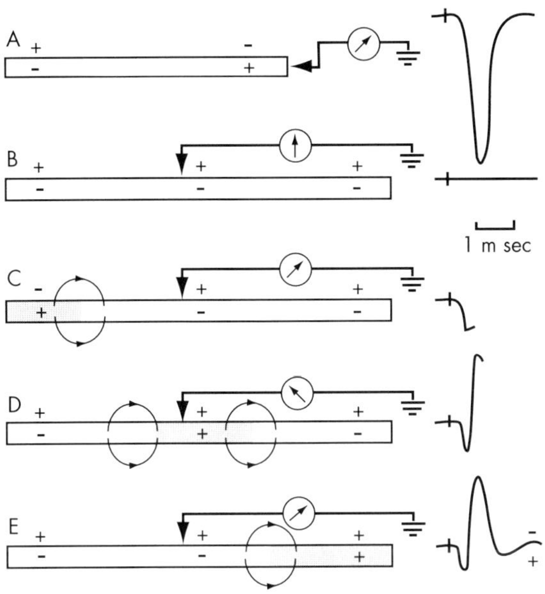

Fig. 1. The action potential spike recordes from outside the neuron (From: Schlag J, 1973).

lowed by a return to the normal resting value (Fig. 1).

When several axons present a synchronised volley of action potentials, which is the case in a nerve, extracellular currents are summed and can be recorded at a site relatively far from the nerve. While the axons of peripheral nerves are parallel, the same is not true in the CNS, which contains a wide range of neuron forms and lengths, and mutual associations of neurons. Lorente de Nô (1947 a, b) described the consequences of these different associations on extracellular currents (Fig. 2).

Excitatory synapses distributed on the dendrites of neuron cell bodies produce an EPSP and a flux of local current. The vertical orientation of dendrites, as shown in figure 3a, could be a source of primary current which can be recorded at a distance if the amplitude of the EPSP is sufficient. If a group of neurons is depolarised simultaneously by a synchronous potential volley, their extracellular currents are summed and can be recorded relatively far away. The distribution of this type of resultant potential was called open field by Lorente de Nô (1947 a, b) (Fig. 2a). If neurons are arranged as a flat surface or a sphere with multiple radiations in all directions, their simultaneous depolarisation by a synchronous volley of action potentials will produce a resultant extracellular current, restricted to a sphere equivalent to a zero or closed field potential (Fig. 2b). This is the "neurophysiological black hole, invisible from the outside" of Allison et al. (1986). In the cerebral cortex, the open field situation is more common, while an intermediate situation, between open, and closed field exists more often in subcortical neurons (Fig. 2c).

EEG recording of the electrical activity of the CNS is made possible by all these basic physiological phenomena.

Anatomical and physiological basis of the main EEG rhythms

The characteristics of the main EEG rhythms are shown in Table 1. In the normal adult, in standard recording conditions, the EEG is composed of a basal rhythm, called the alpha rhythm, which has a frequency between 7 and 14 Hz. Delta and theta rhythms are slower, while beta is faster than alpha rhythm. The same frequency band includes different rhythms with independent anatomical and physiological bases.

Alpha frequency band

The frequency band 7-14 Hz includes three main possible events: spindle oscillations, alpha rhythm and mu rhythm.

Spindles oscillations

Spindle oscillations are 7-14 Hz waves which appear as bursts lasting 1-2 seconds, between the waking state and the onset of slow sleep. Because of their frequency and their detection in cats anaesthetised with barbiturates, these waves had long been taken to be fragments of alpha rhythm. It is now known that their origin and significance are totally unrelated to it. The thalamic origin of spindle oscillations was shown by Morrison and Bassset in 1945, who reported that these waves continue to be recorded in the thalamus after total decortication and cephalic section of the brain stem. Although thalamic reticular cells play an important role in the formation of spindles oscillations, they are included in a circuit composed of, among others, thalamocortical and corticothalamic neurons.

The reticular endothelial (RE) nucleus is a thin sheet of GABAergic neurons covering the lateral ventral surface of the thalamus (Jones, 1985). Its major output is directed primarily to the dorsal thalamus and secondarily to the brain stem, but not to the cerebral cortex. Inputs arise in the thalamus, the cerebral cortex, the rostral part of the brain stem and the basal forebrain. The cortically projecting thalamic nuclei and cerebral cortex are structures that resonate within spindle frequency and so reinforce this oscillation. Steriade (1993) has shown that spindle oscillations are generated in the RE nucleus, and that RE neurons impose rhythmic IPSPs on thalamo-

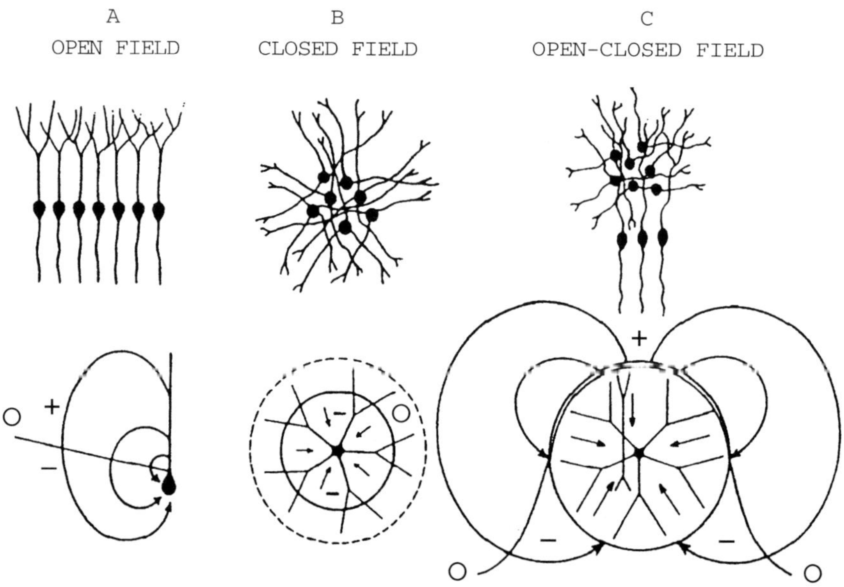

Fig. 2
Extracellular volume currents. Predicted current blood flow and potential fields producted by synchronous depolarization of the cell bodies of a row of neurons with parallel orientation (A), with dendrites arranged radially, cell bodies being clustered in the center (B), and with a combination of open and closed fields (C), In: Reagan D (1989) adapted from Lorente de Nô (1947 a) and Allison et al. (1986).

cortical cells. The latter transfer postinhibitory rebound bursts to the cerebral cortex, where they elicit EPSPs and spike discharges. Thus, spindle oscillations have been interpreted as powerful inhibitors of information destined to the cerebral cortex at the moment of falling asleep (Fig 3).

Alpha rhythm

The alpha rhythm, considered the basic rhythm, and is in the 8-13 Hz frequency band. This rhythm is the longest known EEG rhythm, known since the work of Berger. The international Federation of Societies for Electroencephalography and Clinical Neurophysiology (1974) proposed the following definition of alpha rhythm:

Rhythm at 8-13 Hz occuring during wakefulness over the posterior regions of the head, generally with higher voltage over the occipital areas. Amplitude is variable but is mostly below 50 µV in adults. Best seen with eyes closed and under conditions of physical relaxation and relative mental inactivity. Blocked or attenuated by attention , eseacially visual and mental effort (IFSECN, 1974)

During cerebral maturation, the basal rhythm frequency increases from 4 months to 10 years. Around the age of 4 months there is a detectable posterior basic rhythm with a frequency of 4 Hz. This shows a progressive increase frequency in with average values of 6 Hz at age 12 months, 8 Hz at 3 years and 10 Hz at 10 years.

For a long time, the origin of the alpha rhythm was investigated by studying the spindles obtained under barbiturate anaesthesia. It is now known, however, that even though the frequency band of these two rhythms is superimposable, they have different anatomical and physiological origins. Alpha rhythms appear in conscious adults at rest, are occipital and disappear following visual stimuli, but increase during visual concentration (Mulholland, 1969).

The concept of a thalamic genesis of the alpha phenomenon has been challenged by Lopes da Silva et al. (1973). Alpha waves are generated in the visual cortex by a dipole centered in the dendrites of pyramidal neurons of layers IV and V (Lopes da Silva and Storm van Leeuwen, 1977). These data led to the conclusion that an intracortical system with progressively closer changes along intracortical connections fibres are responsible for the alpha rhythm and that thalamocortical activity has only a modest effect on its generation. Even though this rhythm is considered the basal rhythm, it is not only secondary importance in neuropsychological studies.

Mu rhythm

The mu rhythm is related to the posterior alpha rhythm in frequency and amplitude, but its topography and physiological significance are different. The C3 and C4 electrodes, over the precentral gyrus are in an optimal location for picking up mu rhythm. This rhythm is bilateral but trends to shift from side to side, it is blocked with movement. The prevalence of mu rhythm is about 10 % but differs greatly with age: it is 9 % between birth and 10 years, 14 % between 11 and 20 years and only 4 % after 40 years (Niedermeyer and Koshino, 1975). There are three theories as to the neurophysiological basis of the mu rhythm: 1) neuronal hyperexcitability restricted to the Rolandic cortex; 2) superficial cortical inhibition, which would explain the suppression of

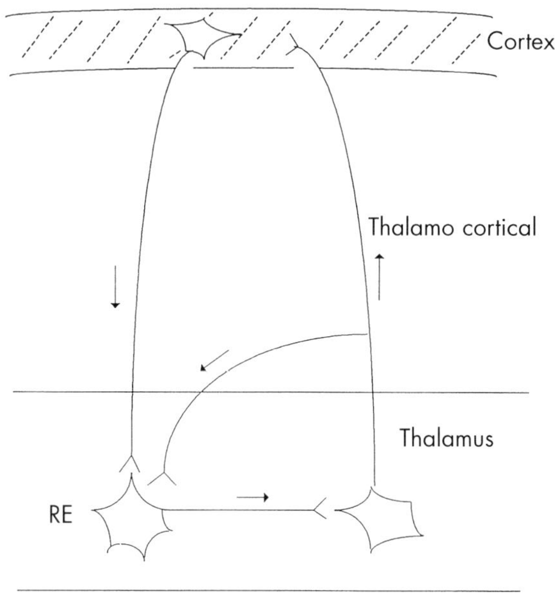

Fig. 3. Circuit of three neural types of spindles oscillations in cortical EEG (from Steriade, 1993).

mu rhythm with motor activity; 3) somatosensory cortical idling turning mu rhythm into an afference-dependent phenomenon (Niedermeyer, 1993).

A review of work on alpha rhythms shows that rhythms having the same frequency can have not only different anatomical and physiological bases, but different functions as well.

Beta frequency band

Beta rhythms are rapid, in the range of 15 — 45 Hz, and involved in the control of states of vigilance and selective attention. The term gamma rhythm was used by Jasper and Andrews (1938) to designate frequencies above 30 Hz, but was abandoned and gamma rhythms are now simply a part of the beta rhythm. Beta rhythm is found in every healthy adult. As with the 7-14 Hz rhythms, this frequency band also appears to include two phenomena, one in the 20-40 Hz range, undoubtedly involved in waking states, while an other, more restricted band at 40-45 Hz results from more selective and sustained attention.

The 15-40 Hz rhythm

The relationship between the EEG and waking states has been known since the work of Moruzzi and Magoun (1949), who showed that when different sites of the reticular formation of the brain stem of deeply anaesthetised animals were stimulated, low-frequency, high voltage EEG rhythms were transformed to rapid, low-voltage rhythms, equivalent to those observed during waking states. Following this finding, considerable work was carried out involving section of the brain stem at different levels, which served as the basis for research on control of states of vigilance by brain stem structures. Recently, Steriade (1993) showed that the neurons involved in ascending activation of the thalamus and cortex are in two cholinergic nuclei of the mesopontine junction: the pontopeduncular tegmentum and the laterodorsal tegmentum. This highly localised region also contains noradrenergic neurons from the locus coeruleus and serotoninergic neurons from the dorsal raphe. Thus, EEG activation in waking states is due to the combined action of cholinergic nuclei via the thalamus and monoaminergic nuclei with diffuse cortical projections, while during paradoxical sleep only monoaminergic nuclei are involved and serotoninergic nuclei remain quiescent (Steriade and McCarley, 1990).

The activating role of these structures exists not only in anaesthetised, but also in conscious animals. Bremer and Stoupel (1959) and Dumont and Dell (1960) showed that stimulating prethalamic fibres increased the field of cortical potentials when the reticular formation itself was stimulated. Thus, in these conditions of double stimulation, a 40-45 Hz cortical EEG rhythm emerges, that is stable, regular and of low voltage.

The 40-45 Hz rhythm

The 40 Hz rhythm is detected in both animals and humans. Thus, Murthy and Fetz (1992) reported a 40 Hz rhythm in motor cortex cells of monkeys during a task requiring fine prehensile skills. Rhythmic 40 Hz activity has been demonstrated over the left central region (C3 electrode) at the onset of self-paced voluntary right finger movements (Pfurtscheller and Neuper, 1992). Similarly, Sheer (1984) observed a 40 Hz rhythm in humans during a complex task and Garreau et al. (1997) reported a frontal distribution and right parietal distribution of the 40-45 Hz frequency band in normal adults during an object permanence test, involving a motor-visual co-ordination task.

Most workers believe the 40 Hz rhythm to have a cortical origin. Llinas et al. (1991) suggested that in guinea pigs it could be generated by interneurons in layer IV of the frontal cortex. Similar recordings were also obtained in the corpus callosum, which would explain the coherence of the 40 Hz rhythm in the cortical areas of both hemispheres.

There is compelling evidence that, in addition to intracortical circuits, subcortical structures are interposed in complex neuronal chains generating the 40 Hz rhythm. A hypothesis according to which corticothalamic projections drive RE thalamic neurons, thus leading to 40 Hz IPSP rebound sequences in thalamic relay cells, which then re-enter the cortex, has been proposed (Llinas, 1990). If this were so, during the waking state, when the 40 Hz rhythm is supposed to occur preferentially, the inhibitory input from RE thalamic neurons would be transmitted back to the cortex. However, the relation between RE and thalamocortical cells in this fast rhythm is not elucidated, especially because RE cells also have access to thalamic inhibitory input from RE cells to thalamic relay neurons; disinhibition may even prevail. The fact is that thalamocortical cells oscillate at 40 Hz, due to both intinsic and extrinsic factors. The presence of 40 Hz oscillatory neurons in the intralaminar centrolateral nucleus (Steriade et al., 1981b), which hare widespread projections to the cerebral cortex (Jones, 1985), including the visual areas, is important for the concept of thalamic conjunction and synchronisation of distant cortical areas. It is also possible that the resonant thalamocorticothalamic circuits are based only on direct excitatory projections, requiring just one interposed synapse in layer VI. Indeed, there is direct built-in frequency amplification in the corticothalamic pathway, as demonstrated by the fact that 30-50 Hz cortical volleys lead to a dramatic increase of EPSPs in target thalamocortical neurons (Lindström and Wrobel, 1990).

The 40 Hz rhythm is potentiated by mesopontine cholinergic systems, whose stimulation directly excites thalamocortical cells (Curro Dossi et al., 1991); indirectly excites thalamocortical cells by inhibiting reticular thalamic cells (Hu et al., 1989).

These findings thus show the importance of the 40 Hz rhythm in processes of selective and sustained attention and its relationship with ascending systems involved in the waking state.

Theta frequecy band

These rhythms cover the range 4-7 Hz and were first recorded in the hippocampus of conscious rabbits (Green and Arduini, 1954) and in cats during paradoxical sleep (Jouvet, 1965). A number of workers, however, have questioned the existence of these rhythms in humans, even when electrodes were implanted in the hippocampus (Halgren et al., 1985), except in certain cases of epilepsy (Arnolds et al., 1980) or during considerable reduction in blood flow to the brain (Ingvar et al., 1976). Nevertheless, work has shown that a theta wave pacemaker would be dependent on cholinergic systems, corresponding to the facilitation of the first phase of memorisation (Traub et al., 1989).

EEG processing methods

Visual interpretation of electroencephalograms has enabled the rhythms observed to be divided into delta (0-3 Hz), theta (4-7 Hz), alpha (8-12 Hz) and beta (beyond 12 Hz). For the past 15 years, analytical methods using the Fourier transform have enabled power spectra of the different frequency bands of the standard EEG to be obtained for each electrode. Since the initial studies, technical progress in both EEG instrumentation and signal processing methods has been considerable, leading to increasing use of the quantitative EEG (EEGq) in psychiatry and neuropsychiatry. Construction isolelectric maps has facilitated the interpretation of the results obtained.

The principle of EEGq acquisition is the same as that of the standard EEG. Only data processing differs, requiring the acquisition of a totally artefact-free record. Apart from its low cost, the major advantage of this method are that it requires no injection or premedication, and that its temporal resolution is of the order of a second or even millisecond when evoked potentials are studied. The increased number of electrodes available and the increased performance of computation has made this method attractive, the more so since the EEG is recorded in the sitting position, in surroundings having any instrumentation other than the head fitting. This affords ideal physiological conditions for executing even complex tasks. Currently, the depth and thus the anatomical origin of the electrical currents can be recorded by combining high resolution 128 Channel EEG recording with 3-dimensional MRI and appropriate computation methods (Gevins et al., 1994). Similarly, the concomitant processing of EEGq and digitised video images obtained during motor tasks enables behaviour and electrical activity to be studied simultaneously.

A more recent application of EEGq concerns spectral coherency (Saltzberg et al., 1986), based on cross-correlation of spectral functions with two electrodes. Coherence is reflects information rather than visual analysis, and enables one to see how the EEGq changes simultaneously at both electrodes. Coherence has been investigated in detail by Thatcher et al. (1994) Bullock et al. (1995) and by Bell (in this volume) to determine the major steps in development and lateralisation in children. As with EEGq, the study of coherence requires totally artefact-free recording.

Thus, the EEG is not only the oldest method for functional cerebral exploration, but has also been used for diagnostic purposes for a long time. Experimental physiology has led to a better understanding of the origin of EEG rhythms and technical progress has enabled the EEG to remain a promising method of the imaging brain, its low cost and noninvasive nature.

References

Adrian ED, Matthews BHC (1934) The Berger Rhythm: potential changes from the occipital lobes in man. Brain 57: 355-385

Allison T, Wood CC, McCarthy G (1986) The central nervous system. In: Coles MC, Donchin E, Porges SW (eds): Psychoneurobiology. Guilford Press, New York, p 5-25

Arnolds DEAT, Lopes da Silva FH, Aitink JW, Kamp A, Boejinga P (1980) The spectral properties of hippocampal EEG related to behaviour in man. Electroencephalogr Clin Neurophysiol, 50: 324-328

Bell MA (1997) The ontogeny of the EEG during infancy and childhood: implications for cognitive development. In: Garreau B (ed) Neuroimaging in child psychiatric disorders. Springer, Paris

Berger H (1929) Über das Elektroenkephalogramm des menshen. Arch Psychiat Nervenk 87: 527-570

Bremer F, Stoupel N (1959) Facilitation et inhibition des potentiels évoqués corticaux dans l'éveil cérébral. Arch Internat Physiol Pharmacodyn, 67: 240-275

Bullock TH, McClune MC, Achimowicz JZ, Iragui-Madoz VJ, Duckrow RB, Spencer SS (1995) Temporal fluctuations in coherence of brain waves. Proc Nat Acad Sci, 92, 25: 11568-11572

Curro Dossi R, Paré D, Steriade M (1991) Short-lasting nicotinic and long-lasting muscarinic depolarizing responses of thalamocortical neurons to stimulation of mesopontine cholinergic nuclei. J Neurophysiol, 65: 393-406

Dumont S, Dell P (1960) Facilitation réticulaire des mécanismes visuels corticaux. Electroencephalogr Clin Neurophysiol, 12: 769-796

Garreau B, Debiais E (1997) Electroencephalographic Study in man during an object permanence task. Submitted to Electroencephalogr Clin Neurophysiol.

Gevins A, Le J, Martin NK, Brickett P, Desmond J, Reutter B (1994) High resolution EEG-124 channel recording, spatial deblurring and MRI integration methods. Electroencephalogr Clin Neurophysiol, 90, 5: 337-358

Green JD, Arduini A (1954) Hippocampal electrical activity in arousal. Neurophysiol 17: 533-537

Halgren E, Smith ME, Stapelton JM (1985) Hippocampal field potentials evoked by repeated vs non repeated words. In: Buzsaki G, Van Derwolf CH (eds),Electrical activity of the achicortex..Akademiai Kiado, Budapest, P 67-81

Hu B, Steriade M, Deschênes M (1989) The effects of brainstem peribrachial stimulation on perigeniculate neurons: the blockage of spindle waves. Neurosci 31: 1-12

International Federation of Societies of Electroencephalography and Clinical Neurophysiology (1974) A glossary of terms commonly used by clinical electroencephalographers, Electroencephalogr Clin Neurophysiol 37: 538-548

Ingvar DH, Sjölund B, Ardo A (1976) Correlation between ECG frequency, cerebral oxygen uptake and blood flow. Electroencephalogr Clin Neurophysiol 41: 268-276

Jasper HH, Andrews HL (1938) Electroencephalography. III: Normal differentiation of occipital and precentral regions in man. Arch Neurol Psychiat, 39: 96-115

Jones EG (1985) The thalamus. Plenum Press, New York

Jouvet M (1965) Paradoxical sleep: a study of its nature and mechanisms. In: Akert K, BallyC, Schadé JP (eds) Progress in Brain Research, Vol 18, Sleep mechanisms. Elsevier, Amsterdam, p 20-57

Kandel ER, Schwartz JH, Jessell TH (1991) Principles of neural sciences. Elsevier, Amsterdam

Lindström S, Wrobel A (1990) Frequency dependent corticofugal excitation of principal cells in cat's dorsal lateral geniculate nucleus. Exp Brain Res 79: 313-318

Llinàs RR (1990) Intrinsic electrical properties of mammalian neurons and CNS functions. In: Fidia Research Foundation Neuroscience Award Lectures. Raven Press, New York, p 175-194

Llinàs RR, Grace AA, Yarom Y (1991) In vitro neurons in mammalian cortical layer 4 exhibit intrinsic oscillatory activity in the 10 to 50 Hz frequency range. Proc Nat Acad Sci, 88: 897-901

Lopes da Silva FH, Storm van Leeuwen W (1977) The cortical source of alpha rhythm. Neurosci Lett, 6: 237-341

Lopes da Silva FH, Van Lierop THMT, Schrijer CFM, Storm van Leeuwen W (1973) Organization of thalamic and cortical alpha rhythm: spectra and coherences. Electroencephalogr Clin Neurophysiol, 35: 627-639

Lorente de Nô R (1947 a) Action potentials of the motoneurons of the hypoglossus nucleus. J Cell Comp Physiol 29: 207-289

Lorente de Nô R (1947 b) A study of nerve physiology. In: Studies of the Rockfeller Institute, 16: 132

Morison RS, Bassett DL (1945) Electrical activity of the thalamus and basal ganglia. J Neurophysiol 8: 309-314

Moruzzi G, Magoun HW (1949) Brain stem reticular formation and activation of the EEG. Electroencephalogr Clin Neurophysiol, 1: 455-473

Mulholland T (1969) The concept of attention and the electroencephalographic alpha rhythm. In: Evans CR, Mulholland TB (eds) Attention in neurophysiology. Butterworth, London, p 100-127

Murthy VN, Fetz EE (1992) Coherent 25-35 Hz oscillations in the sensorimotor cortex of the awake behaving monkey. Proc Nat Acad Sci 89: 5670-5674

Niedermeyer E, Koshino Y (1975) Mù-Rhythmus: Vorkommen und klinische Bedeutung. Z. EEG-EMG 6: 69-78

Pfurtscheller G, Neuper C (1992) Simultaneous EEG 10 Hz desynchronizationand 40 Hz synchronization during finger movements. Neuroreport

Regan D (1989) Human brain electrophysiology: evoked potentials and evoked magnetic fields in science and medicine. Elsevier, Amsterdam

Saltzberg B, Burton WD, Burch NR, Fletcher J, Michaels R (1986) Electrophysiological measures of regional neural interactive coupling: linear and non-linear dependence relationships among multiple channel electroencephalographic recordings. Internat J Biomed Comput 18: 77-87

Schlag J (1973) Generation of brain potentials. In: Thompson RF, Patterson MM (eds) Bioelectric recording techniques: Part A. Cellular Processes and brain potentials. Academic Press, New York, p 33-65

Sheer D (1984) Focused arousal 40 Hz and dysfunction. In: Ebert (ed), Selfregulation of the brain and behavior. Springer, Berlin, p 64-84

Steriade M (1993).Cellular substrates of brain rhythms. In: Niedermeyer E, Lopes da Silva F (eds) Electroencephalography: basic principles, clinical applications, and related fields.Williams and Wilkins, Baltimore, p 27-62

Steriade M, McCarley RW (1990) Brainstem control of wakefulness and sleep. Plenum Press, New York

Steriade M, Curro Dossi R, Paré D, Oakson G (1991) Fast oscillations (20-40 Hz) in thalamocortical systems and their potentiation by mesopontine cholinergic nuclei in the cat. Proc Nat Acad Sci, 88: 4396-4400

Thatcher RW (1994) Cyclic cortical reorganization: origins of human cognitive development. In: Dawson G, Fisher KW (eds) Human behavior and the developing brain. Guilford, New York, p 232

Traub RD, Miles R, Wong RK, Schulman LS, Schneiderman JH (1987) Models of synchronized hippocampal bursts in the presence of inhibition. II Ongoing spontaneous population events. J Neurophysiol, 58: 752-764

4. Frontocentral electrical brain activity in normal boys: impact of EOG correction on retest stability, topography and condition effects of slow negative cortical potentials

C. DUMAIS-HUBER, A. ROTHENBERGER

Because research on slow cortical potential (SCP) in general, and particularly the one involved in frontocortical, activity, can be seriously impeded by ocular artefacts which may bias the results, it was clearly important to exclude the possibility that differences in SCPs between groups in a clinical study and apparently reflecting a brain-behaviour relationship could in fact be explained by an oculomotor-behavioural association. Therefore, slow negative potential (SNP) and postimperative negative variation (PINV) measures obtained without and with electrooculogram (EOG) correction will be reported side by side. It must be stressed that our intention was not to compare uncorrected and EOG-corrected data directly, but rather to find out whethers/and if so, how, an additional EOG correction would modify our SCP findings and their interpretation. We believe this objective meets the main concerns of many clinical researchers, especially if children and/or patients are to be examined. In this context, the issue of EOG correction is not meant to present innovative techniques for basic research, and does not raise such questions as how changes in EOG variance criteria for trial selection affect the correction coefficients computed. Rather, the present paper is aimed at validating to some extent "ready for use" EOG correction programmes, showing concrete examples of the influence of the EOG on the SCP data obtained in clinically oriented experiments in healthy children.

Despite its importance, EOG correction is all too often neglected in event-related potential (ERP) studies: instead, the conventional "rejection method", which excludes EEG segments heavily contaminated by eye movement and exceeding a given amplitude, continues to be used in routine analysis. A major practical drawback of the rejection method is that it may lead to an unaccept *loss of trials* (especially in clinical studies dealing with unco-operative patients), which in turn would yield a poor signal-to-noise ratio and bias the information processing to be investigated. In addition, the rejection method does not tap the problem of *subthreshold* residual EOG activity. EEG contamination by eye movement is particularly invidious when the EOG activity is time-locked to the stimuli presented and risks modifing ERP wave forms considerably. Further more, in the influence of longitudinal studies, for which there is an urgent need in clinical research, variation of the influence of eye movement over time may introduce bias in the results and be detrimental to data interpretation.

This prompted us to evaluate the possible impact of EOG correction on retest stability, frontocentral topography and condition effects.

Methods

Healthy boys

Within a large scale longitudinal study on central nervous control mechanisms and the course of child psychiatric disorders, 32 healthy boys 9-16 years of age, mean IQ 114 as evaluated by the PSB, (Horn, 1969) were willing to take part in the experiment; on average they were 12.1 years-old (SD 2.0). Overall, 21 (mean age 12.2 years; mean IQ 113) were submitted to a second examination four weeks after the first.

Task procedure

The children, comfortably seated in a reclining chair, kept their eyes closed during the recording session. They were submitted to a paired stimuli reaction time task (S1-S2-R paradigm) in which each trial consisted of a warning stimulus (S1: 1000 Hz sine tone, 4 s duration, rise and decay time 2 and 6 ms, respectively) followed by an imperative stimulus (S2: aversive white noise, maximum duration 3 s if not stopped), both presented binaurally through headphones with an intensity of 70 dB. This means that the interstimulus interval (ISI) between the onset of S1 and S2 was 4 s. Upon hearing S2, they were to press a button as promptly as possible. The intertrial-interval varied pseudorandomly between 8 and 10 seconds.

The experiment was run under two conditions: in the control (C) condition, the subject could effectively stop S2, whereas this was made impossible in the non-control (NC) condition in which S2 lasted 3 s irrespective of any adequate motor reaction. The trials were distributed into 3 blocks of 36 pairs of stimuli each. Block 1 had 36 trials presented under the control condition; block 2 was a block of transition in which the first half contained C trials and the second NC trials; Block 3 was composed of 31 NC trials and 5 C serving motivational purposes.

Data acquisition

EEG activity was recorded via 15 (for the objective of this paper we looked at only Cz and Fz) sintered Ag/AgCl cup electrodes (impedance under 3 k; 10-20 system locations); the linked mastoids (shunted via a 10 k resistor) served as a reference. Vertical and hor-

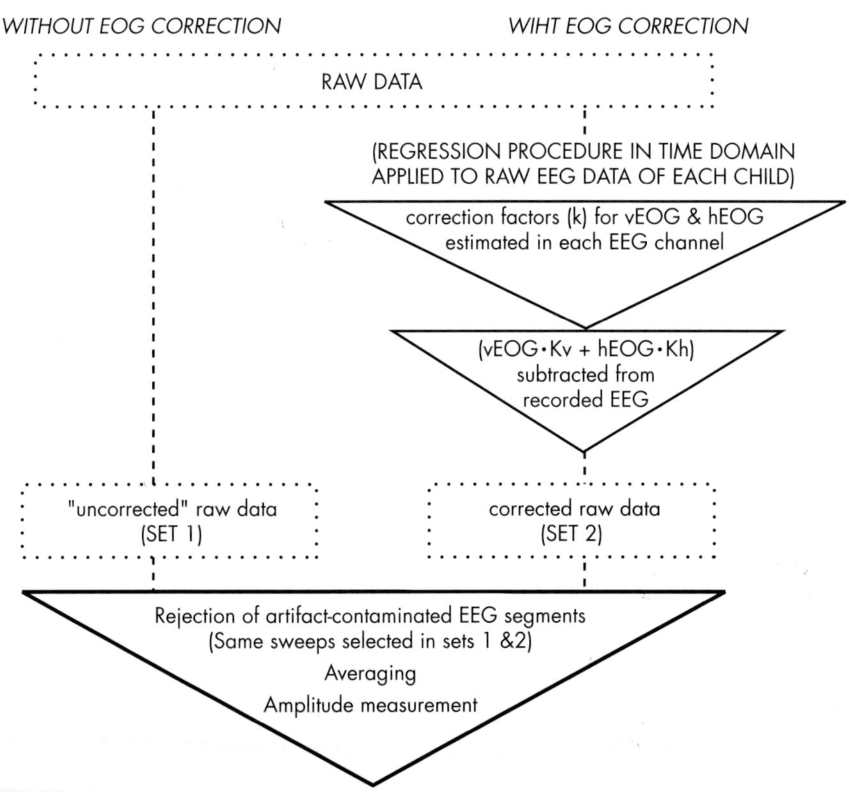

Fig. 1
Simplified flow diagram of the steps involved in data analysis with and without EOG correction of raw EEG data.

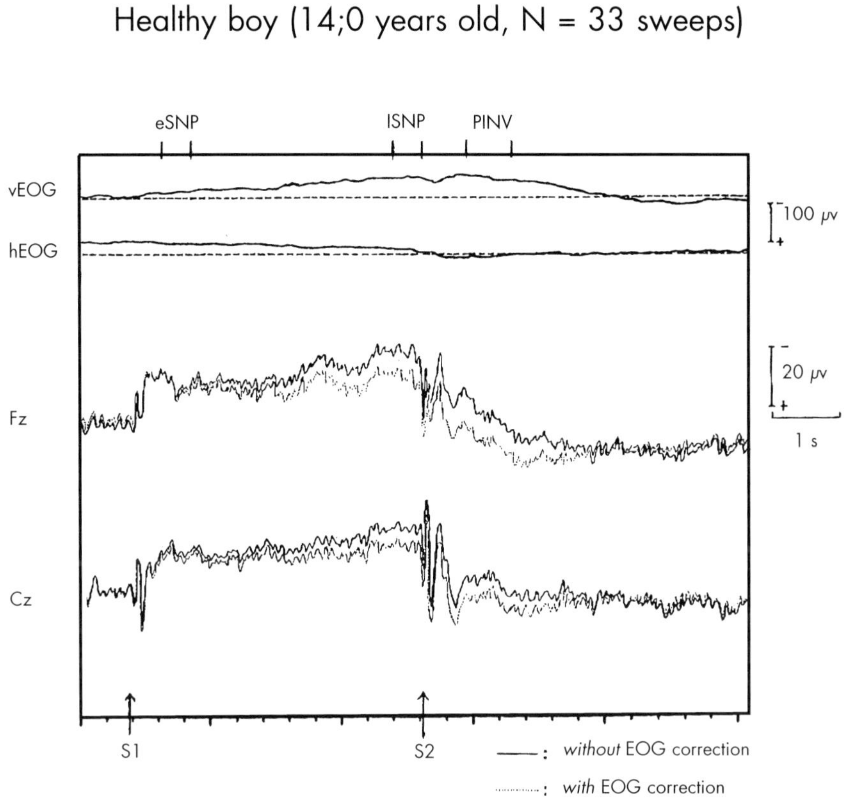

Fig. 2
Impact of EOG correction on average wave forms recorded from one healthy boy in the control condition. For the Fz and Cz derivations, the solid traces represent recordings made prior to EOG correction and the dotted traces result from the off-line removal of ocular activity. The dashed line in the two upper traces refers to the "technical" zero line used as a reference level by the EOG correction procedure. EOG and EEG channels have different scales, as illustrated.

izontal EOGs were recorded in a bipolar fashion from electrodes above and below the right eye and at the outer canthi. Electrodermal activity and ECG were also recorded, and reaction time data were collected. The EEG and EOG signals were amplified and filtered by a Nihon Kohden electroencephalograph (model 4321G), with a lower frequency limit at 0.03 Hz (5 s time constant). The upper cut off frequency was 120 Hz for EEG channels and 70 Hz for EOG channels.

Signals were then digitised by a Compaq 386 computer, sampling rate 500 Hz. The EEG sweeps heavily contaminated with ocular movements (EOG activity greater than 150 µV) and muscle artefacts were rejected, along with the first uncontrollable trial associated with multiple button presses; EEG segments were also excluded if signals were out of the amplifier range. The analysis of selected sweeps was carried out twice: *once after EOG correction* of the EEG raw data and once *without* this correction, to test the impact of the procedure. For comparability, the *same* EEG segments were rejected from the EOG-corrected and uncorrected raw data sets before averaging (Fig 1). Of course, when using EOG correction it would have been possible to save some of the sweeps excluded on the basis of the traditional rejection criteria. However, the resulting differences between EOG corrected and uncorrected data could not have been interpreted in terms of EOG the influence of correction alone, one would have needed also to take the differences in sweeps into account. By explicitly equalising the EEG segments, our approach differs from most other studies in which different methods of data treatment were compared. For instance, when Verleger (1993) nicely demonstrated what may happen if blinks are ignored, rejected or corrected, the number of EEG sweeps necessarily varied according to the method of data treatment chosen.

For EOG correction, we resorted to an *off-line* regression-based algorithm performed in a *time domain* ("OASYS 88.1", "Ocular Artifact SYStem", distribution and copyright by Base-Line, SofAS-Software for Applied Science, Hessenplatz 3, 60487 Frankfurt/M, Germany), which is based on the work of Möcks (Gasser et al., 1985, 1986) and developed by himself.

Averages were computed off-line for each condition. Mean amplitudes were measured relative to a 500 ms pre-S1 baseline within the following time windows: 450-850 ms after S1 (early SNP), 400 ms interval prior to S2 (late SNP), 600-1200 ms after S2 (PINV). Our choice of a time window starting 600 ms after S2 was justified by the need to measure this last component *after* execution of the motor response, to avoid confounding effects. Measures were not only reported for Fz and Cz recording sites independently; the difference between them ("Cz-Fz") was also included as an indicator of frontocentral brain dynamics.

Considering the 3 blocks of trials mentioned previously, measures had to be weighted according to the respective number of sweeps accepted in each average wave form before they could be submitted to statistical analysis. The weighting procedure uses the following operation:

$$\frac{(\text{eSNP-blockA} \times \text{Nr sweeps-blockA}) + (\text{eSNP-blockB} \times \text{Nr sweeps-blockB})}{(\text{Nr sweeps-blockA} + \text{Nr sweeps-blockB})}$$

where blockA and blockB refer to block 1 and block 2 (2.1) in the C condition, but to block 2 (2.2) and block 3 in the NC condition.

To test for differences between recording sites as well as experimental conditions, a Wilcoxon matched pairs signed rank test was conducted for each SCP measure within control and patient groups separately. To compare different groups of subjects, we used a Mann-Whitney U-test.

Results

General influence of EOG correction

From figure 2 it is possible to get a visual impression of the influence of eye movement artefact removal at the individual and group level, as it shows the SCP measures recorded in a healthy boy, an ADHD boy and the group of healthy boys. As expected, the curves indicate that the signal recorded over Fz is more affected by the correction procedure than that recorded over the vertex (Cz).

Table 1 reveals that correlations between the vertical EOG and EEG amplitudes were much reduced, if not absent, after EOG correction had been performed.

Another aspect of EOG correction is that the corrected EEG data yield SNP and PINV measures whose standard deviations are smaller than for uncorrected data, as seen in table 3.

A) CONTROL CONDITION:

Recording site	eSNP without/**with** EOG correction	ISNP without/**with**	PINV without/**with**
Fz	0.39*/ **0.08**	0.73***/**0.24**	0.79***/ **0.45****
Cz	0.26 /**−0.08**	0.62***/**0.36***	0.41** / **0.14**
(Cz-Fz)	−0.29 /**−0.10**	−0.17 /**0.22**	−0.54***/**−0.27**

B) NON-CONTROL CONDITION:

Recording site	eSNP without/**with** EOG correction	ISNP without/**with**	PINV without/**with**
Fz	0.26 /**−0.14**	0.72***/**0.34**	0.71***/ **0.24**
Cz	0.30*/ **0.06**	0.58***/**0.35***	0.39* / **0.02**
(Cz-Fz)	−0.08 / **0.14**	−0.11 /**0.10**	−0.43** /**−0.22**

*p<.05, **p<.01, ***p<.001 (Spearman, one-tailed)

Table 1
Correlations between vertical EOG and EEG amplitudes without vs with EOG correction in 32 boys.

Test-retest reliability

Correlation coefficients that were relatively low for data recorded at Fz in the NC condition increased after EOG correction (Table 2). It can also be seen that the mean amplitude difference "Cz-Fz" calculated for PINV seemed to be particularly stable, even without EOG correction.

A) CONTROL CONDITION:

Recording site	eSNP without/**with** EOG correction	ISNP without/**with**	PINV without/**with**
Fz	0.72***/**0.72*****	0.45 /**0.41**	0.54** /**0.55****
Cz	0.61** /**0.69*****	0.47 /**0.32**	0.36 /**0.48**
(Cz-Fz)	0.48 /**0.45**	0.66***/**0.54****	0.80***/**0.69*****

B) NON-CONTROL CONDITION:

Recording site	eSNP without/**with** EOG correction	ISNP without/**with**	PINV without/**with**
Fz	0.49 /**0.59****	0.20 /**0.46**	0.35 /**0.65*****
Cz	0.64***/**0.58****	0.51**/**0.61****	0.60** /**0.73*****
(Cz-Fz)	0.63** /**0.68*****	0.35 /**0.24**	0.74***/**0.79*****

**p<.01, ***p<.001 (Spearman, one-tailed)

Table 2
Influence of EOG correction on test-retest reliabilities dor eSNP, ISNP and PINV amplitudes: correlation coefficients at four-week retest interval in 21 boys.

Topography and condition effects

Considering the whole group of 32 healthy boy, the early SNP (eSNP) was more pronounced over Fz (Wilcoxon for Fz vs Cz, p<.01 in the C condition; p<.1 in the NC condition), whereas the late SNP (lSNP) showed a maximum over Cz (p<.01 in the NC

Recording site	Condition	eSNP [μV] without/ **with** EOG correction	lSNP [μV] without/ **with**	PINV [μV] without/ **with**
Fz	C x̄	-15.1/**-15.3**	-11.4/**-8.9**	0.1/**-0.4**
	(s)	(7-6)/**(5.9)**	(8.2)/**(5.2)**	(12.5)/**(7.9)**
	NC x̄	-12.4/**-13.1**	-9.6/**-7.8**	-1.8/**-2.0**
	(s)	(5.7)/**(4.7)**	(8.0)/**(5.4)**	(9.8)/**(6.3)**
	C vs NC p	**/*	NS/NS	NS/NS
Cz	C x̄	-12.5/**-12.6**	-12.4/**-10.8**	-3.6/**-4.3**
	(s)	(5.8)/**(5.1)**	(8.1)/**(6.3)**	(10.9)/**(8.6)**
	NC x̄	-11.1/**-11.6**	-11.6/**-10.4**	-3.2/**-3.2**
	(s)	(4.9)/**(3.7)**	(9.5)/**(7.6)**	(10.0)/**(8.1)**
	C vs NC p	T/NS	NS/NS	NS/NS
(Cz-Fz)	C x̄	-2.6/**-2.7**	-1.0/**-1.9**	-3.7/**-3.9**
	(s)	(4.9)/**(2.9)**	(5.3)/**(5.0)**	(8.2)/**(7.6)**
	NC x̄	-1.3/**1.5**	-2.0/**-2.6**	-1.4/**-1.2**
	(s)	(3.5)/**(4.7)**	(3.8)/**(5.4)**	(8.3)/**(8.0)**
	C vs NC p	NS/NS	NS/NS	T/*

T<.10, *p<.05, **p<.01 (two-tailed)

Table 3
Effect of experimental condition (C vs NC) for eSNP, lSNP and PINV amplitudes (without and with EOG correction) in 32 boys. Significance levels by the Wilcoxon test.

condition). Within the post-S2 time window the negative wave recorded was larger over Cz than over Fz reaching significance level in the C condition (Wilcoxon, p<.05). This was not the case for the PINV in the NC condition, as frontocortical areas were also activated, leading to activity distributed more broadly over frontocentral areas. Consequently, the PINV amplitudes recorded over frontocortical areas in the NC condition did result in a less negative mean amplitude difference "Cz-Fz" when S2 became uncontrollable (Wilcoxon for C vs NC, p<. more broadly 01 without EOG correction; p<.05 with EOG correction).

In both uncorrected and EOG-corrected data (Table 3), eSNP amplitudes were significantly smaller in the NC condition; the difference Cz-Fz for PINV was less negative in this NC condition, suggesting recruitment of frontocortical activity. No condition effect was documented for lSNP before or after EOG correction.

Some advantages of adding an off-line EOG correction to the more traditional method of artefact rejection were also demonstrated in a clinical study (Dumais-Huber 1993) of 20 healthy controls, 20 children with ADHD (N = 20) and 20 patients with tic disorder. Concerning topography effects, the subtraction of appropriately weighted EOG from EEG recordings uncovered the central maximum of lSNP which was apparently concealed by EOG activity in uncorrected data. Frontal predominance of eSNP was retained in both conditions. Condition effects and group differences relating to activation patterns also remained unchanged after EOG correction, indicating that these effects, e.g. PINV increase over Fz in the NC condition, more diffuse activation pattern and different time course of PINV dynamics in children with ADHD, were not merely caused by EOG contamination.

Discussion

By recruiting only boys, we excluded one possible source of variation, namely sex.. Although the influence of this factor on the genesis of the SCP has been investigated very little, some workers have found differences attributable to sex (Delse et al., 1970; Knott and Peters, 1973).

From a methodological point of view, it is important to stress that the SNPs recorded may derive not only from a contingent negative variation (CNV) wave developing in a S1-S2-R paradigm but also from a sustained negative wave elicited by the continuous S1 tone presented to the subjects. However, since this sustained potential has been found to start developing 150 ms post stimulus (Picton et al., 1978), it should exert an equal influence on both eSNP and lSNP, whose amplitudes were measured within much later time windows. Consequently, their topographical distribution would be expected to be similar. As this was not the case, the sustained potential cannot be viewed as the main or exclusive determinant of the SNPs at measured; thus, it is reasonable to describe the obtained eSNP and lSNP data as partly reflecting orienting and anticipation (Dumais-Huber and Rothenberger, 1992).

In general, EOG correction improved the quality of EEG signals not only by subtracting eye movement-related artefacts but also by enhancing the signal-to-noise ratio; it removed practically all positive correlation between vertical EOG and EEG amplitudes and considerably reduced the standard deviations of the SNP and PINV. Nevertheless, a regression-based EOG-correction algorithm may also remove some EEG activity present at the EOG electrodes.

Test-retest reliability

As expressed by Roth et al. (1975), the experiments designed in different laboratories to study *CNV* waves are sufficiently similar to be associated with comparable retest coefficients, despite variations in the parameters used for SNP measures. Comparison of our data with the few reports available on SNP reliability in normal subjects indicates that the retest coefficients we obtained, ranging from 0.50 to 0.80 at four-week retest interval, are reasonably high. Timsit-Berthier et al. (1978) reported CNV reliabilities of 0.55. Whereas a retest coefficient of 0.80 was reported by Cohen (1969),over a 2-8 day retest interval, much lower coefficients were indeed found by Straumanis et al. (1969): 0.32 at Cz in 20 college students, retested on the same day. Roth et al. (1975) also tested college students, not children, like us; they calculated reliabilities of 0.68 for the CNV amplitudes at 1 week retest interval. This value was interpreted by the authors as intermediate between the reliabilities respectively found for tests assessing personality traits (0.61-0.91) and psychological states (0.15-0.21).

Importantly, there are some limitations to the comparison of our retest coefficients with these values from the literature, because the latter were not given for both eSNP (orientating) and lSNP (anticipation), as in our study: Indeed, the ISI intervals usually chosen (between S1 and S2) were too short to allow differentiation between an early and a late SNP component. Nevertheless, since it is reasonable to assume that the retest coefficients of various SNP components will be close to one another, the literature still provides a basis for evaluation of our findings. We agree with Simons and Miles (1990) that the issue of ERP reliability has not been assessed sufficiently by researchers; they emphasise the need to evaluate ERP reliability by mentioning the considerable variation that may arise between the coefficients obtained for different components, the exogenous components being more reliable than the endogenous ones, and for different parameters, the amplitude measures being more reliable than latency measures. Stability of the PINV component has not been similarly investigated in earlier studies, so that no reference value is available. The retest coefficients we obtained for PINV fell within the range of values observed for the retest coefficients of SNP.

Overall, our retest coefficients are compatible with those documented in longitudinal analyses of the standard EEG (Woerner et al., 1987) and visual evoked potentials [VEPs] (Rothenberger et al., 1987) in school-age children. Even after a retest interval of 5 years, these workers reported satisfactory stabilitiy of the parameters chosen (0.58-0.75 for / ratios of resting EEG; 0.39-0.49 for VEPs). Thus, our results attest to the adequate reliability of the electrophysiological measures chosen for investigating cognitive processes in children and adolescents, even in longitudinal studies, especially after EOG correction, which led to higher retest coefficients.

Topography and clinical condition effects

The data we gathered in healthy boys support the different topographical distributions predicted for the early and late components of the SNP, eSNP having its maximum over Fz and lSNP over Cz. This finding which *applied to both conditions as well as uncorrected and EOG-corrected data* is in agreement with the observations in the literature (Grünewald-Zuberbier and Grünewald, 1982). The fact that frontal dominance of eSNP was retained after EOG correction argues against the simplified view that eye movements would essentially cause artefactual activity to be recorded over Fz in the form of additional negativity which would then be subtracted by the EOG correction procedure. Systematic use of EOG correction in routine analysis of slow cortical potentials becomes all the more important when one considers that the observed central dominance of lSNP appeared to have been partly concealed by ocular activity and was slightly more pronounced after removal of eye movement artefact. One more argument in favour of EOG correction is that it helps to improve data quality: this was indicated by higher retest coefficients and may also be reflected in the general lowering of standard deviations after EOG correction.

As regards the assumption of frontal predominance of PINV in the literature (Elbert et al., 1981; Rockstroh et al., 1989), both uncorrected and EOG corrected data revealed activation of frontocortical areas in NC condition.

Conclusion

In general, we have demonstrated the usefulness of running an EOG correction on the raw EEG data to account for the influence of eye movements, which may fluctuate markedly from one recording session to another. This disturbing contamination of EEG signals especially in studies aimed at clarifying frontal lobe function — could introduce a bias in the comparison of slow cortical potentials between as well as within sessions and prevent formulation of reasonable interpretations of the results in terms of underlying cognitive processes (Dumais-Huber 1993). We showed that EOG correction improved the quality of EEG signals not only by subtracting eye movement related artefacts without distortion of the wave forms but also by enhancing the signal-to-noise ratio; it removed practically all positive correlation between vertical EOG and EEG amplitudes and considerably reduced the standard deviations of the SNP and PINV. The increased stability of these parameters contributes to better extraction of topograpic effects. Thus, the advantages of adding an off-line EOG correction to the more traditional method of artefact rejection include increased reliability of SNP and PINV measures at retest, an important prerequisite for longitudinal studies.

References

Cohen J (1969) Very slow brain potentials relating to expectancy: The CNV. In: Donchin E, Lindsley DB (eds.), Averaged Evoked Potentials, NASA SP-191. US Government Printing Office, Washington DC, p 143-198

Delse F, Marsh G, Thompson L (1970) The contingent negative variation as a pre-motor potential. Psychophysiology 6: 619

Dumais-Huber C (1993) Electrical brain activity and stimulus control: a study on the regulatory processes of the frontal cortex in psychiatric disordered children. Doctoral Thesis, University of Heidelberg, Germany

Dumais-Huber C Rothenberger A (1992) Psychophysiological correlates of orienting, anticipation and contingency changes in children with psychiatric disorders. J. Psychophysiol 6: 225-239

Elbert T, Birbaumer B., Rockstroh B, Lutzenberger W, Bippus W, Breidt R (1981) Slow cortical potentials under conditions of uncontrollability. A comparison between patients with frontal lobe lesions and healthy controls. Proc. Int. Conf. Event-Related Potentials (Sixth International Conference on Event-Related Slow Potentials of the Brain, Lake Forest, Illinois), p 27

Gasser T, Sroka L., Möcks J (1985) The transfer of EOG activity into the EEG for eyes open and closed. Electroencephalogr Clin Neurophysiol 61: 181-193

Gasser T, Sroka L, Möcks. J (1986) The correction of EOG artifacts by frequency dependent and frequency independent methods. Psychophysiology 23: 704-712

Grünewald-Zuberbier E, Grünewald G (1982) Event-related EEG changes in children with different abilities to concentrate. In: A. Rothenberger (ed.), Event-related potentials in children, Elsevier, Amsterdam, p 295-316

Horn W (1969) Prüfsystem für Schul- und Bildungsberatung P-S-B. Hogrefe, Göttingen/Toronto/ Zürich

Knott JR, Peters JF (1973) Sex, stress and interstimulus interval. In: McCallum WC, Knott JR (eds.), Event-related slow potentials of the brain: their relations to behavior Electroencephalogr Clin Neurophysiol (suppl 33): 191-193

Picton TW, Woods DL, Proulx GB (1987) Human auditory sustained potentials. I. The nature of the response. Electroencephalogr Clin Neurophysiol 45: 186-197

Rockstroh B, Elbert T, Canavan A, Lutzenberger W, Birbaumer N (1989) Slow cortical potentials and behaviour. Urban & Schwarzenberg, Baltimore

Roth WT, Kopell BS, Tinklenberg, JR, Huntsberger GE, Kraemer HC (1975) Reliability of the contingent negative variation and the auditory evoked potential. Electroencephalogr Clin Neurophysiol 38: 45-50

Roth WT, Rothbart RM, Kopell BS (1978) The timing of CNV resolution in a memory retrieval task. Biol Psychol 6: 39-49

Rothenberger A, Woerner W, Blanz B (1987)Test-retest reliability of flash-evoked potentials in a field sample: a 5 year follow-up in school children with and without psychiatric disturbances. In: Johnson R, Rohrbaugh JW, Parasuraman R (eds.), Current trends in event-related potential research. Electroencephalogr Clin Neurophysiol (Suppl 40): 624-628

Simons RF, Miles MA (1990) Non familial strategies for the identification of subjects at risk for severe psychopathology: issues of reliability in the assessment of event-related potential and other marker variables. In: Rohrbaugh JW, Parasuraman R, Johnson R (eds.), Event-Related Brain Potentials, Basic Issues and Applications. Oxford University Press, New York/Oxford, p 343-365

Straumanis JJ, Shagass C, Overton DA (1969) Problems associated with application of the contingent negative variation to psychiatric research. Nerv Ment Dis 148: 170-179

Timsit-Berthier M, Delaunoy J, Xhenseval B, Timsit M (1978) Reliability of contingent negative variation in psychopathology. In: Otto DA (ed.), Multidisciplinary Perspectives in Event-Related Brain Potential Research. US Government Printing Office, Washington DC, p 373-375

Verleger R (1993) Valid identification of blink artefacts: are they larger than 50 V in EEG records? Electroencephalogr Clin Neurophysiol 87: 354-363

Woerner W, Rothenberger A, Lahnert, B (1987) Test-retest reliability of spectral parameters of the resting EEG in a field sample: a 5 year follow-up in school children with and without psychiatric disturbances. In: Johnson R, Rohrbaugh JW, Parasuraman R (eds.), Current trends in event-related potential research. Electroencephalogr Clin Neurophysiol (Suppl. 40): 629-632

5. Cerebral development and MRI

C. RAYBAUD, N. GIRARD

The development of the brain in the first months of life is characterised by morphological changes (growth and shape) and by histological changes (cellularity and myelination). Morphology is of course inexquisitely depicted by magnetic resonance imaging (MRI), but the maturational changes — water and lipid contents, cellularity — are also reflected in MRI. Since the development of the brain follows a constant, species specific course, identification of the normal milestones is possible, as is an understanding of the disease processes leading to impairment of cerebral function in the growing child. To understand the potential of MRI in this clinical context, it is necessary to recall the basic principles of MRI of the brain, and the steps in the cerebral development.

Magnetic resonance imaging of the brain

MRI basically uses two parameters to image the brain, T1 (longitudinal relaxation time) and T2 (transverse relaxation time), to produce so-called T1 weighted images and so-called T2 weighted images respectively, so-called proton-density (PD) images being a mixture of both.

On T1 weighted images of the mature brain, the CSF (water) appears dark (because it has a long T1), the white matter bright (short T1) and the grey matter has different degrees of intermediate signal, depending on the structure considered.

In neonates, the CSF (water) is dark, but the white matter, devoid of myelin and therefore more hydrated than in older individuals, appears much darker than the grey matter.

On T2 weighted images of the mature brain the CSF is bright (because of its long T2), the white matter is dark (short T2), and the grey matter has intermediate signals. Again, in neonates, if the CSF is bright, the contrast between white matter (also bright) and grey matter (darker) is the reverse of that in the adult.

This evolution, on T1 and T2 weighted imaging, reflects at least in part the maturation of the brain. In fetuses and at birth the cortex and the white matter contain 90 % of water, and little lipid or protein. In adults, the grey matter contains about 85 % of water, with more lipid and protein, but the white matter contains only 75 % of water, against 18 % of lipids. These alterations accounts for the changing images of the brain.

Imaging through the magnetic resonance phenomenon consists of making images which shows the different behaviour of protons (H+) according to their molecular environment (other elements such as carbon, sodium, phosphorus etc., could be used, but the overwhelming abundance of hydrogen makes proton imaging easier). Protons are first polarised (aligned) by a strong constant magnetic field, then excited (i.e., brought to a higher energy level) by a radiofrequency (RF) pulse. The time taken for their return to the initial energy state (relaxation time) depends on the magnetic influence of the nuclei around them, that is, on the various energy transfers between the nuclei of the tissue. Because the two relaxation parameters used for imaging , the T1 and T2 reflect energy transfers between neighbouring nuclei, they depend on the physicochemical composition of the tissues, the strength of the main magnetic field, the temperature, on the various energy transfers and loss from RF pulse to tissues, etc. This means that the images obtained reflect a relative intensity of the resonance signal between different structures at a given moment and in given circumstances, and that they are by no means quantitative data, unlike X-Ray CT images.

To image with the magnetic resonance phenomenon, one registers the strength of the resonant RF (echo) that elicited by the exciting RF. The energy level of the excited tissue depends on how frequently excitation is repeated (defined as the repetition time, TR); the intensity of the resonant signal depends on the time elapsed between excitation and registration of the echo (echo time, TE). To obtain specific imaging patterns according to T1 or T2, specific TR and TE sequences are used, resulting in so-called T1 weighted images (sequences with short TR and short TE) and so-called T2 weighted sequences (long TR, long TE).

To get rid of the T1 effect, T2 weighted sequences should have a TR at least three times as long as the T1 relaxation time. This T1 depends on the tissue composition; it is extremely long in neonates, and this means that *during the early maturation of the brain, the images and the imaging parameters of the sequences, are changing with time* and have therefore to be adapted to this stage of maturation. In a mature child, the TR of T1 and T2 weighted sequences is, as in the adult, approximately 600 ms and 3000 ms, respectively. However, in neonates not yet myelinated, the brain contains more water and therefore the T1 is prolonged to 1800-3500 ms; the TR for T2 weighted sequences should be prolonged, ideally to 10000 ms, TE should be increased as well as. Prolonging the TR for T1 weighted sequences and the TE for T2 weighted sequences improves the quality of the images, but prolongs the imaging time, and compromises may be accepted.

The nature of the signal should also be understood. On T1 weighted images, white matter appears dark (long T1) because it contains 90 % water, while in the mature brain, the white matter appears brighter than the grey, because it contains more myelin (18 %). This phenomenon is explained by the fact that the signal from the free protons in the water is changed by transfer of energy from the bound protons of the membrane molecules (magnetisation transfer), knowing that myelin is an accumulation of layers of oligodendrocytic membranes. Also, even before the development of myelin, multiplication of cells, with all their membranes (glia, neuronal fibres, intracellular organelles), will increase this signal (make it brighter) on T1 weighted sequences (Boorstein et al., 1994; Campi et al., 1996; Fralix et al., 1991; Grossman et al., 1994, Hajnal et al., 1992; Hiehle et al., 1995; Koenig et al., 1990, Koenig et al., 1991; Kucharczyk et al., 1994; Mathews et al., 1994; Wolff and Balaban, 1989; Wolff and Balaban, 1994).

On the other hand, this magnetisation transfer phenomenon is almost non existent with T2 weighted sequences, while the accumulation of membranes whose protons do not resonate decreases the signal on T2 weighted images: the white matter is bright on T2-weighted imaging in the neonate, and dark in mature children.

Other types of sequence may be used for specific goals: calcification and haemorrhages are better shown by so-called susceptibility (gradient echo) sequences. Metal (usually iron compounds) is better seen on T2 weighted gradient echo images. Saturation (i.e. masking) of the signal coming from the bound protons while registering only the signal from free protons (so-called magnetisation transfer sequences) on T1 weighted images enhances the contrast of tissue change against background. It can be used to demonstrate hamartomatous tissue lesions such as those of tuberous sclerosis or neurofibromatosis type 1, or to increase the relative contrast of gadolinium compound enhancement (to show a defective blood-brain barrier) with as compared with the normal tissue (Elster et al., 1994; Finelli et al., 1994; Grossman et al., 1994; Hiehle et al., 1995; Kurki et al., 1994; Mathews et al., 1994,Tanttu et al., 1992). Using such a technique with on T2 weighted images is also useful for assessing abnormal myelin content in the tissues.

Diffusion sequences (Cowan et al., 1994; Ono et al., 1994) are used for Brownian motion of protons: in nerve fibres, this motion is free along the axis of the firer, but limited across it. Motion can therefore be detected strongly only along the axis in normal fibers. Detected in any other direction, it means that the fibre's structure is altered, by either destruction of the fibres themselves, or accumulation of fluid outside the fibres.

Finally, specific sequences may be used to show the pulsatile movements of the CSF. Knowing that the CSF physiology depends normally on the rigidity of the cranial vault, the morphological relationships between the peripheral brain tissue and the central or basal of accumulation CSF, the systolic wave, the elasticity of brain tissue and the functional maturation of arachnoid granulations which resorb the fluid in the dural sinuses, it is evident that the CSF dynamics change from the fetus (with an extensible, still membranous skull within the pressure of the amniotic fluid) to the neonate (with membranous sutures and fontanelles) and to the mature child (with closed sutures); this can be illustrated by various MRI techniques.

Thus in MRI, many tools are available for illustrating not only the "steady state" image of the mature brain, but still more the changing pattern of the maturing brain from the fetus or the premature infant to the grown child. These tools help to show normal and abnormal phenomena: they are sensitive to many physicochemical energy transfers between the protons bound to various molecular compounds and the free-water protons. Depending on the stage of maturation MRI may show mainly cellularity (neurons, astrocytes, oligodendrocytes), the expanding network of the fibres, myelination, and metal deposition in certain nuclei or fibre bundles. All these phenomena occur concurrently, making a composite global image of the brain that is never quantitative, but only expresses the greater or lesses contrast between the various elements obtained at a given stage of evolution. Because the maturation of different structures develops at different rates, the contrast between them will change with time, and the same type of signal change may express different phenomena, depending on the stage of maturation.

The main steps of cerebral development

The developement of the brain is a continuous process which begins with differentiation of the neural ectoderm (3rd week), closure of the neural tube and early dilatation of cerebral vesicles (end of the 4th week), to the completion of cerebral growth, which is nearly attained by the 5th year of life. Two phases are usually distinguished during gestation; organogenesis, during which the brain acquires its basic shape, covers the embryonic period (the first two months); histogenesis, during which the brain grows and becomes organised, covers the fetal period from the 3rd to the 9th month. The actual developmental processes are more complex: histogenesis obviously begins during morphogenesis; morphological changes such as the formation of the corpus callosum extend to the 20th week; the histogenetic period itself can be subdivided according to which type of cell lineage develops (neuronal, astrocytic or oligodendrocytic precursors); myelination of the cerebral fibres bundles begins during the end of gestation, but goes on until adolescence; and the "adult" size of the brain is not attained until the 5th year.

Organogenesis the shaping of the brain covers the embryonic period: after implantation of the egg (1st week) and differentiation of the embryo into two (2nd week) then three (3rd week) layers, the neural tube forms (neurulation, 4th week), its cranial end dilates and becomes segmented to form three, then five, vesicles (paired hemispheric telencephalon, diencephalon, mesencephalon, pontocerebellar metencephalon, myelencephalon) (5th to 7th week), and commissural fibres of the anterior commissure, corpus callosum and hippocampal commissure develop (from week 7 to week 20). Failures of these processes result in neurulation disorders (myelomeningocele, encephalomeningocele, Chiari malformations), diverticulation disorders (holoprosencephaly with or without facial abnormalities), cystic malformations of the posterior fossa posterior (Dandy-Walker, Dandy-Walker variant, Blake's retrocerebellar pouch), and "callosal" (in fact commissural) agenesis (complete, partial, segmental).

While the end result of a distorted organogenesis brain malformation is significant for MRI, because precise diagnosis and extensive investigation of the abnormal brain are possible, the organogenetic processes leading to the malformation are beyond the reach of MRI, because of the small size of the embryo at that stage, its situation and its mobility. Nevertheless, at least during the second half of the gestation, the fetal brain can be adequately examined, and normal or abnormal features identified.

General principles of histogenesis

Histogenetic growth of the brain is characterised by development, around the lumen of the neural tube, of a germinal zone or germinal matrix within which the cells multiply and differentiate according to a predetermined timetable, and by migration towards the periphery of the cells produced by the germinal matrix (Mickel and Gilles, 1970; Rakic, 1971; Sarnat and Sarnat, 1994; Volpe, 1995).

The first step is the developement of the radial glia. Radial glial cells develop in the germinal matrix and, by a to-and-fro movement between the depth and surface of the tube, establish a cytoplasmic connection between the ventricular and meningeal surfaces. These cytoplasmic links persist throughout gestation, and act as guidelines for the cells which will eventually migrate from the germinal matrix to the periphery. They form a radial pattern (hence their cells) which lays the ground for the basically columnar development and organisation of the brain.

The second step is the period of multiplication, differentiation, and migration of the neuroblasts from the germinal matrix to the periphery. It starts during the 7th week, and is effectively finished at midgestation (20th week). After division in the germinal matrix, neuroblasts migrate outwards, following the cytoplasmic guides of the radial glia. They may remain in the vicinity of the ventricular lumen, constituting the basal ganglia, or migrate towards the meningeal surface of the brain to build up the cortical plate. Cortical neurons migrate in three waves, each going beyond the previous one ("the inside-out" process). Therefore, the deeper neurons are "older", more mature; and the neurons of each successive wave can establish connections with the more mature neurons of the underlying wave.

As stated above, differentiation and migration of the neurons in the brain are achieved at midgestation. From that time on, neurons will develop fibres (axons and dendrites) and establish synapses. Within the cortex, this results in the organisation into six layers, because of the development of intracortical, tangential layers of fibres), which is apparent at week 23. Under the cortex, it results in development of the white matter. During the whole process of migration of neuroblasts, fibres extend from one hemisphere to the other, initially through the anterior end of the third ventricle (commissural plate), then progressively from front to back, over the roof of the ventricle, to form the anterior commissure, corpus callosum, and fornix with the hippocampal commissure, the septum pellucidum remaining in the middle, bordered by these three structures.

The whole stock of neurons is therefore constituted at midgestation. A selection is made from this stock, the "unnecessary" cells (neurons without a target) disappearing (programmed cell death): this gives in the first specialization pattern of the grey matter.

At this point (20-23 weeks), the brain weighs about 80 g. Its surface is smooth, only the depression of the sylvian (lateral) fissure being apparent. Although histogenesis is far from being achieved at this stage, it is the time when early premature neonates can be born (which means that further histogenetic processes are at great risk), and also to the time when the brain can be imaged by MRI in utero.

The next step is the development of the glia. The cells of the germinal matri now differentiate into glial cells, first astrocytes, then oligodendrocytes. Astrocytes are essentially the supporting cells of the neurons. Oligodendrocytes elaborate myelin, which is to develop mainly at the end of the gestation and after birth. These astrocytes and oligodendrocytes migrate from the germinal matrix to the periphery in a manner similar to that of the neurons. The "migrant layer" can be seen in the white matter between the germinal matrix and the cortex, histologically and MRI (Fig. 1, Fig. 5). This layer of developing glia is more central at first, and then moves to the subcortical zone by weeks 30-32. Towards the normal end of gestation (40 weeks) the germinal matrix progressively attenuates and disappears at term. However, in contrast to neurons, glial cells retain their potential regeneration for thoughout life, and astrocytes formscar tissue even when neuronal fibres have been destroyed.

The final step of maturation is myelination of the brain. Myelinogenesis accompanies the development of the fibres network of the brain. Myelin favours conduction of the action potential along nerve fibres (saltatory conduction) and saves time, energy, and space. Myelin is, basically, nothing more than a plasmic membrane wrapped in concentric layers around an axon (Norton, 1981); up to 100 layers may wrap one axon. Oligodendrocytes are glial cells specialised for the production of myelin, each one being able to participate in the myelination of up to 50 or 70 different axons; this means that the destruction of one oligodendrocyte will affect many axons and that even if cellular multiplication allows replacement of destroyed oligodendrocytes, the repair of myelination may not be as good as it would other wise have been.

Oligodendrocytes need the presence of axons to produce myelin (except in rare abnormal cases such as status marmoratus). Multiplication of oligodendrocytes begins in the last weeks of gestation (myelination gliosis) and continues to adolescence, when turnover equilibrium is reached. Myelin consists of lipids (cholesterol, galactolipids, phospholipids) and proteins (PLP or proteolipid protein, and MBP or myelin basic proteins). An appreciation of the chemical composition is essential for understanding the effects of myelination on MRI. Galactolipids, and especially galactocerebrosides, produce a strong "magnetisation transfer" effect on the neighbouring free protons (hydrogen nuclei) of water, and therefore act as a strong contrast agent on T1-weighted imaging, shortening the T1 relaxation time, and appearing as a bright signal (white) on T1-weighted images. Conversely, wrapping of the oligodendrocytic membrane around the axon is accompanied by a loss of cytoplasm, the membranes being attached to each other by myelin basic protein. The protons of the cell membranes have no signal, and therefore myelination is expressed on T2 weighted images, by a loss of signal, myelinated areas appearing blacker), since the cytoplasm (and therefore the water) has disappeared between the myelin layers.

Myelination of the nervous system develops in the sensory before the motor pathways then in the association areas. It develops along the spinal cord before the hindbrain, and then in the forebrain. In the cerebral hemispheres, the primary sensorimotor, visual cortex, auditory and hippocampal cortex, already show myelination at birth. White matter myelination is expressed later, but again first in these four primary systems, and from the centre of the brain to the periphery, the cortex. It should again be emphasised that MRI does not give quantitative images, and that the progress of myelination in one area can be appreciated only by comparison with other areas; since myelination of different portions of the brain proceeds not only at different times, but also at different rates, it can on MRI a structure may appear as strongly myelinated as surrounding brain at a given time, and yet seem less myelinated later on, because the surrounding tissue is catching up.

Surface morphology of the brain

In the same way as organogenesis necessarily results from cellular multiplication, histogenetic development of the brain leads to significant morphological changes. The change in volume is striking: it is: 80 g at 23 weeks in utero, 350 g at birth, 800 g at 12 months, 1300 g at four or five years and 1350 to 1450 g in healthy young adults.

Still more conspicuous are the changes on the surface of the brain: totally smooth (except for a widely open lateral fissure) at 23 weeks, with only primary fissures (callosal and cingulate, calcarine and hippocampal fissures, early central sulcus) at 26 weeks, the brain then develops a more convoluted surface with secondary sulci (the 1st temporal sulcus is apparent at 28 weeks) and tertiary sulci. Except for details, the convolution of the brain surface is complete at birth (although the weight of the brain is only a quarter that of the mature brain). The pattern of gyri and sulci is species-specific, constant and recognisable from one human brain to another, like a face. It is related in part to tangential growth of the cortex (the number of neurons does not increase, but there is a tremendous increase in the number of fibres and supporting glia), in part to the predetermined pathways of the projection long association and commissural fibres; the appearance of the medial surface of the brain in callosal agenesis is different from that in normal).

Development of the brain vasculature

Finally the specific timetable of development of the various cell lineages of the brain, leading to its particular appearance at certain stages of developmental, must to be correlated with the parallel times- table of development of the vascular system of the brain, since this may explain specific destructive lesions of the developing brain. During the first weeks, when the neural tube is still open, nutrients diffuse from the amniotic fluid. When it closes, it becomes surrounded by dense connective tissue, the meninx primitiva, which contains vascular loops from which nutrients also diffuse through the surface of the nervous tissue. Between the 5th and 7th weeks, the meninx primitiva sends expansions into the ventricular lumen to form the early choroid plexuses, from which nutrients also diffuse through the ventricular surface of the brain. Then, because the brain mantle becomes thicker and thicker, intracerebral vessels develop, first in the periventricular region, where the germinal matrix actively produces the cells for the brain, then in the basal ganglia and the deep layers of the cortex, and only later in the more superficial cortical layers. Layers of "young" neurons are not vascularised, because aerobic metabolism appears only with synaptic activity. Fetal intracerebral vessels consist of endothelial cells only, without ement membrane or muscular sheath, which appear only at the end of the gestation, they are called "sinusoid capillaries". They persist in the germinal matrix throughout gestation, and are therefore still there in preterm infants. Fetal and infantile arteries form a widely connected network not only on the surface of the brain, but probably also within the parenchyma, explaining why young infants may be more vulnerable to blood perfusion pressure disorders than to vascular occlusions, especially since the metabolic needs of the neonatal brain are very high, and hardly satisfied by the heart working at its maximum capacity.

Specific vulnerability periods of the brain

The pattern of development of the brain in time specific stages of cellular multiplication (radial glia, neuroblasts, astrocytes, oligodendrocytes and myelination) with time specific stages of metabolic need and vascularity, all resulting in time specific morphological changes, explains that insults affecting the brain during its development produce time-specific lesions, depending on when they occur.

Physical insults, such as irradiation or metabolic damage to the whole brain during histogenesis affects the germinal matrix and results in a micrencephaly, which different from the genetically determined micrencephalia vera.

Infectious or anoxic destruction of the radial glia may interrupt the migration pathway of neuroblasts, resulting in heterotopic nests of grey matter (Sarnat, 1992).

An early defect in the cerebral mantle, during the phase of neuroblast migration, will alter the migration pattern, produce a hole in the brain, and change the convolutional pattern, explaining at least some types of schizencephaly. The specific sensitivity of the deep layers of the cortex during the period of cortical layering (weeks 20-23) may explain their destruction, with consequent cortical disorganisation, in cases of micropolygyria, together with a distorted convolutional pattern. Later destruction of the cerebral mantle, extending to the periventricular matrix, may explain encephaloclastic porencephaly, with no glial scarring at the site of destruction, the astrocytes of the germinal matrix having been destroyed, resulting in a fluid filled cavity, yet with good preservation of the adjacent brain.

The vulnerability to changes in blood pressure of the sinusoid capillaries in the persisting germinal matrix of the preterm infants can explain the frequency of haemorrhages there.The high metabolic needs of the brain in the perinatal period, which the heart is scarcely able to satisfy, explain the topography of necrosis in cases of periventricular leukomalacia. The end- territory of the arterial perforators is the furthest from the heart, and therefore the most sensitive to drops in blood pressure. This is still more true at the junction of the territories of the anterior, middle and posterior cerebral arteries, that is in the wall of the ventricular trigone (Banker and Larroche, 1962; Garcia-Alix et al., 1994; Larroche et al., 1986; Paneth et al., 1990; Rorke, 1992; Thornberg et al., 1995; Volpe, 1992; Yoshioka et al., 1992).

Because at the end of gestation, the most active cellular lineage is that of oligodendrocytes (myelination gliosis), higher metabolic needs make these cells more sensitive to anoxia: even if the anoxic-ischaemic deficit is not sufficient to produce tissue necrosis, it may selectively affect the oligodendrocytes, producing telencephalic leucoencephalopathy (Gilles, 1985) with a myelination defect but no axonal destruction in the same locations as periventricular leukomalacia, and thus especially in the wall of the ventricular trigone.

During maturation of the cortex, selective necrosis of certain populations of neurons may occur when anoxia affects the metabolic chain (Garcia-Alix et al., 1994; Sheldon et al., 1996; Thornberg et al., 1995; Vannucci, 1990; Volpe, 1995; Young et al., 1990) with production of toxic metabolites such as glutamate. This results in laminar necrosis of the cortex. In a similar way, selective bilateral, largely symmetrical necrosis of the neurons may occur in the basal ganglia or the thalami: paradoxical hypermyelination then may develop in spite of the neuronal loss, to produce status marmoratus. Beside anoxia, other insults, such as infection with cytomegalovirus, may produce different lesions in the brain depending on the moment they develop.

Imaging maturation of the brain

To make illustration of the maturational changes easier, the description of the images will be given according to a precise calendar, addressing the fetal period (gestational weeks 23, 28, 32, 36) and the postnatal period (birth, months 1, 4, 6, 10, 18), knowledging that gestational age may be quite approximative. During the fetal period, MRI is systematically correlated with the atlas of anatomy of the fetal brain by Fees-Higgins and Larroche, the current reference for maturation of the fetus (Fees-Higgins and Larroche, 1987).

CEREBRAL DEVELOPMENT AND MRI

The following images have been chosen according to a precise chronology (see text), with constant anatomical landmarks, and the same types of imaging (T1- and T2 weighted).

The normality of the patients has been inferred from the morphological features, comparison with those of other patients of the same gestational age, and from follow-up. Of course, these patients were not thought to be normal at the beginning (MRI would not have been performed if they were; it would be ethically unacceptable). For the series of fetuses, there is necessarily a range of error in the estimation of the gestational age. Clinical data have been correlated with the anatomical atlas of Fees-Higgins and Larroche (1987).

Postnatal images have been dated according to the birthdate, corrected for preterm neonates according to the gestational age at birth (which raises the same uncertainty as fetal age).

As in the text of the chapter, brains are illustrated at the following ages: for fetal brains, at weeks 23 (Fig. 1), 28 (Fig. 2), 32 (Fig. 3), and 36 (Fig. 4). A preterm neonate of 30 weeks gestational age is also illustrated (Fig 5), to compare with - and validate-imaging in utero. For the infant brain, the ages chosen are birth (Fig. 6), 1 (Fig. 7), 4 (Fig. 8), 6 (Fig. 9), 10 (Fig. 10) and 18 months (Fig. 11) after normal term.

Three imaging planes have been used: mainly the axial plane (labelled A; for example, Fig. 6 A means: term neonatal brain, axial), coronal, labelled C; sagittal, labelled S. T1-weighted images have been labelled simply A, C, S; T2-weighted images A', C', S'.

Finally, to identify the level of the images, each slice has been numbered 1, 2, 3, etc.,according to the morphological features illustrated. In the axial plane (A and A'), the slices pass through the posterior cranial fossa (A1, A'1), the trigones of the ventricules (A2, A'2), the basal ganglia, internal capsules, and genu and splenium of the corpus callosum (A3, A'3), and the centrum semiovale (A4, A'4). In the coronal, numbering is from front (C1, C'1) to back (C3, C'3). In the sagittal plane, numbering is from the midline (S1, S'1) laterally (S3, S'3).

Thus, the Fig. 8 A'3 means: 4 months of age, axial, T2-weighted, basal ganglia and capsules. Fig. 11 S1 means: 18 months, sagittal, T1-weighted, midline.

This applies to all brains illustrated in the following pages, except for the small fetal brains when so many slices could not be obtained at the given age.

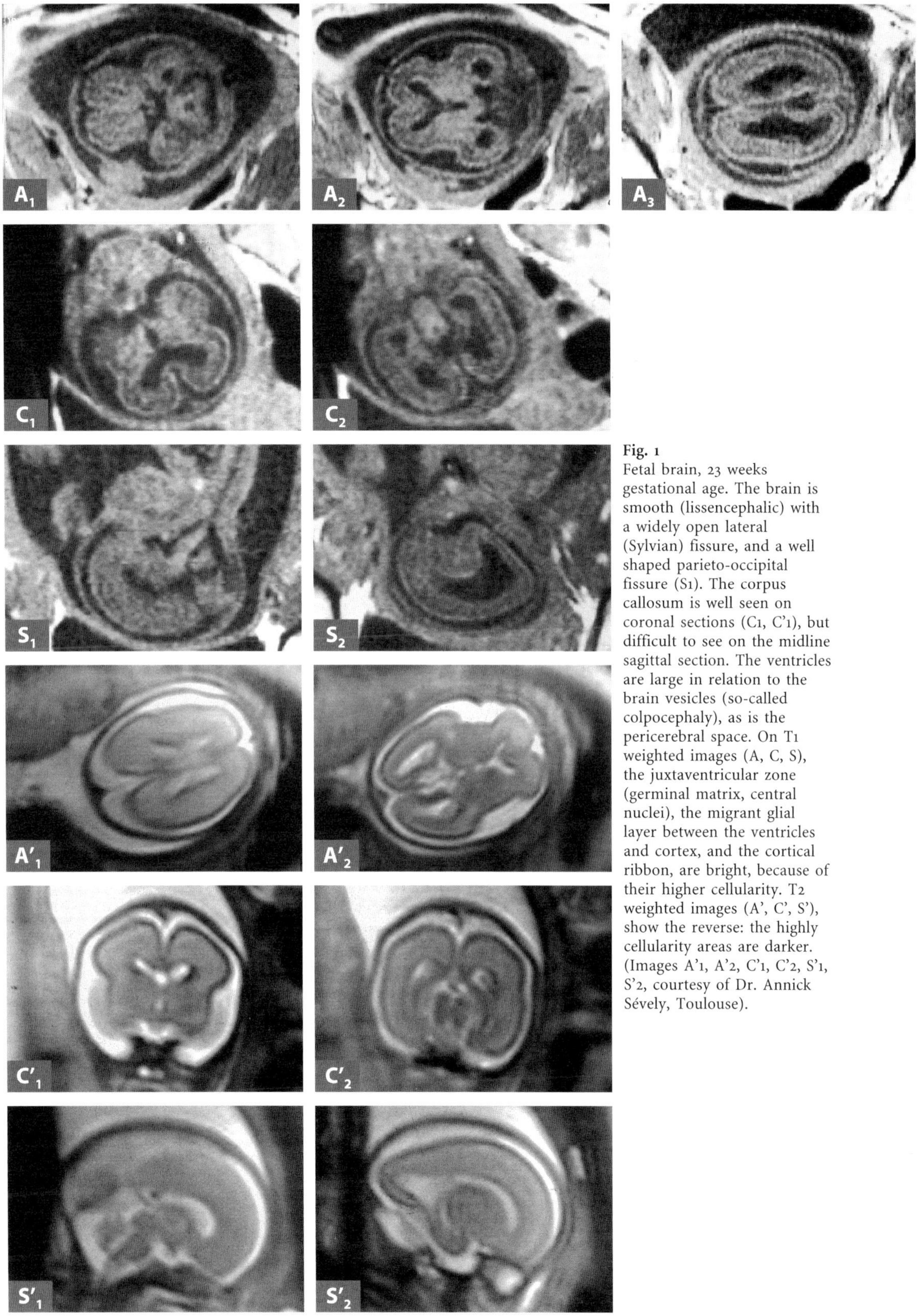

Fig. 1
Fetal brain, 23 weeks gestational age. The brain is smooth (lissencephalic) with a widely open lateral (Sylvian) fissure, and a well shaped parieto-occipital fissure (S1). The corpus callosum is well seen on coronal sections (C1, C'1), but difficult to see on the midline sagittal section. The ventricles are large in relation to the brain vesicles (so-called colpocephaly), as is the pericerebral space. On T1 weighted images (A, C, S), the juxtaventricular zone (germinal matrix, central nuclei), the migrant glial layer between the ventricles and cortex, and the cortical ribbon, are bright, because of their higher cellularity. T2 weighted images (A', C', S'), show the reverse: the highly cellularity areas are darker. (Images A'1, A'2, C'1, C'2, S'1, S'2, courtesy of Dr. Annick Sévely, Toulouse).

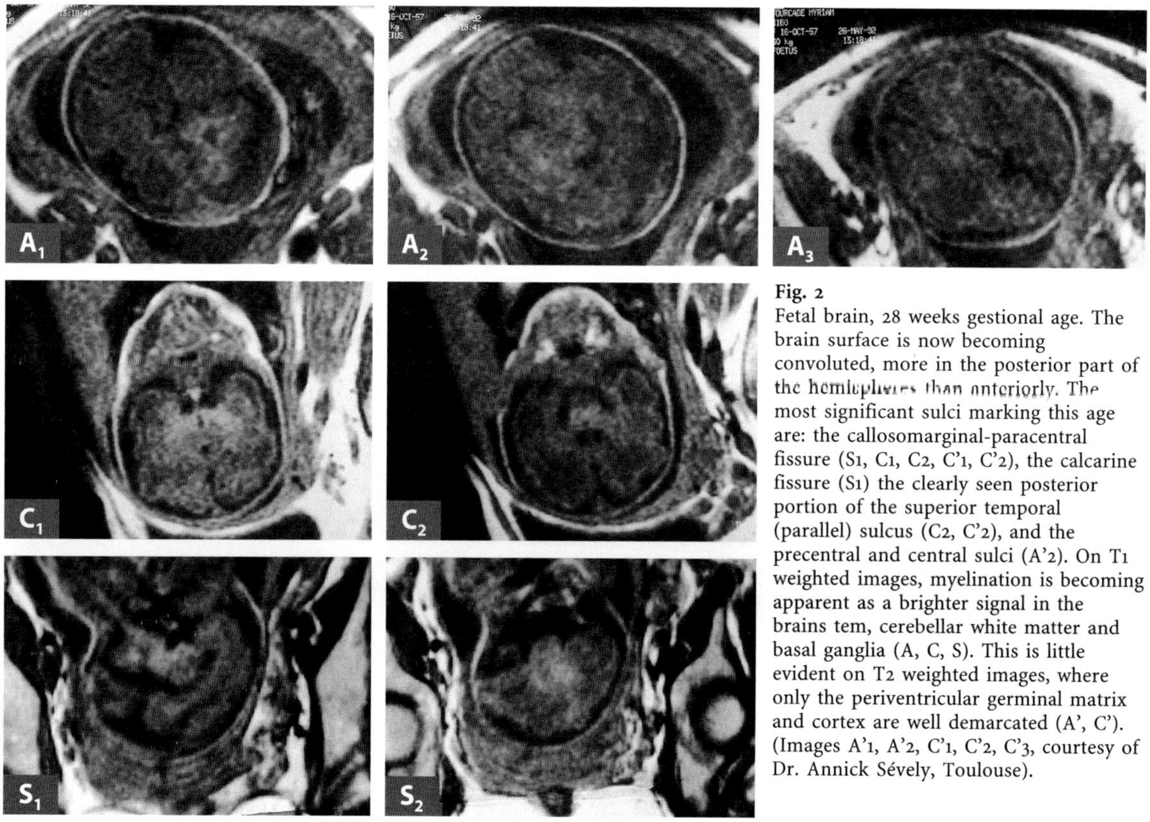

Fig. 2
Fetal brain, 28 weeks gestional age. The brain surface is now becoming convoluted, more in the posterior part of the hemispheres than anteriorly. The most significant sulci marking this age are: the callosomarginal-paracentral fissure (S1, C1, C2, C'1, C'2), the calcarine fissure (S1) the clearly seen posterior portion of the superior temporal (parallel) sulcus (C2, C'2), and the precentral and central sulci (A'2). On T1 weighted images, myelination is becoming apparent as a brighter signal in the brains tem, cerebellar white matter and basal ganglia (A, C, S). This is little evident on T2 weighted images, where only the periventricular germinal matrix and cortex are well demarcated (A', C'). (Images A'1, A'2, C'1, C'2, C'3, courtesy of Dr. Annick Sévely, Toulouse).

T1-weighted imaging of the fetal brain

Week 23 (Fig. 1)

The antero posterior dimension of the brain is 75 mm, the transverse 65 mm. The ventricles are large compared with the thickness of the mantle. Organisation of the six-layered isocortex is just complete but no gyrus or sulcus is present and the brain has a vesicular appearance with depression of the insula. The germinal matrix is present, active, producing glial cells, mostly astrocytes at this stage and between this germinal matrix and the cortex, a layer of "migrant cells" is interposed in the white matter. There is practically no myelination at this stage, and the T1 signal expresses the cellularity of the brain. Therefore, the more cellular areas appear bright against the less cellular From the periphery to the centre, they consist of the cortical ribbon (bright), the subcortical white matter (darker), the intermediate "migration" layer (bright), the deep white matter (darker), the periventricular germinal matrix and the central grey matter, the basal ganglia and thalamus. The CSF within the ventricles is dark, as is the CSF around the brain. The pericerebral space is large, the brain is not abutting the vault (Girard and Raybaud, 1992; Girard et al., 1995).

Week 28 (Fig. 2)

The antero-posterior dimension of the brain is 80 mm, the transverse 70 mm. The overall morphology of the brain is not very different from that at 23 weeks, except that sulci are now more apparent, a well defined superior temporal sulcus being a specific marker of the 28th week. The ventricles are still large (10 mm at the trigone) as is the pericerebral space. The periventricular cellular areas (germinal matrix, basal ganglia, thalamus) are well defined, as is the cortical ribbon but the intermediate layer of "migrant cells" is no longer evident, supposedly because of more homogeneous dispersion of the glial cells. From histology, we know that myelination has already begun in the basal structures of the brain, and the brighter signal there on T1 weighted sequences expresses the high cellularity as well as the beginning of myelination.

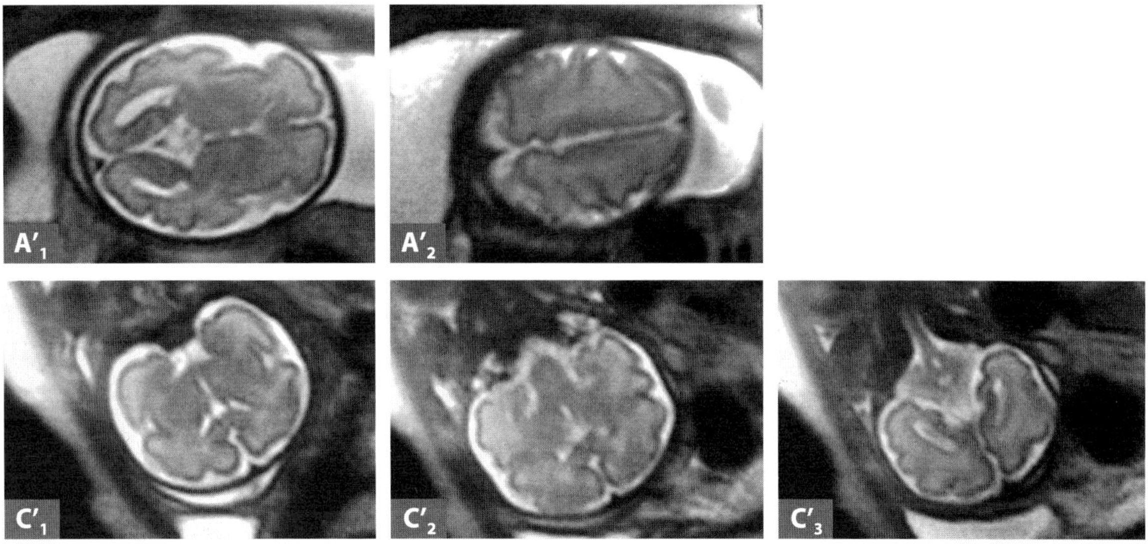

Week 32 (Fig. 3)

The brain now measures 100 mm from front to back, and 80 mm across. Because the white matter has grown significantly relative to the grey matter and the CSF spaces, the cortex appears relatively thinner, and the ventricular trigones small. The cortex is now convoluted, with the primary and secondary sulci, still shallow and can still be seen as a bright ribbon between the peripheral CSF and the subcortical white matter. This bright signal in the cortex, and in the central nuclei, now expresses evolving myelination. In the posterior cranial fossa the cisterna magna is large, because the cerebellum, although well developed as far as the folia are concerned, is still small in the relatively large posterior cranial fossa.

Week 36 (Fig. 4)

The brain now measures 110 mm antero-posteriorly, and 90 mm in the transverse diameter. However, the cortical ribbon has not enlarged since week 23, and is therefore hardly visible against the rest of the brain, the more so because the pericerebral fluid space is disappearing. In the same way, the ventricles now appear small in relation to the brain. Myelination is becoming apparent against the white matter, mainly in the basal ganglia mostly but also the dorsal, tegmental regions of the brain stem.

T2-weighted imaging of the fetal brain (Fig. 1 and 2)

Basically, T2 weighted images appear the reverse of the T1-weighted images: the CSF is bright, the central nuclei and the periventricular germinal matrix are darker, as is the cortex. However, the intermediate layer of "migrant cells", interposed in the white matter is not as apparent as on T1 weighted images, probably for technical reasons (poor signal-to-noise ratio) in the obstetric conditions (fetal head within the amniotic fluid, within the maternal abdomen, with respiratory, vascular and intestinal motion artefacts), since this layer is clearly seen in premature infants of the same fetal age (Fig. 5). T2 weighted images are extremely useful for detecting the cortex as a low signal interposed between the high signal of the peripheral CSF and the underlying white matter, and thereby for early diagnosis of cortical abnormalities.

Imaging the infant brain

Although it weight only a quarter of the mature brain, the neonatal brain (at normal term) already has its permanent shape, except for a few details: incomplete frontal operculation of the lateral fissure, thin corpus callosum and relatively small cerebellum. Its tissue composition is as yet still close to that of the fetal brain: 90 % of water in the grey matter

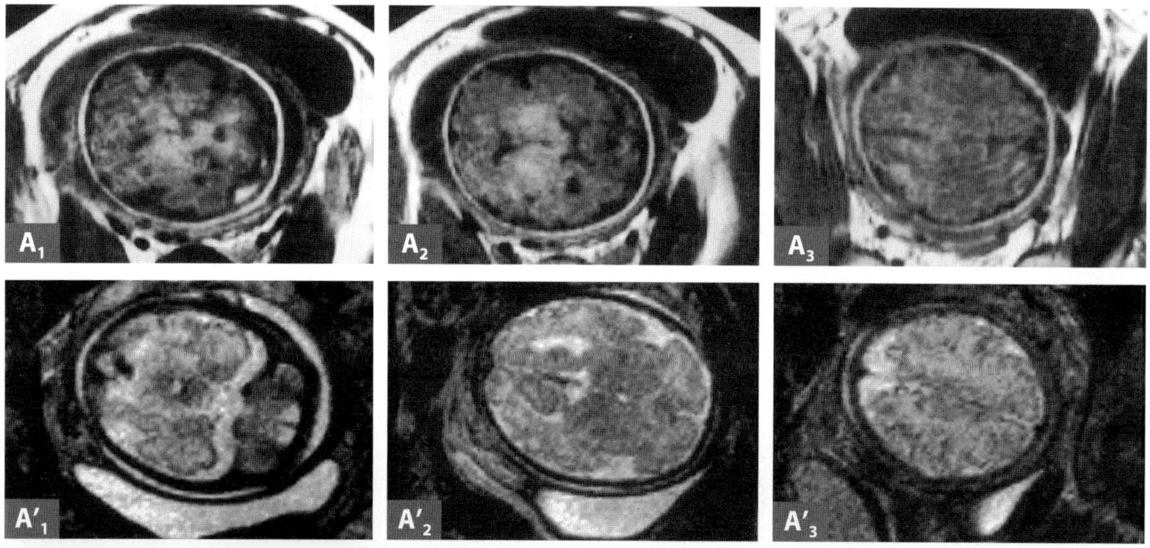

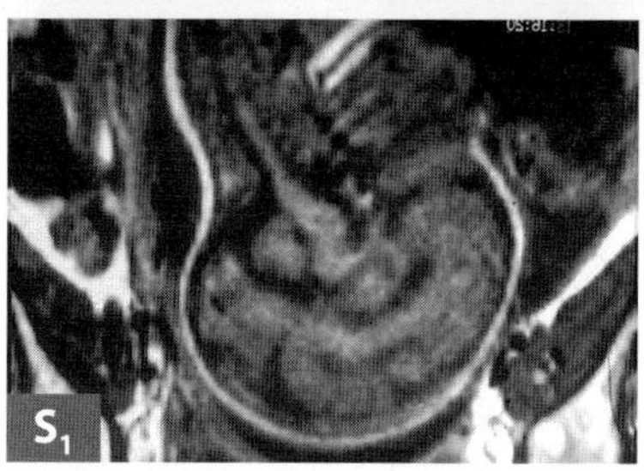

Fig. 3. Fetal brain, 32 weeks gestional age. Although still shallow, many sulci and therefore gyri, are now seen on the cerebral surface. The 3rd ventricle (S1) is well individualised, with optic chiasm, pituitary gland, and massa intermedia. On the T2 weighted sagittal section (S'1), the internal cerebral vein can be seen. The ventricles are becoming generally smaller in relation to the rest of the brain (there is some asymmetry in these cases, which are not actually completely normal). The pericerebral space is smaller. Developing myelination of the central structures is clearly seen as a bright signal on T1 weighted images (espacially A1, A2, S1), and now also on T2 weighted images as a dark (low) signal in the dorsal brain stem (A'1, S'1), and basal ganglia (A'2, S'2).

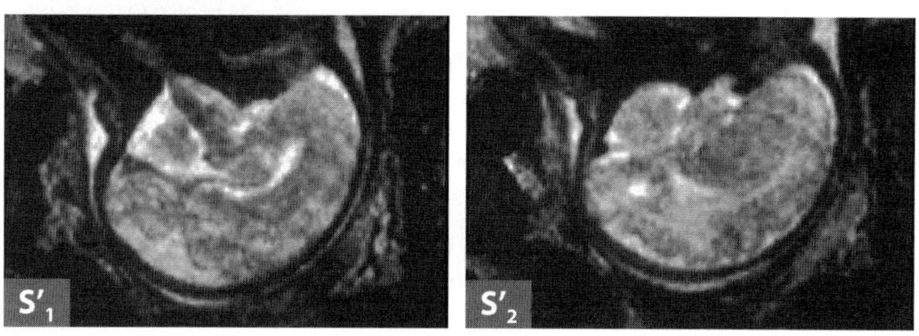

and in the white. The myelination process has begun in the last weeks of gestation, but is still rudimentary. As stated above, the myelination develops in the sensory system before the motor system and in the latter before the association areas, and in the spinal cord before the hindbrain, then in the forebrain; in the forebrain, the grey matter appears myelinated before the white matter and in the latter myelination develops from the centre to the periphery. Although the cortex and white matter do not appear connected in this respect, the early myelination process involves primarily four functional unites, the olfactory-hippocampal, visual, auditory, and primary sensorimotor systems. This pattern does not reflect any functional precocity of these systems relative to the association areas, but simply the phytogenetic heritage, since in rudimentary mammals, such as the shrew, only these functional units are present, without any association cortex (Barkovich et al., 1988; Brody et al., 1987; Girard et al., 1991; Holmes, 1986; van der Knaap and Valk, 1995).

From a technical point of view, and whatever type of sequence is used properly adapted to the stage of maturation of the brain), imaging of the infant brain is usually performed with both T1- and T2-weighted images. On T1 weighted images multiplication of interfascicular oligodendrocytes (myelination gliosis) and the progressive expansion of their membranes which will make up the myelin, create a strong magnetisation transfer effect which shortens T1, and therefore induces a very strong T1 signal, without changing T2: the changes expressed on T1 weighted images are not only myelination itself but also the cellular changes preceding it. For a given stage of de-

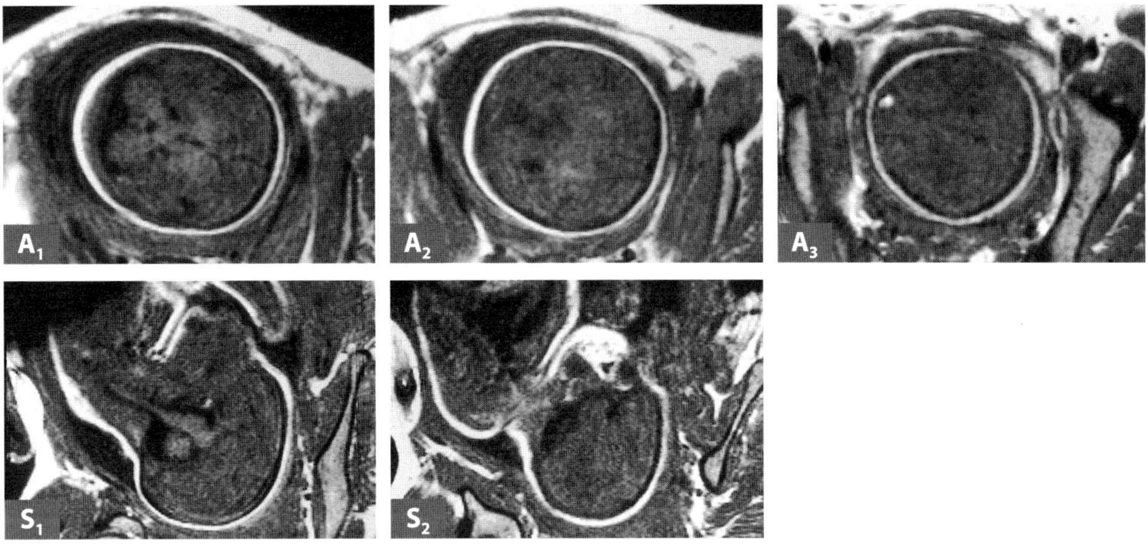

Fig. 4. Fetal brain, 36 weeks gestational age. The relative volume of the brain has markedly increased, so that the ventricles are now small, and the pericerebral space very thin. The thickness of the cortex (2 - 4 mm) has not changed since midgestation, and the cortex is now barely visible, because myelination there is more advanced than in the white matter. The content of the posterior cranial fossa are now clearly demarcated, with a large cisterna magna, present throughout the whole fetal period. Because of the advancing myelination, the dorsal brain stem is brighter, as are the central portions of the basal ganglia. The reason, the morphological features are not as evident as in earlier stages, although the brain is larger than in the previous illustrations (figures 1 to 3), is that the relative decrease in the volume of the fluid spaces makes the parenchyma more compact, and not so well delineated.

velopment, maturation always seems more advanced on T1-weighted images than on T2-weighted ones, because on the latter, only completed maturation is apparent as loss of signal from the parenchyma. Therefore, T2-weighted imaging shows what is already myelinated; T1-weighted shows what is still myelinating.

At birth

At birth (Fig. 6), the brain weight approximately 350 g. Its maximum longer anteroposterior diameter is 115 mm, its maximum transverse (biparietal) diameter 95 mm, the bifrontal ventricular distance is 25 mm and the width of the ventricular trigone 7 mm. On T1-weighted images the white matter throughout is strongly contrasted against the grey matter, giving very low signal (dark). The cortex is diffusely brighter but its brightness is more pronounced in the sensorimotor and premotor areas (central and precentral cortex), the primary visual area (calcarine cortex), the primary auditory cortex (planum temporale) and the hippocampal formation.

In the centre of the forebrain, the grey matter nuclei and internal capsules are diffusely bright (contrasting with a 30 weeks gestation premature infant, in whose brain the internal capsules are darker, less myelinated than the surrounding nuclei (Fig. 5), with no evident limits between the grey and white matter of the capsule. In the posterior cranial fossa, the brain stem is bright, more in the tegmentum than in the pons, and the cerebellar arbor vitae is also bright.

On T2-weighted images white matter is bright. The cortex and the nuclear grey matter in the centre of the brain are darker. Because of the more advanced maturation there, the sensorimotor, visual, auditory and hippocampal cortex is darker than the rest of the cortex but, in contrast with the T1 weighted images the internal capsules, especially the anterior limbs, appear rather poorly myelinated at this stage against the central nuclei. Maturation of the brain stem and the cerebellar arbor vitae is more advanced.

At one month

At one month after normal term (Fig. 7), changes in signal are more apparent on T1 weighted images than on T2 weighting. with T1 weighting, contrast between the white matter (dark) and the grey matter (brighter) has diminished diffusely. Within the internal capsule, the posterior limb appears very bright, expressing the more advanced maturation of the pyramidal tract. In the cortex, the four primary

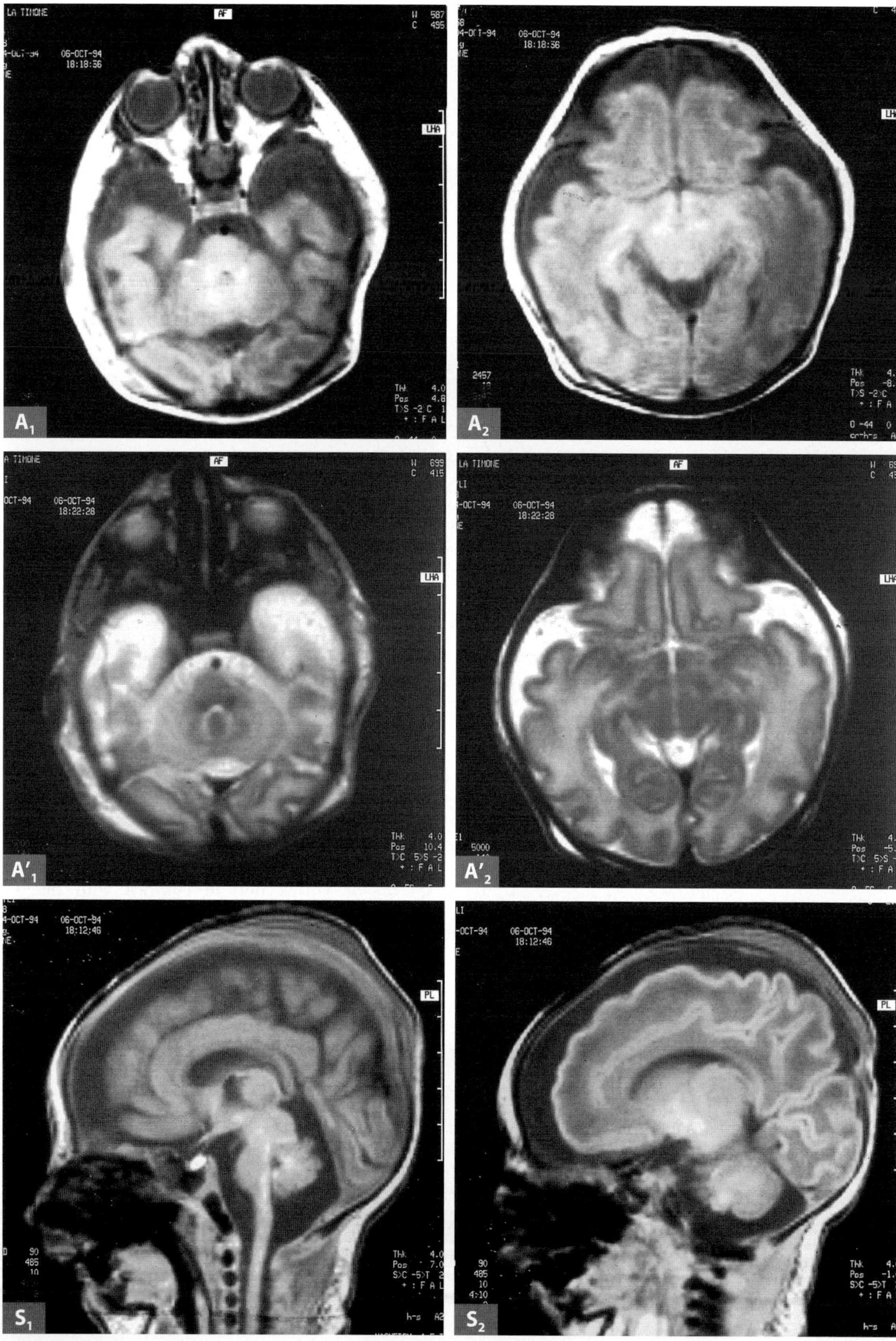
A₁
A₂
A′₁
A′₂
S₁
S₂

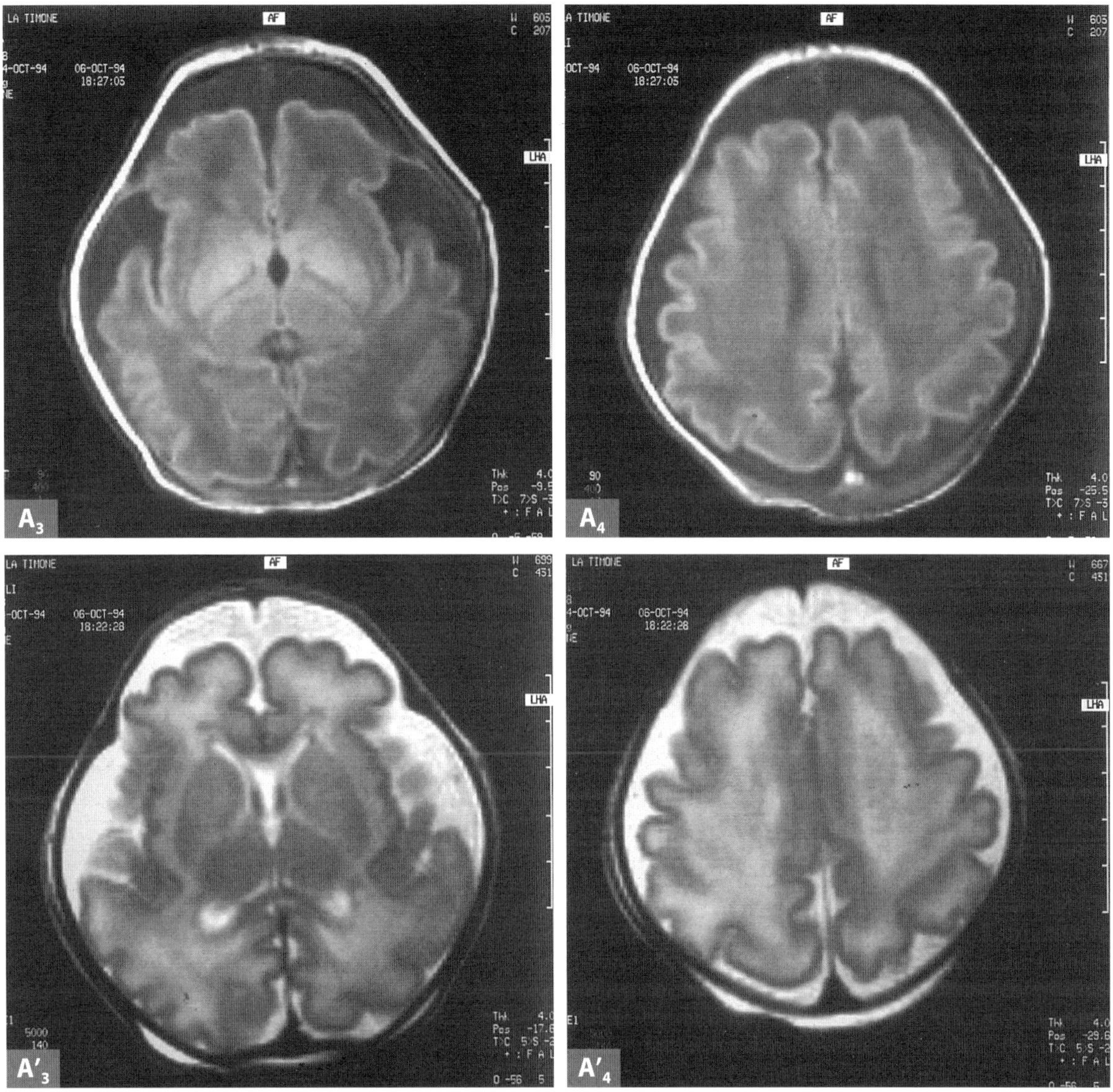

Fig. 5. Premature neonate, 30 gestational weeks. The images are considerably better than those obtained in utero, because of artefacts generated by the thickness of the mother's abdomen, and the movement of bowels, diaphragm and surrounding large vessels. The morphology of the brain is close to that of the term neonate, except that the sulci are shallow, and that only fissures (primari sulci) and secondary sulci are well demarcated. This brain is intermediate between those brains of figures 2 and 3: the pericerebral space is large, the more so because amniotic pressure is absent in this born neonate. On T1 weighted images the more advanced myelination is well seen as brighter signal in the brain stem (A1, A2, S1) and the grey matter of the basal ganglia (A3), and hypothalamus (A2, S1) and in specific cortical areas, namely the hippocampus (A2), sensori motor cortex (A4, S2), planum temporale (A3) and calcarine fissure (S2). In the white matter, the subcortical white matter appears slightly brighter, because of the migrant glial layer is now reaching the periphery. On T2 weighted images (A'1 to A'4), the same features are more or less apparent, but signal intensity is reversed. At this stage, the corpus callosum (A'3) is clearly more mature (darker) than most of the white matter, as in the fornix also. The internal capsule, on the other hand, is clearly less myelinated than the adjoining grey matter nuclei (A3, A'3). The relatively very bright signal of the pituitary gland (S1), which will change little over the years, indicates that the highly hydrated brain parenchyma generally gives a very low T1 signal at this stage.

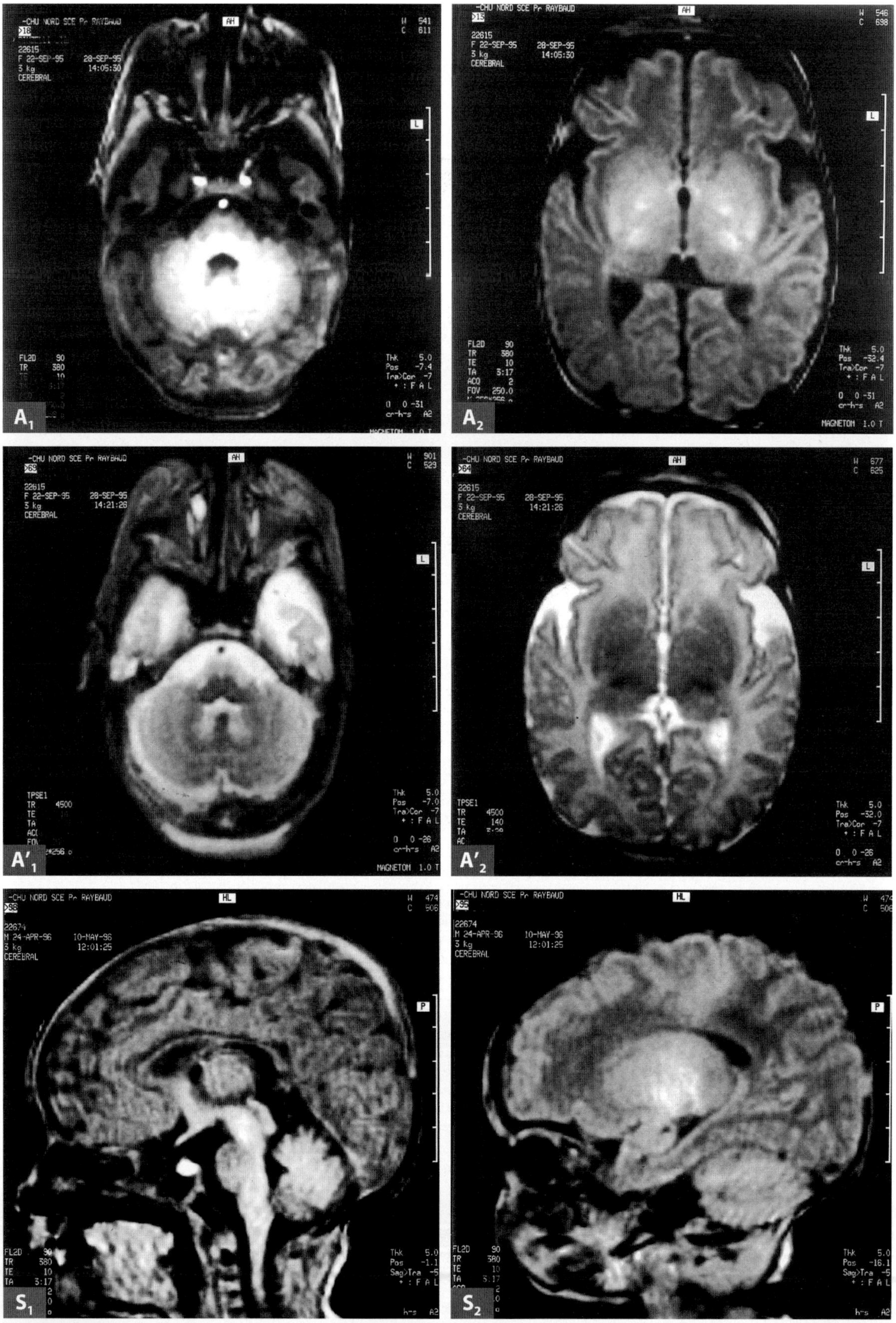
A1
A2
A'1
A'2
S1
S2

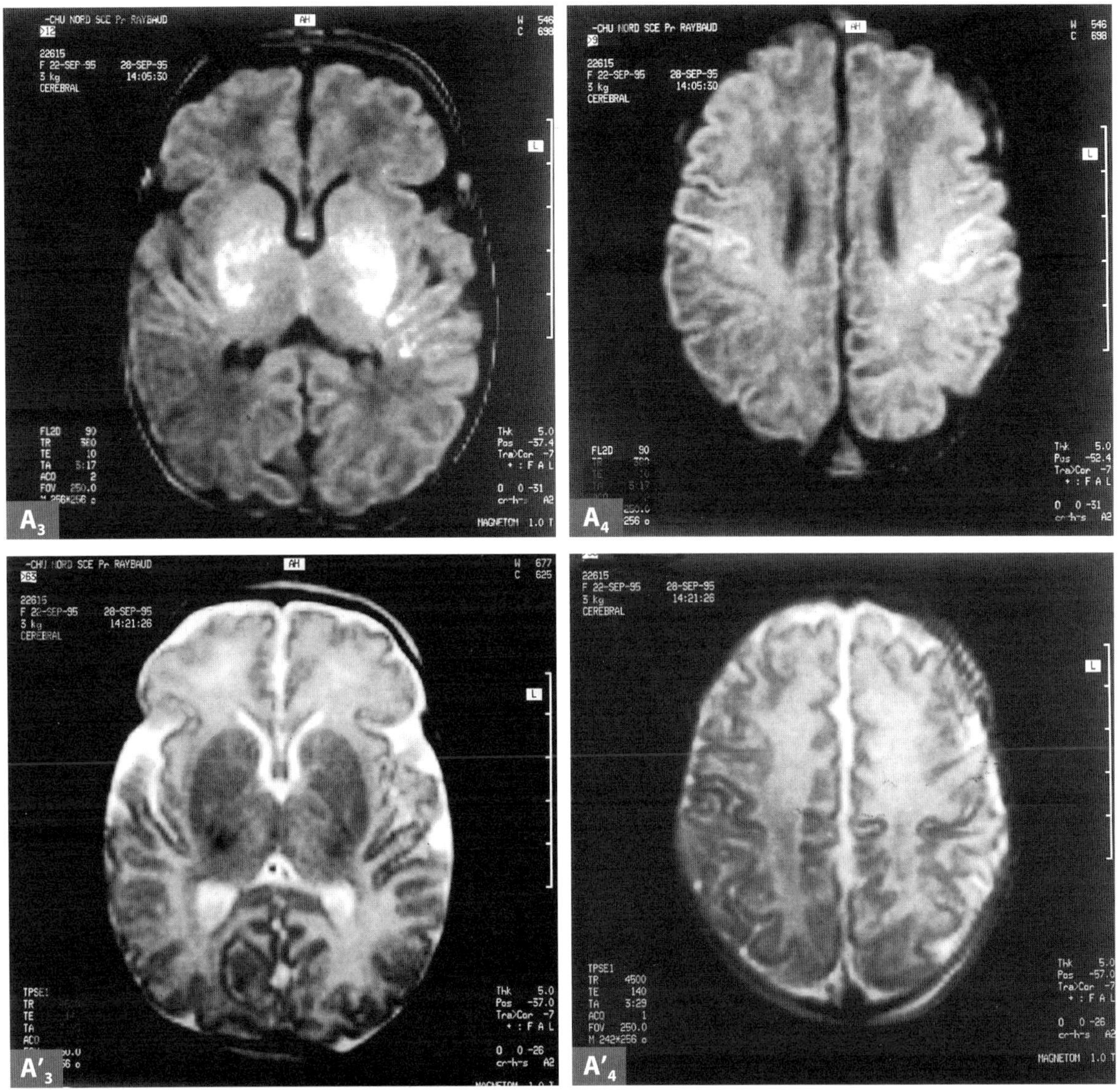

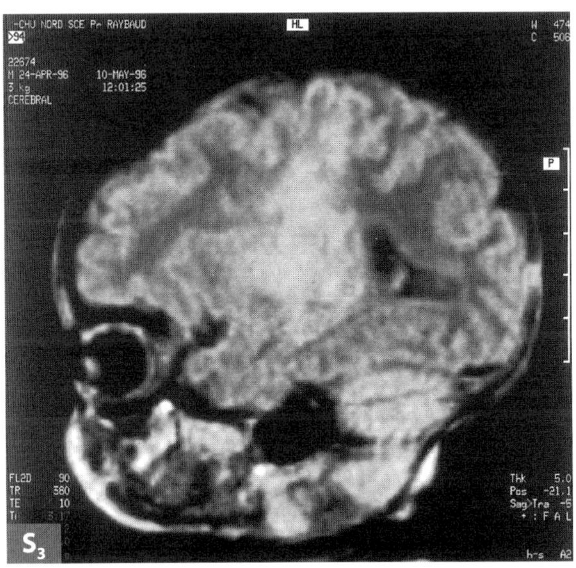

Fig. 6. Term neonate, between 40 and 42 weeks gestational age. There is a very strong contrast between the white matter (dark on T1 and bright on T2-weighting) and the grey matter. Morphologically, the cortex has completed its sulcation and gyration. On T1 weighted images, the whole posterior cranial fossa appears bright, because of its advanced myelination (A1). Myelination also appears advanced in the posterior part of the lentiform nucleus, and in the anterolateral part of the thalamus (A2, A3, S2). It has also clearly advanced in the sensori motor cortical areas (A), the planum temporale (A3) and in the inner parts of the occipital lobe (A2, A3, S2). On T2-weighted images (A'1 to A'4), the pattern is reversed (low instead of high signal), but comparison in a single child, demonstrates that the maturational changes always appear more advanced and more diffuse on T1-weighted imaging (myelination in progress) than with T2 weightening (myelination completed). As compared with the pituitary gland , the brain is still highly hydrated, giving low signal on T1-weighted images.

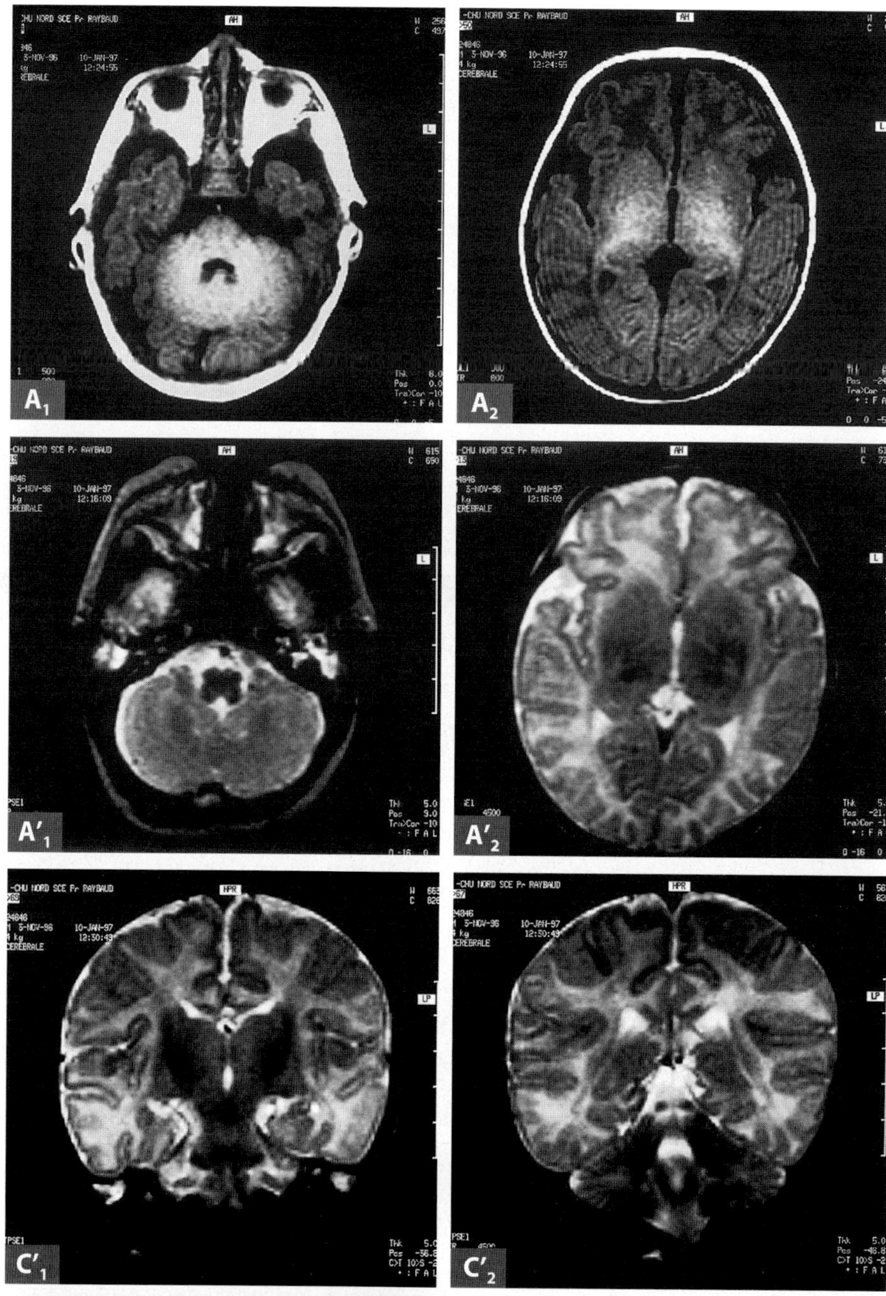

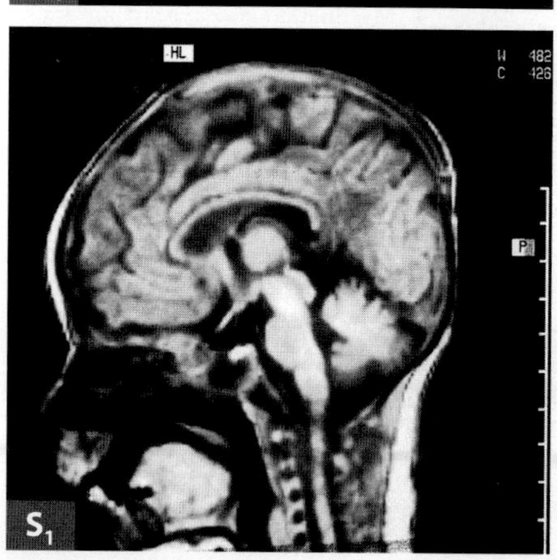

Fig. 7
Infant brain, one month after term. On T1 weighted images, there is strong contrast between the grey and white matter, but within the latter, some fibre bundles now give higher signal: the posterior limbs of the internal capsules (A3), thalamo-occipital tracts (optic radiations) (A2, A3), thalamotemporal tracts (acoustic radiations) (A3), and the subcortical white matter in the sensori motor area (A4). On T2 weighted imaging, things have evolved in the same direction but not to the same extent: myelination in progress is expressed more on T1 weighted images (bright), because of the magnetisation transfer effects (see text), than the completed myelination (loss of signal) is shown on T2 weighted images. On the whole, the

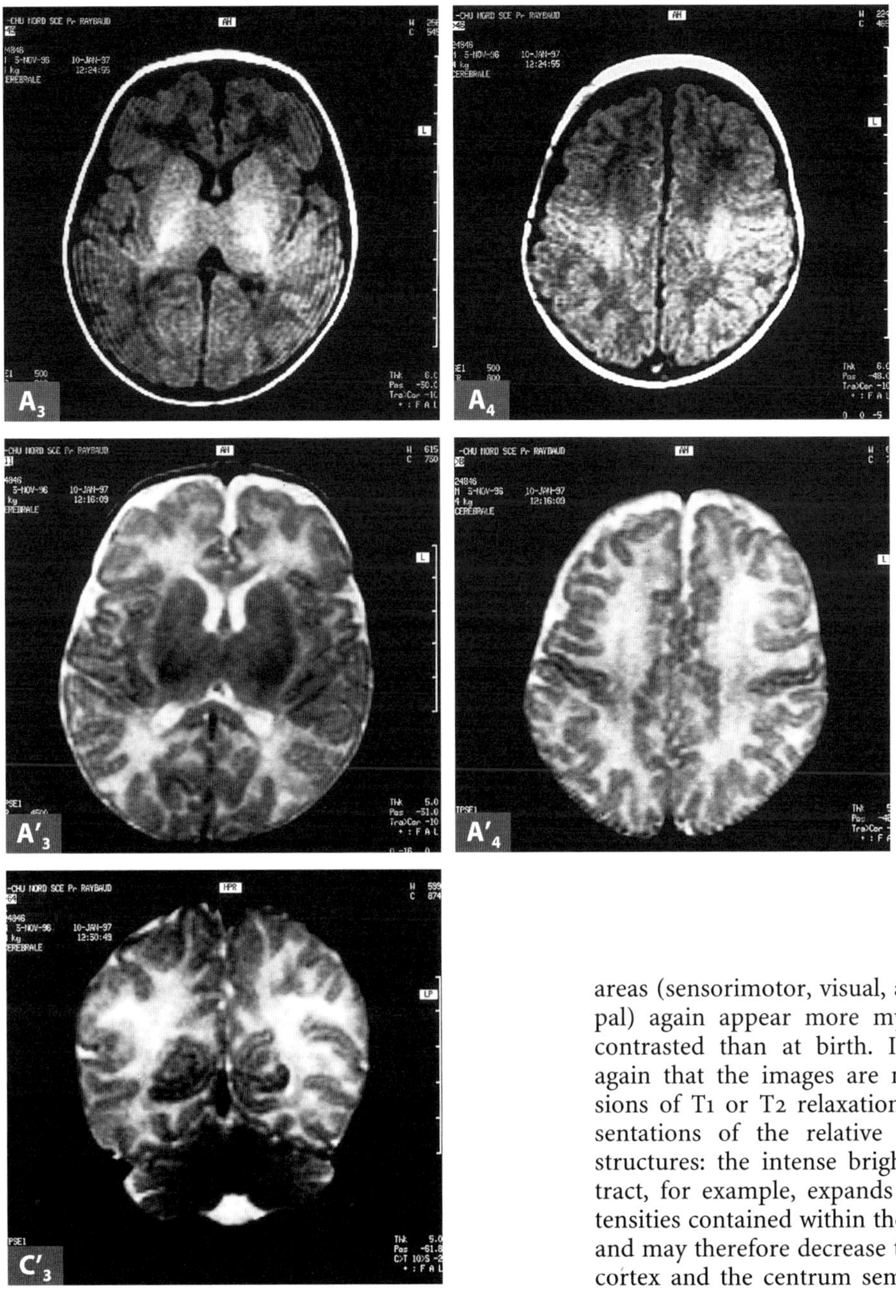

hydration of the brain, as appreciated by comparison with the T1 signal of the pituitary gland, is decreasing.

Myelination of the cortex is more advanced in the sensori motor area, as shown on T1-weighted images (A4) and still more with T2 weightening (A'4) and in the planum temporale (A2, A'2, A3, A'3). T2 weighted coronal sections demonstrate, as lower signal, the more advanced myelination of the upper sensori motor cortex (C'2), of the calcarine (striate) cortex (C'3) and of the whole corticospinal tract (C'2). The corpus callosum now appears clearly against the surrounding brain on a midline T1 weighted sagittal image (S1) but is still much thinner than in more mature brains.

areas (sensorimotor, visual, auditory and hippocampal) again appear more myelinated, although less contrasted than at birth. It should be remember again that the images are not quantitative expressions of T1 or T2 relaxation times, but only representations of the relative brightness of different structures: the intense brightness of the pyramidal tract, for example, expands the range of signal intensities contained within the greyscale of the image, and may therefore decrease the contrast between the cortex and the centrum semi ovale, to some extent this depends upon the characteristics of individual imagers.

T2 weighted images one month post-term are essentially unchanged as compared with images at birth.

At four months

At four months (Fig. 8) changes are apparent on both T1- T2 weighted images. On T1 the former, contrast between the cortex and the subjacent white matter has disappeared, the diffuse myelination of the peripheral white matter catching up with the cortical signal. But the corona radiata converging toward the internal capsules from the whole brain now

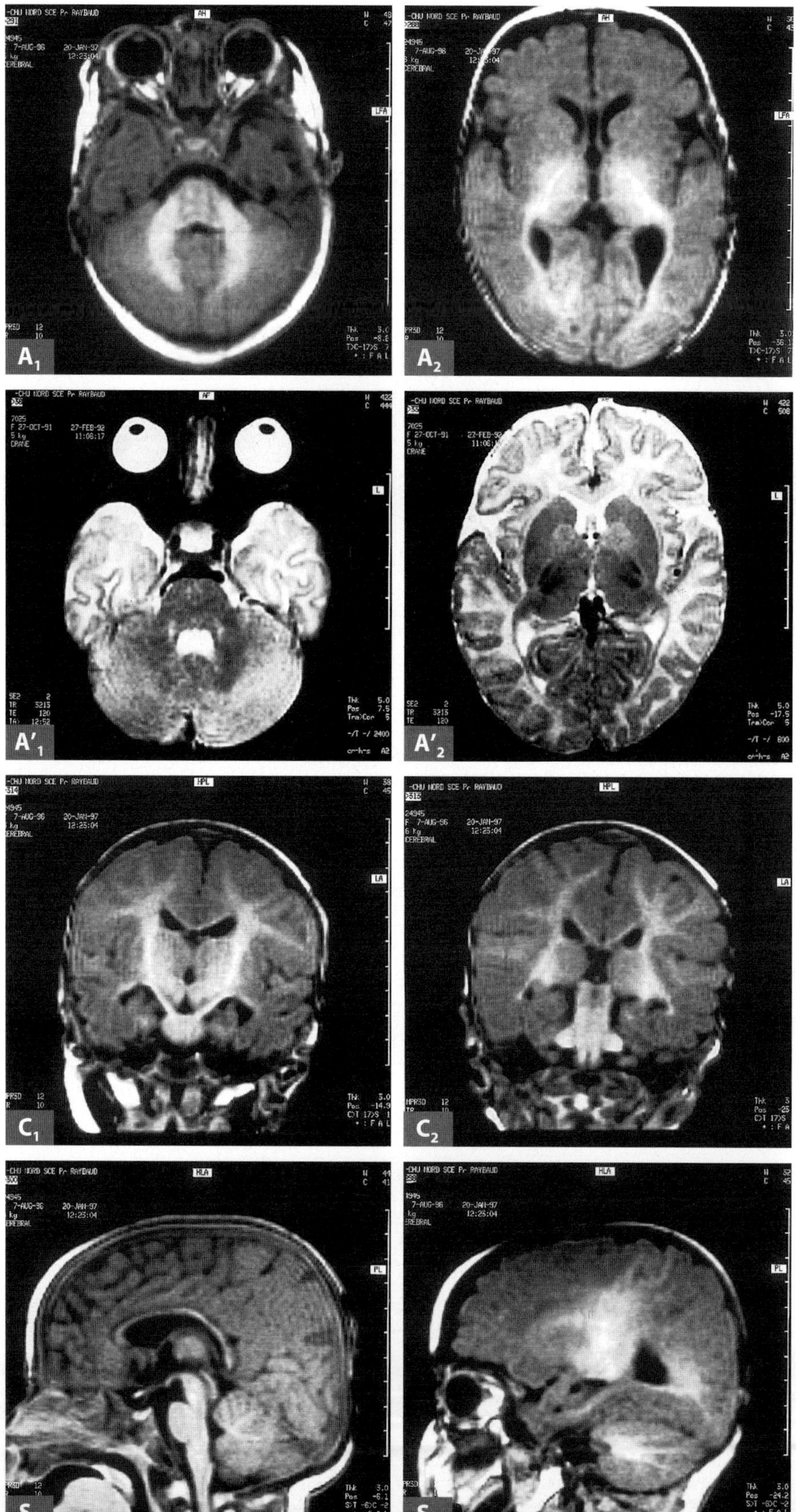
A1
A2
A'1
A'2
C1
C2
S1
S2

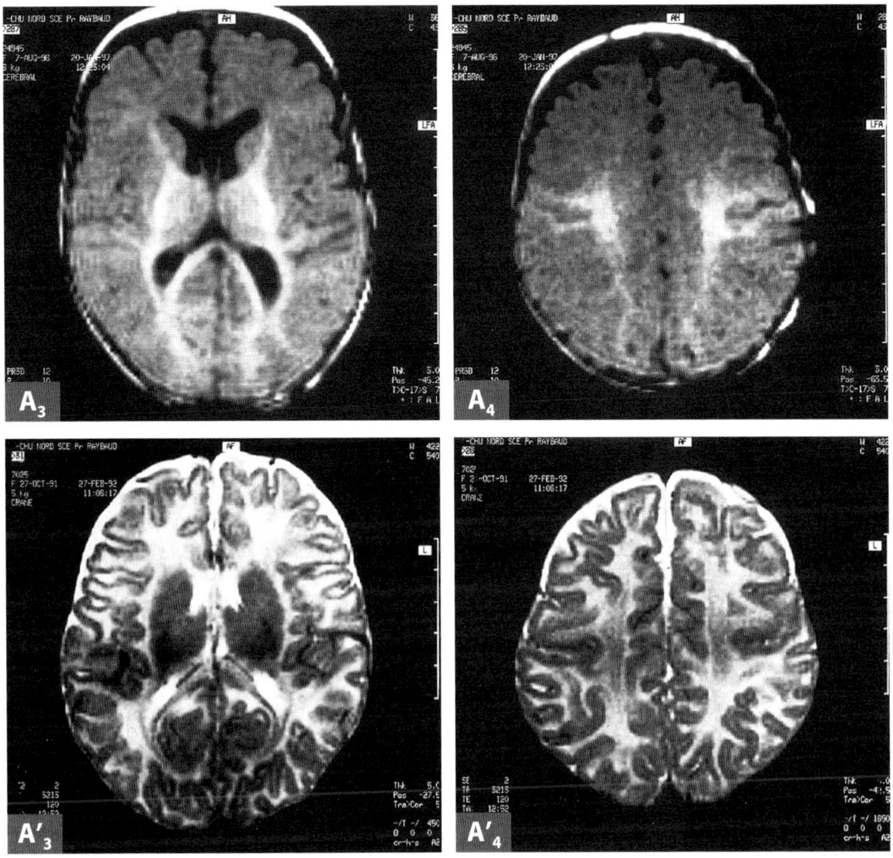

Fig. 8. Infant brain, 4 months after term. On T1 weighted images, the features are clearly different from previously. At the periphery, contrast is lost between the cortex and white matter, meaning that maturation of the latter is now matching that of the former. Moreover, some bundles appear now much brighter: the corticospinal tracts in the posterior limbs of the internal capsules (A2, A3, C1) and toward the sensori motor cortex (A4, C1, S2), the thalamo-occipital tracts (optic radiations) (A2, A3, C2, S2, S3), and the superior longitudinal (arcuate) fasciculus (S3). The posterior part of the corpus callosum also appears brighter (A3, S1), but is still thin.
On T2 weighted images, the general features have not changed much since the previous stages except that the optic radiations should now be clearly visible along the lateral walls of the trigones of the ventricles. Because this area of white matter is anatomically more exposed to anoxia-ischaemia, being the deep end-territory of the watershed zone between the anterior, middle and posterior cerebral arteries, any change in myelination there is the earliest and the most sensitive index of anoxic insult to the brain, especially since the myelin-producing cells, the oligodendrocytes, are the glial cells most sensitive to anoxia, particularly in the maturing brain, where their metabolic activity is very high, making them very vulnerable to metabolic deficits.

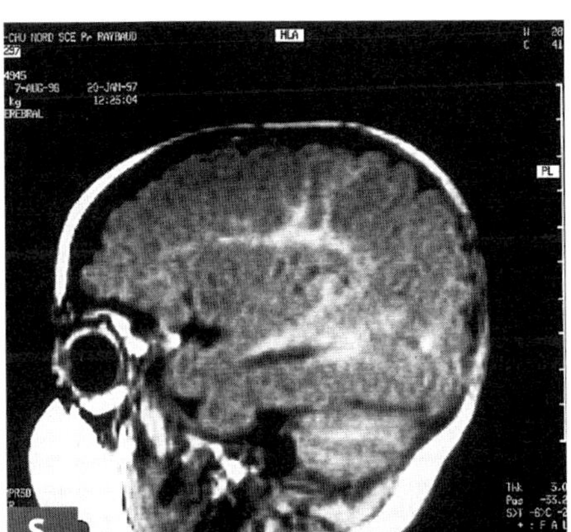

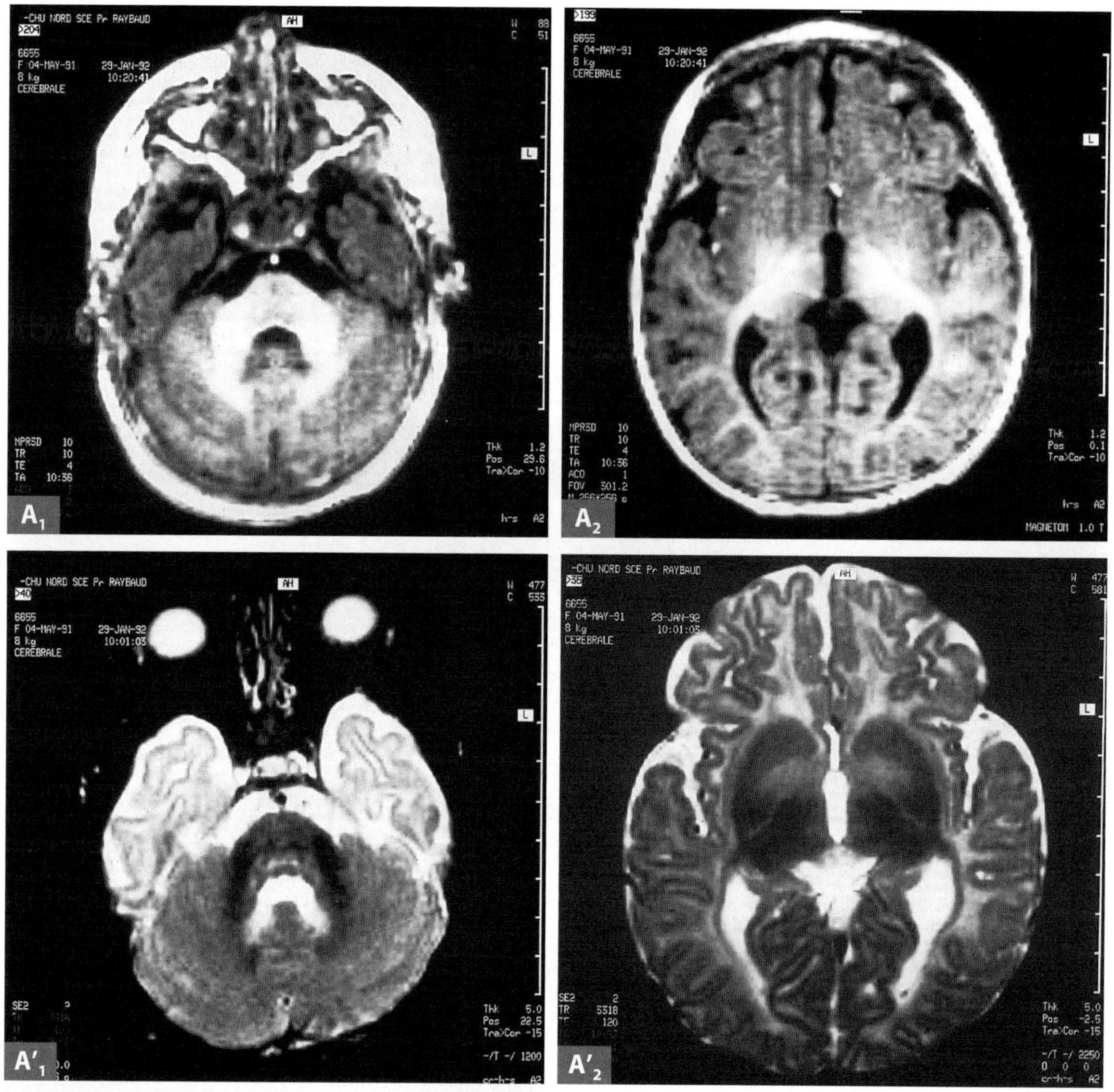

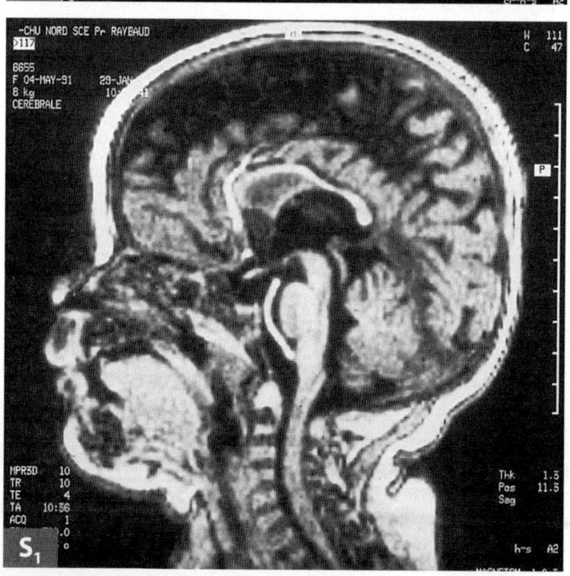

Fig. 9. Infant brain, 6 months after term. On T1 weighted images, the features are closer to those of the mature brain, especially in the posterior part of the hemispheres,where the white matter now is brighter than the cortex. In the frontal lobes, myelination is advancing mainly in the corona radiata (on each side of the frontal horns) (A3). The genu of the corpus callosum is becoming brighter (A3, S1), but the corpus callosum is still generally thin. The T1 signal of the brain overall at this stage is not different from that of the pituitary gland.
On T2 weighted imaging, the features still lag behind, remaining not very different from those of a 4 month brain. Although the maturation process in this child is normally advanced, the MRI examination is not completely normal; the enlarged CSF space over the frontal and temporal lobes, so-called external hydrocephalus manifested clinically by an enlarged head, is presumably related to a temporary delay of the maturation of the arachnoid granulations in the dural venous sinuses over the cerebral convexity.

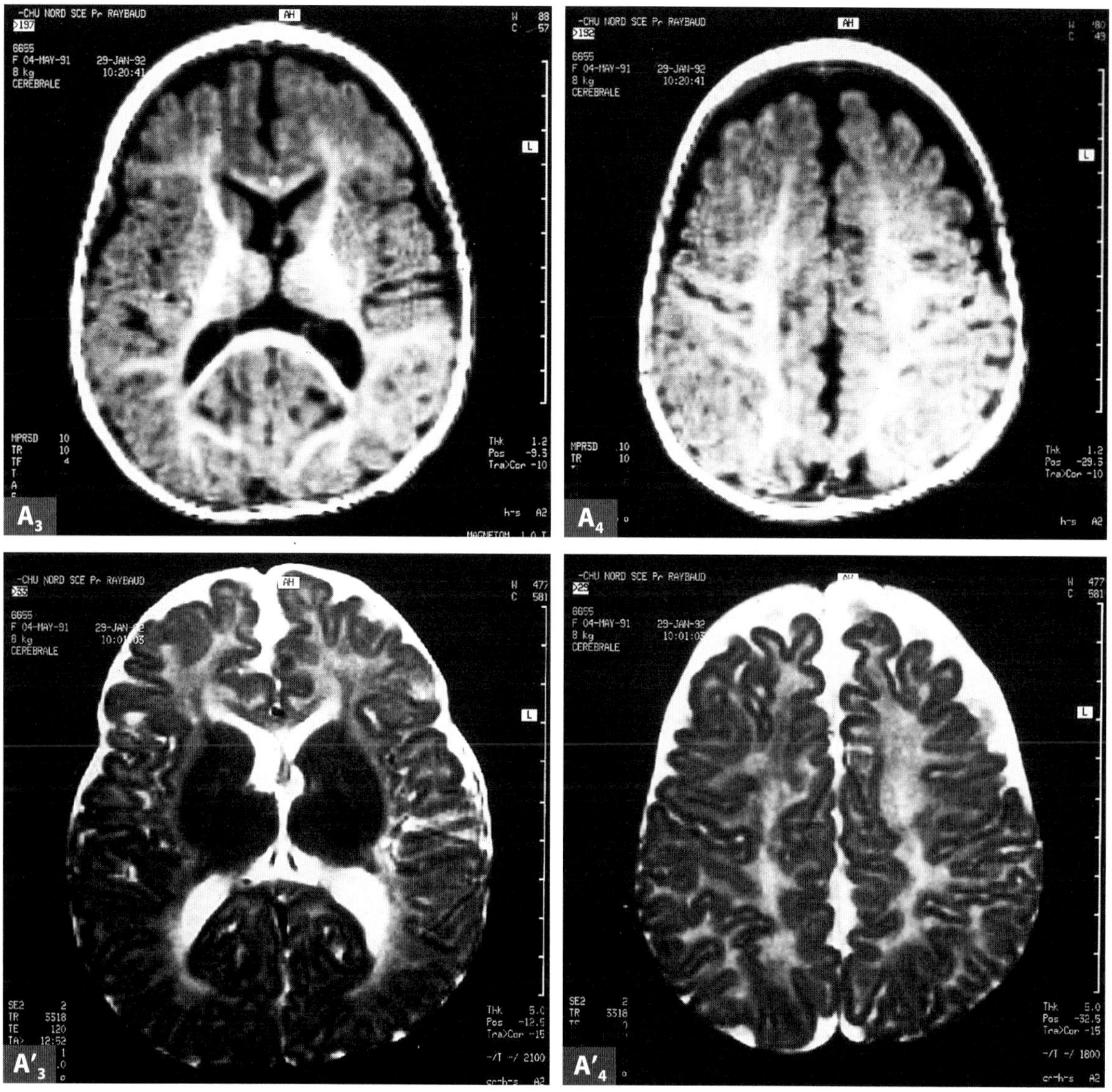

gives very high signal and, in the sensorimotor subcortical white matter, extends to the cortex itself. In the same way, tracts projecting from the lateral geniculate bodies to the medial occipital cortex along the lateral walls of the trigones of the ventricles (optic radiations) appear bright against the darker white matter, as do the acoustic tracts running towards the planum temporale. Therefore, at this stage, the forebrain appears uniformly grey except for these specific bundles of the corona radiata.

On T2 weighted images, specific changes have occured since the one month brain: the internal capsules cannot now be distinguished from the adjacent grey nuclei, and the optic radiations are clearly apparent on the lateral wall of the trigones of the ventricule. The cortex is more diffusely myelinated and the white matter in the centrum semiovale is more heterogeneous with advancing myelination, especially in the sensorimotor area.

At six months

At six months (Fig. 9) on T1 weighted images the appearance is getting closer to its mature state one: most of the white matter is brighter than the grey matter, except for the immediately subcortical zone. The corpus callosum appears bright.

On T2 weighted images, on the other hand, the contrast in the images is not very different from how it was at four months: only the posterior corpus callosum appears obviously dark.

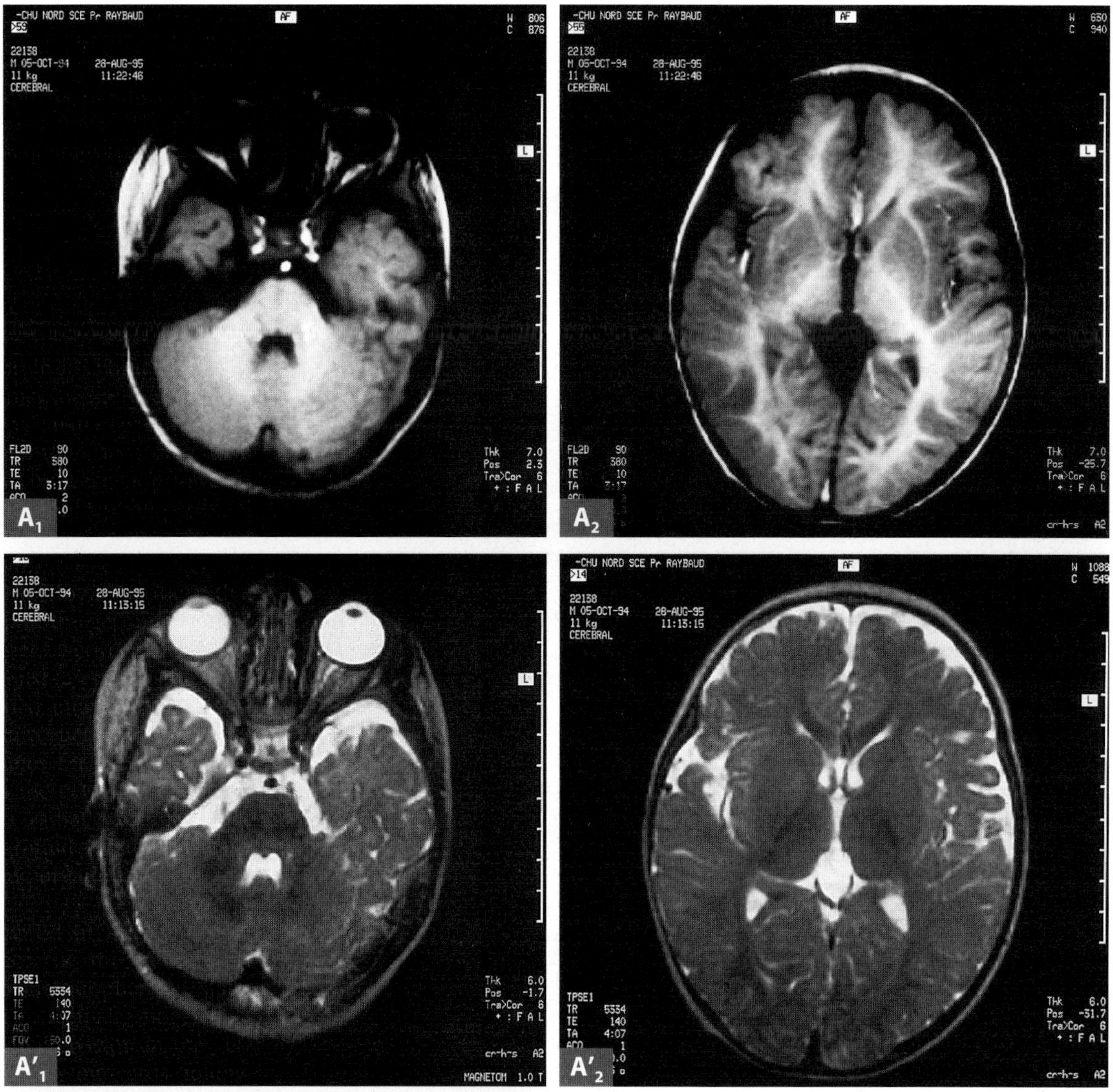

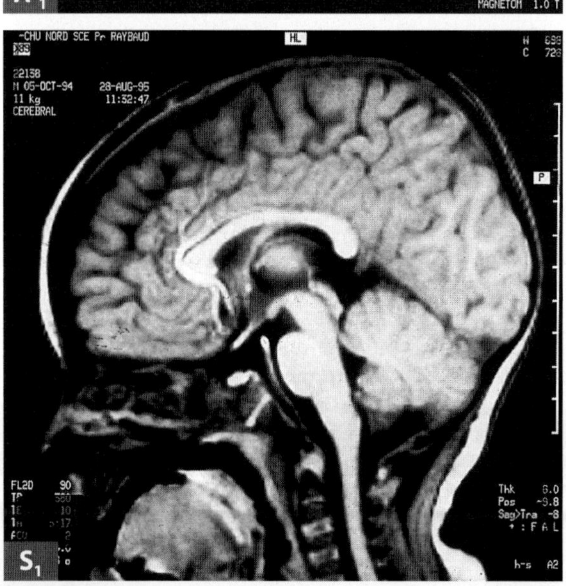

Fig. 10. Infant brain, 10 months after term. On T1 weighted images, the features are now those of a completely mature brain, although the brain will not be completely mature, histologically, until pubertaly period. The white matter is diffusely brighter than the grey (A1 to A4, S1) and in the grey latter, there is a gradation between the corpus striatum (caudate nucleus and putamen), darker, the pallidum, slightly brighter, and the thalamus (A3, A4). The corpus callosum is much thicker (S1) and well shaped, in a clockwise fashion: rostrum, genu, body, isthmus and splenium.
On T2 weighted images, the white matter is still clearly behind, with diffuse myelination of the white matter under the cortical association areas, resulting in loss of contrast between grey and white matter (Fig. 9). The central grey matter nuclei still give an evenly low signal.

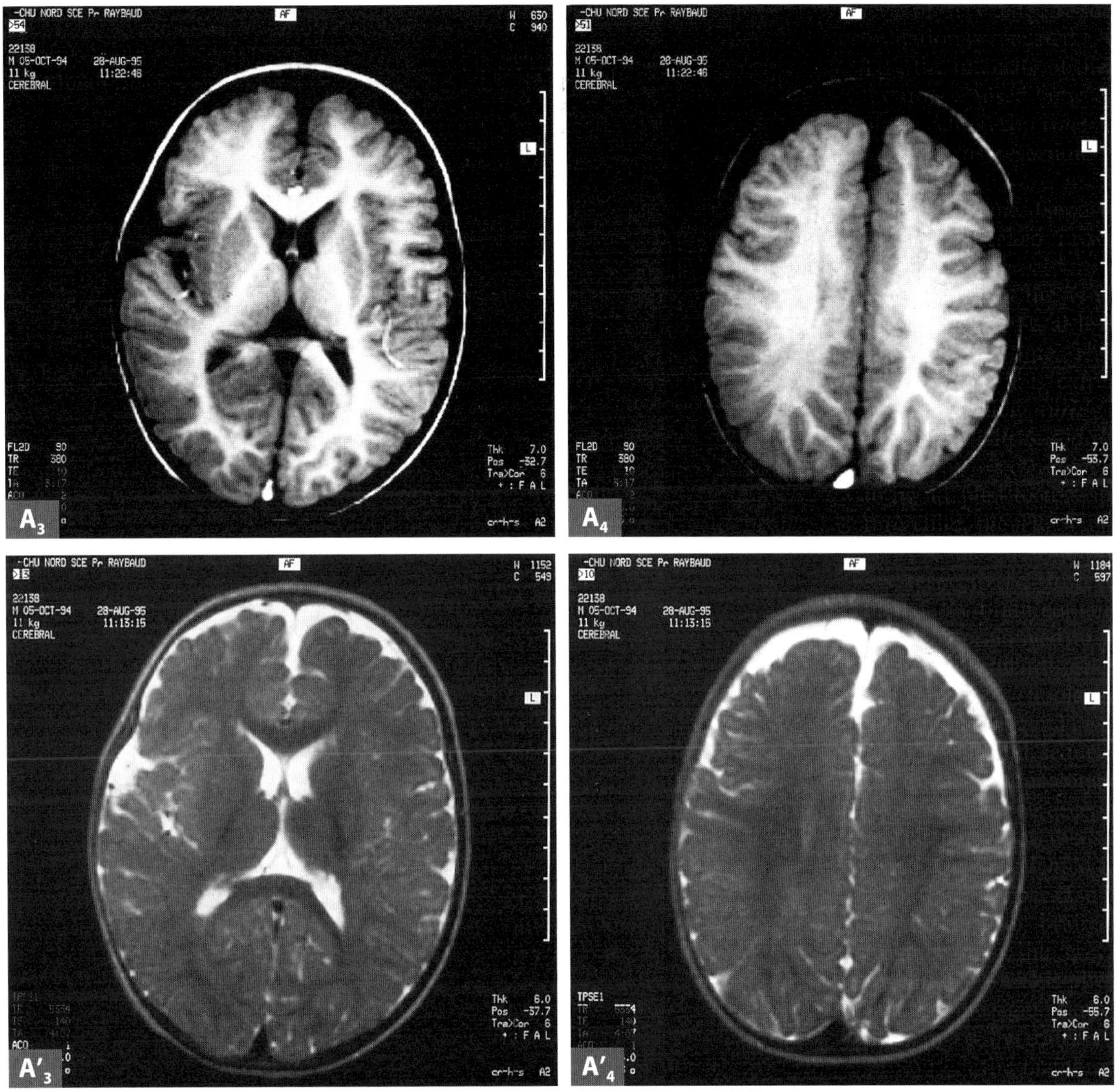

At ten months

At ten months (Fig. 10) the "mature" contrast of the brain is obtained on T1 weighted images: the white matter is brighter than the grey matter and no specific fibre bundle can still be identified.

On T2-weighted images, the maturation of white matter is catching up with that of the grey, so that all contrast is lost, the whole brain appearing uniformly grey, the maturation process being more advanced posteriorly than in the frontal lobes.

At eighteen months

At 18 months (Fig. 11) the images of the brain are show practically the adult pattern: bright white matter against the intermediate signal of the grey matter on T1 weighted images, very dark white matter against less-dark grey matter on T2 weighted images. Although the adult picture has been reached, this does not mean that myelination of the brain is mature; histologically, myelination will not reach the steady-state turnover stage until adolescence , but this histological progression is not expressed on images after 18 months. This continuing maturation may explain why in abnormal brains, the normal appearance may be obtained after a delay of several years: this would mean not that the insult is repaired, but that the imaging sequences used are not sufficiently sensitive beyond a certain point of maturation which is the 18 months stage in the normal brain). Thus the concept of "delayed" myelination, based purely on imaging data may be misleading,

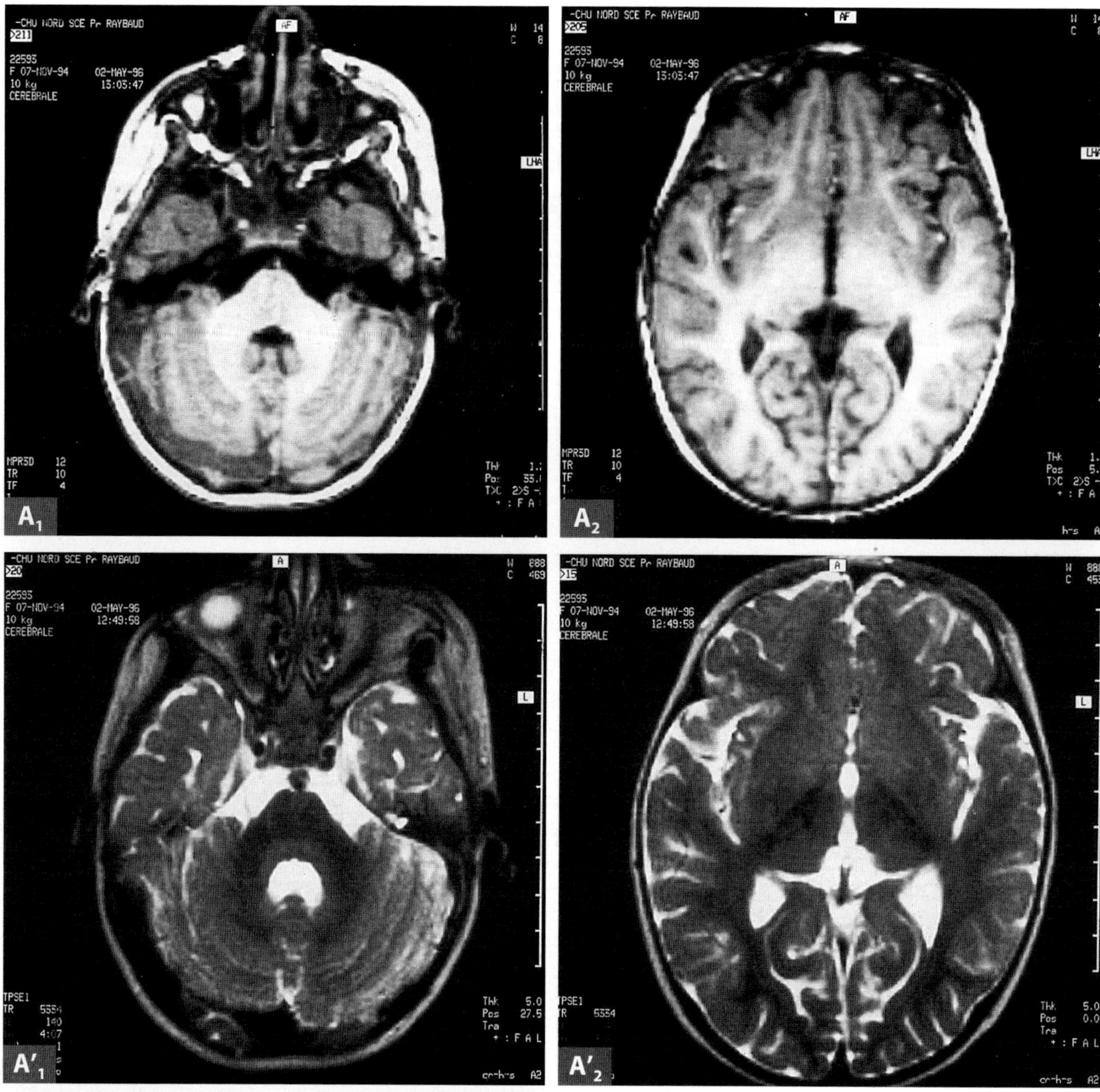

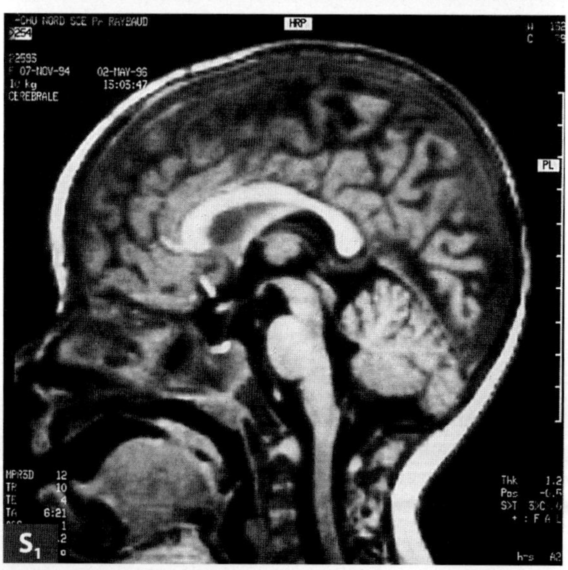

Fig. 11. Brain of a 18 month old child. Basically, the contrast between the different structures of the brain is the same as in on older child (although histologically myelination is not complete), on both T1- and T2-weighted imaging.
On T1-weighted images, there is no difference from the features seen in a 10-month infant.
On T2-weighted images, contrast between grey matter and white matter is now reversed as compared with before: the white matter now is darker than the grey be it cortex or the basal ganglia. Further contrast will, however, appear in latter years, related not to myelination, but rather to the deposition in some structures (corpora striata, optic radiations, red nuclei, etc.), of iron containing salts.

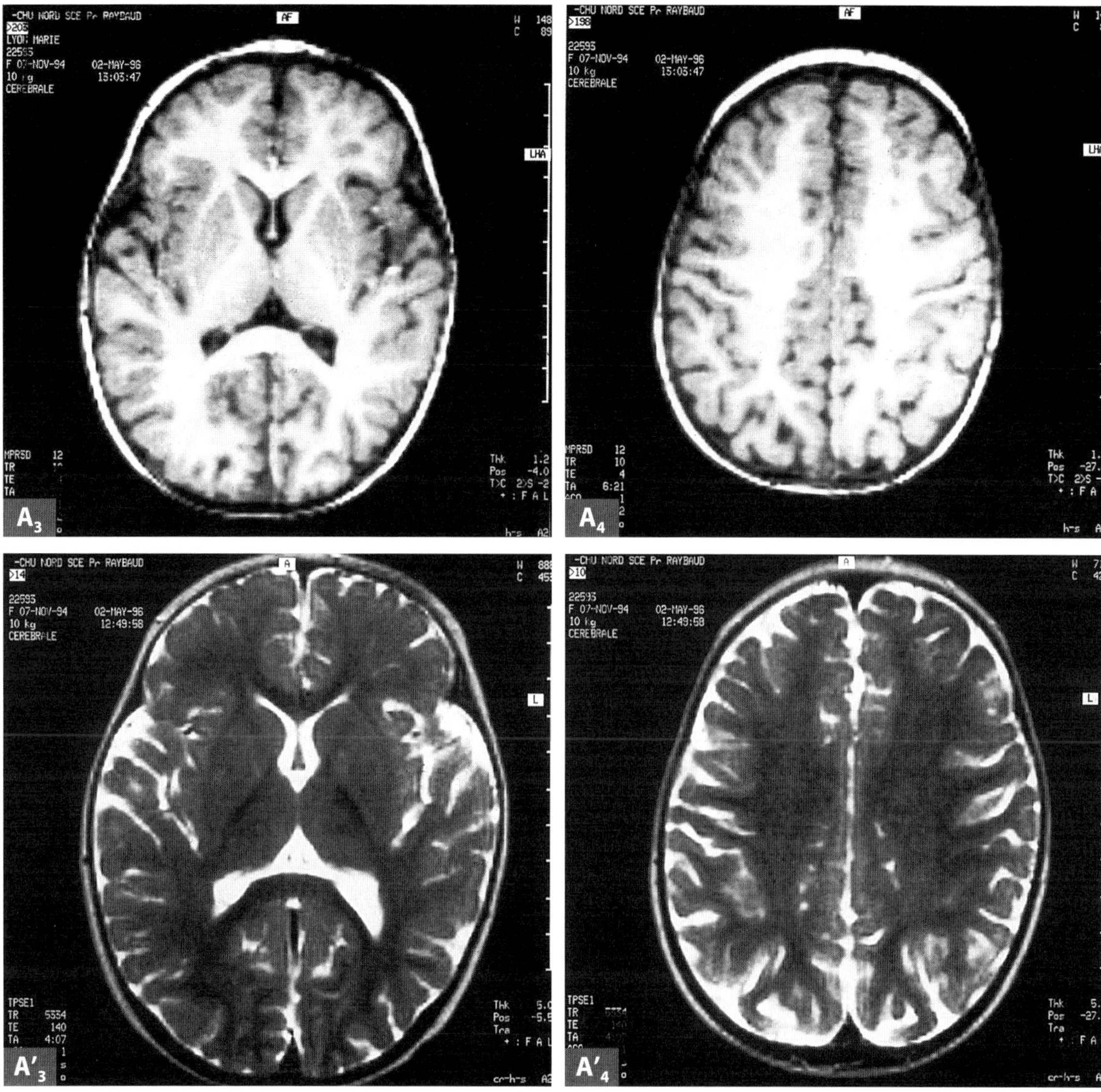

and should be replaced by the concept "unknown myelination status".

Even in the normal brain, further contrast develops over the years, no longer related not to myelination, but to deposition of iron salts in specific structures: commissural bundles, optic radiations, striatum, red nucleus and substantia nigra, for exemple. This iron deposition may confer a slight higher signal on T1 weighted images, and causes further loss of signal on T2-weighted.

Thus, in addition to the morphological changes, maturation of the brain can easily be followed by MRI during the first 18 months of life. The images obtained result from the relative T1 contrasts and T2 contrasts of the various different brain structures, giving in a composite representation of the relative stages of their maturation. The precise steps of brain myelination are known from histological studies to develop over a long period extending from the last trimester of gestation to adolescence, the changes demonstrated by MRI are apparent only from the late fetal stage to 18 months. This means that the mature MRI appearance does not express really mature myelination, and that MRI offers only a relatively limited window on to the maturation process, giving no information about whatever develops beyond a normal 18 months brain or in cases of "delayed" (? incomplete or ? arrested) myelination beyond the stage corresponding to the normal 18 months brain. However, given the importance of the changes and of the particular vulnerability of the brain during that period, this "narrow" window is extremely useful for understanding acute changes and of their sequelae. Finally, T1- and T2- weighted imaging express two different phenomena, myelination gliosis and myelin elaboration on T1 weighted, laid down myelin on T2 weighted imaging. This explains why there is a delay of several weeks between the time when morphological milestones are reached on T1- and T2- weighted images, the T1- weighted changes occuring earlier. As a consequence, insults to the brain may cause different changes on T1- and T2- weighted images, the latter appearing always to be more sensitive.

Clinical MRI and brain development

MRI is now definitely the most accurate and most sensitive means of analysing the maturing brain. At whatever age, it gives exquisite demonstration of morphology, in any desired plane, producing images of "brain slices" less than one millimetre thick, with an excellent signal-to-noise ratio, and therefore with excellent contrast between grey matter and white matter. More subtle differences in signal within the brain parenchyma can also be demonstrated, and the comparison with histological examination of the developing brain has shown a quite good correlation between the tissue organisation during development and the images obtained in routine clinical practice. As compared with the other neurodiagnostic means currently available in this age range namely ultrasonography and X-ray CT (Levenne et al., 1992; Pidcok et al., 1990; Roth et al., 1993; Rutherford et al., 1994; Wiklund et al., 1990a; Wiklund et al., 1990b) the yield of MRI is much more productive (Barkovich and Truwit, 1990; Keeney et al., 1991a; Keeney et al., 1991b; Martin et al., 1990; Truwit et al., 1992). However, MRI poses technical problems: in spite of improvements of data acquisition and processing times, MRI is still a relatively slow technique (imaging on X-ray CT may take only a couple of seconds), and bringing a young infant out of the incubator in the intensive care unit, down to the magnet of the MRI Unit, by itself poses medical problems easily avoided by the use of ultrasonography. But if a lesion can be partially characterised by ultrasonography, and somewhat better by CT, the changes it induces in the brain may be clearly illustrated only by MRI. The ideal approach then would be early MRI to show brain lesions more thoroughly, and one or more delayed MRI studies to analyse the effects of the initial insult upon the brain, in the most usual indication for examination of the neonatal brain, hypoxic-ischaemic insult.

For established developmental disorders, such as brain malformations MRI remains the essential diagnostic tool in two sets of circumstances. In utero, when abnormalities have already been identified more or less satisfactorily by ultrasonography, MRI brings more certainty to diagnosis helping the decision making process about the continuance or termination of pregnancy, and more detail about tissue abnormalities which are, not usually, seen on ultrasonography. In the infant, MRI shows abnormalities so well that it affords certainty in identification of the malformation, and therefore classification among possible genetic disorders (Chiari malformations, holoprosencephalies, callosal ageneses, true micrencephaly, migration disorders such as agyria-pachygyria, laminar heterotopias, nodular heterotopias, and possibly schizencephaly) and acquired fetopathies (at least some kinds of schizencephaly, micropolygyria, encephaloclastic porencephalies, ischaemic or haemorrhagic). It allows prognostication concerning neurological function, intelligence and epileptic diseases in many instances.

Infections of the fetal brain, such as the so-called TORCH infections: toxoplasmosis, rubella, cytomegalovirus, Herpes, etc.), can also be assessed in utero, looking for local destructions or atrophy, or after birth, facilitating evaluation of the effect of the infection upon the brain (hydrocephalus with aqueducal stenosis, cavitation, atrophy, growth defect, myelination defects).

The investigation of neuroectodermal syndromes (at this age, almost always neurofibromatosis type I, tuberous sclerosis and, more rarely, Sturge-Weber disease) has been transformed by MRI, not so much in utero, only a few cases of tuberous sclerosis having been diagnosed in utero, as after birth. In neurofibromatosis type 1 (von Recklinghausen's disease), as well as tumours, especially in the optic pathways, which could be detected by CT, MRI has demonstrated a range of abnormalities which were invisible on CT and, because they are prominent in children and disappear with age, were little known to neuropathologits as well. These include spots of high T2 signal in the basal ganglia, thalamus, brain stem and cerebellum, which are not tumours, vary with time and eventually disappear (Aoki et al., 1989); and generalised lack of low signal on T2-weighted imaging of the white matter, which spares only the subcortical arcuate fibres and could represent diffusely defective myelination of the brain. If this were true, it could be at least part of the explanation for the frequent learning disabilities of affected patients. In infants with tuberous sclerosis, MRI allows diagnosis of the disease even in the absence of other clinical features which tend to appear later. The subependymal nodules, and the appearances of the tubers adjacent to the cortex or deeper in the white matter, are sufficiently characteristic on T1-, T2- and proton density weighted images as to be pathognomonic; magnetisation-transfer sequences without contrast medium considerably enhance the sensitivity of MRI and therefore provide a thorough assessment of hamartomatous abnormalities of the brain. Finally, Sturge Weber disease also is investigated inadequately by MRI after the diagnosis is made clinically from the port wine angioma in the territory of the first division of the trigeminal nerve: the extent of cortical involvement, effects on the parenchyma, to some extent the alleged but unproved "early" or "accelerated" myelination, ischaemic areas, petechial haemorrhage, and the developing atrophy, which carry a poor long term prognosis.

In progressive encephalopathies, either epileptic which are not so frequent, but more suggestive when epilepsy is myoclonic, or nonepileptic, MRI has become an essential diagnostic element, together with the clinical feature, including the family history and biological studies. Progressive encephalopathies are metabolic and classified as mitochondrial cytopathies, peroxisomal, lysosomal disorders or storage diseases, spongiform encephalopathies of undetermined origin; their morphological patterns on MRI suggest, in many instances, the nature of the disease, e.g. Alexanders disease, adrenoleucodystrophy, Pelizaeus-Merzbacher disease, metachromatic leucodystrophy, Canavan's disease, etc., and have even led, together with MR. Spectroscopy, to characterisation of new disease entities (van der Knaap and Valk, 1995).

Besides these severe, but relatively infrequent diseases, the most important clinical problem in the everyday practice of neonatology, is the precise assessment of the lesions and of prognosis in hypoxic-ischaemic encephalopathies of preterm and term neonates. When the initial lesions are devastating, with diffuse oedema leading to multicystic encephalomalacia, significant periventricular leukomalacia, hemisphere haemorrhage, there is no need for further investigation and ultrasonography, perhaps complemented by CT, is sufficient (Levene et al., 1992; Pidcok et al., 1990; Roth et al., 1993; Rutherford et al., 1994; Wicklund et al., 1990a; Wicklund et al., 1990b). The clinical problem is more difficult when clinically the neonate, , seems to recover satisfactorily from the perinatal insult; ultrasonographic and CT images are not significantly abnormal, but, with its sensitivity, MRI may demonstrate specific abnormalities which cannot be shown by other diagnostic means (Barkovich and Truwit, 1990; Keeney et al., 1991a; Keeney et al., 1991b; Martin et al., 1990; Triwit et al., 1992). Acute abnormalities include small areas of infarction or of haemorrhage. Subacute abnormalities appear when the growth of the brain is compromised — so — called atrophy, which neuropathologically is a different from what is called atrophy in senescence, for example — or when development of myelination is disturbed (Cioni et al., 1992; Kuenzle et al., 1994; Shaywitz et al., 1995) . By following a cohort of patients with a relatively mild perinatal insult and good recovery, with repeated clinical and MRI examination over the years, it has been demonstrated that MRI has excellent prognostic value (Girard et al., 1997). MRI is performed about four months of age (corrected age for preterm infants), because this is the time when in normal children the optic radiations should appear clearly myelinated in the walls trigones of the ventricles, and because the latter, anatomically and haemodynamically, the parts of the brain most exposed to hypoxic-ischaemic insults. A cohort of 60 patients has been followed for between 2 and 5 years. The apparearances sought on MRI are normalty, diffuse injury of the brain parenchyma (mild periventricular leukomalacia), atrophy, focal cortical or subcortical lesions, myelination disorders; when isolated, cases of so-called external hydrocephalus were classed as normal. The neurodevelopmental conditions has been defined as normal, cerebral palsy, mental retardation, sensory defects, epilepsy and cognitive impairment, including attention defects and learning disabilities.

Of 25 children with normal MRI (10 normals, 15 with external hydrocephalus without parenchymal lesions), 22 (88 %) were clinically normal; three had clinical abnormalities: dysphasia, attention deficit with hyperactivity and cognitive impairment each in one case and in these cases repeat MRI demonstrated myelination disorders; the initial normal MRI can be explained by the fact that the lesions were outside the areas myelinated at that time, and without detectable necrosis: only the oligodendrocytic cell lineage was involved (Gilles's telencephalic leucoencephalopathy). Six children had a focal lesion on the initial MRI; four of these had demonstrated motor and / or sensory or cognitive impairment on later clinical examinations, but two were clinically normal, either because the lesion was in a clinically "silent" area or because cerebral plasticity (dendritic and synaptic development) compensated for the deficit. All but four of the 29 infants with diffuse brain damage had clinical impairment, including motor deficits, visuoperceptual impairment, cognitive impairment, mental retardation and epilepsy. MRI in these cases demonstrated mild periventricular leukomalacia, lesions in the basal ganglia or thalamus, abnormal myelination and / or atrophy. Normal development in the remaining four cases may again be related to compensatory brain plasticity.

Thus, MRI appears have excellent predictive value in infants who make an apparently good clinical recovery from a perinatal hypoxic-ischaemic insult: of those who have a normal MRI examination around four months of age, 88 % remained clinically normal, while of those who have diffuse changes on

MRI, although seemingly in good condition, at this time, 86 % eventually showed neurodevelopmental disorders, especially intellectual impairment. This should be compared with a previous study which demonstrated a high incidence of myelination abnormalities in an unselected group of children with partial epilepsy (Peretti et al., 1989).

Conclusions

We have thus seen that MRI has proved to be extremely sensitive to parenchymal changes in the brain and is therefore well suited to demonstrating the successive steps in brain maturation. Technically, MRI is possible as early as midgestation. With the usual sequences used, maturation appears complete by 18 months of age, while histological studies show maturation to continue to adolescence before reaching a steady state. Therefore imaging now does not currently encompass the whole period of myelination; recognising this limitation should stimulate the development of other imaging sequences to expand this time-window. In spite of this limitation, MRI has proved extremely promising in clinical practicing as the best tool in instances of moderate brain injury during cerebral development, for predicting the functional outcome not only neurologically, but intellectually as well, knowing that cognitive, sensory or attention disorders are necessarily prone to interfere with development of a normal, socially adapted personality.

References

Aoki S, Barkovich AJ, Nishimura K, Kjos BO, Machida T, Cogen P, Edwards M, Norman (1989) Neurofibromatosis types 1 and 2: cranial MR findings. Radiology 172: 527-534

Banker BQ, Larroche JC (1962) Periventricular leukomalacia of infancy. Arch Neurol 7: 386-410

Barkovich AJ, Kjos BO, Jackson DE, Norman D (1988) Normal maturation of the neonatal and infant brains: MR imaging at 1,5 T. Radiology 166: 173-180

Barkovich AJ, Truwit CL (1990) Brain damage from perinatal asphyxia: correlation of MR findings with gestational age. An J Neurol Radiol 13: 67-78

Boorstein JM, Wong KT, Grossman RI, Bolinger L, Mc Gowan JC (1994) Metastatic lesions of the brain: Imaging with magnetization transfer. Radiology 191: 799-803

Brody BA, Kinney HC, Kloman AS, Gilles FH (1987) Sequence of central nervous system myelination in human infancy: an autopsy study of myelination. J Neuropathol Exp Neurol 46: 283-301

Campi A, Filippi M, Gereveni S, Ciboddo G, Comi G, Scotti G, Dousset V (1996) Multiple white matter lesions of the brain. Int J Neuroradiol 2: 134-140

Cioni G, Bartalena L, Biagioni E, Boldrini A, Canapicchi R (1992) Neuroimaging and functional outcome of neonatal leukomalacia. Behav Brain Res 49: 7-19

Cowan FM, Pennock JM, Hanrahan JD, Manji KP, Edwards AD (1994) Early detection of cerebral infarction and hypoxic ischemic encephalopathy in neonates using diffusion-weighted magnetic resonance imaging. Neuropediatrics 25: 172-175

Elster AD, King JC, Mathews VP, Hamilton CA (1994) Cranial tissues: appearance at gadolinium-enhanced and nonenhanced MR imaging with magnetization transfer contrast. Radiology 190: 541-546

Fees-Higgins A, Larroche JC (1987) Development of the human fetal brain. INSERM-CNRS, Masson, Paris

Finelli DA, Hurst GC, Gullapali RP, Bellon EM (1994) Improved contrast of enhancing brain lesions on post-gadolinium, T1-weighted spin echo images with use of magnetization transfer. Radiology 190: 553-559

Fralix TA., Ceckler TL., Wolff SD., Simon SA., Balaban RS. (1991). Lipid bilayer and water proton magnetization transfer: effect of cholesterol. Magn Reson Med 18: 214-223

Garcia-Alix A, Cabanas F, Pellicer A, Hernanz A, Sitris TA, Quero J (1994) Neuron-specific enolase and myelin basic protein: relationship of cerebrospinal fluid concentrations to the neurologic condition of asphyxiated full-term infants. Pediatrics 93: 234-240

Gilles FH (1985) Perinatal neuropathology. In: Davis RL., Robertson DM. (eds). Textbook of neuropathology. Williams and Wilkins, Baltimore, p. 243

Girard N, Raybaud C, DuLac P (1991). MRI study of brain myelination. J Neuroradiol 18: 291-307

Girard NJ, Raybaud CA (1992) In vivo MRI of fetal brain cellular migration. J. Comput. Assist. Tomogr. 16: 265-267

Girard N, Raybaud C, Poncet M (1995) In vivo MR study of brain maturation in normal fetuses. An J Neurol Radiol 16: 407-413

Girard N, Millet V, Bartoli JM, Lacroze V, Leboucq N, Raybaud Ch, Unal D (1997) Prognostic value of MR imaging of the brain in four months infants, after perinatal neurologic insult. Intern. J Neuroradiol In press

Grossman RI, Gomori JM, Ramer KN, Lexa FJ, Scnall MD (1994) Magnetization transfer: theory and clinical applications in neuroradiology. Radiographics 14: 279-290

Hajnal JV, Baudoin CJ, Oatridge A, Young IR, Bydder GM (1992) Design and implementation of magnetization transfer pulse sequences for clinical use. J Comput Assist Tomogr 16: 7-18

Hiehle JF, Grossman RI, Ramer KN, Scarano FG, Cohen JA (1995) Magnetization transfer effects in MR-detected multiple sclerosis lesions: comparison with gadolinium-enhanced spin echo images and nonenhanced T1-weighted images. An J Neurol Radiol 16: 69-77

Holmes GL (1986) Morphological and physiological maturation of the brain in the neonate and young child. J Clin Neurophysiol 3: 209-238

Keeney SE Adcock EW, McArdle CB (1991a) Prospective observations of 100 high-risk neonates by high-field (1,5 Tesla) magnetic resonance imaging of the central nervous system: I. Intraventricular and extracerebral lesions. Pediatrics 87: 421-430

Keeney SE, Adcock EW, McArdle CB (1991b) Prospective observations of 100 high-risk neonates by high-field (1,5 Tesla) magnetic resonance imaging of the central nervous system: II. Lesions associated with hypoxic-ischemic encephalopathy. Pediatrics 87: 431-438

Koenig SH, Brown RD III, Spiller M, Lundbom N (1990) Relaxometry of brain: why white matter appears bright in MRI? Magn Reson Med 14: 482-495

Koenig SH (1991) Cholesterol of myelin is the determinant of gray-white contrast in MRI of brain. Magn Reson in Med 20: 285-291

Kucharczyk W, Macdonald PM, Stanisz GJ, Henkelman RM (1994) Relaxivity and magnetization transfer of white matter lipids at MR imaging: importance of cerebrosides and pH. Radiology 192: 521-529

Kuenzle C, Baenziger O, Martin E, Thun-Hohenstein L, Steinlin M, Good M, Franconi S, Boltshauer E, Largo RH (1994) Prognostic value of early MR imaging in term infants with severe perinatal asphyxia. Neuropediatrics 25: 191-200

Kurki T, Niemi P, Valtonen S (1994) MR of intracranial tumors: combined use of gadolinium and magnetization transfer. An J Neurol Radiol 15: 1727-1736

Larroche JC, Bethmann O, Baudoin M, Couchard M (1986) Brain damage in the premature infant early lesions and new aspects of sequelae. Ital J Neurol Sci S5: 43-52

Lenn NJ (1987) Neuroplasticity and the developing brain: implications for therapy. Pediatr. Neurosci. 13: 176-183

Levene M, Dowling S, Graham M, Fogelman K, Galton M, Philips M (1992) Impaired motor function (clumsiness) in 5 year old children: correlation with neonatal ultrasound scans. Arch Dis Child 67: 687-690

Martin E, Boesch C, Zuerrer M, Kikinis R, Molinari L, Kaelin P, Boltshauer E, Duc G (1990) MR imaging of brain maturation and developmentally handicapped children. J Comput Assist Tomogr 14: 685-692

Mathews VP, King GC, Elster AD, Hamilton CA (1994) Cerebral infarction: effects of dose and magnetization transfer saturation at gadolinium-enhanced MR imaging. Radiology 190: 547-552

Mickel HS, Gilles FH (1970) Changes in glial cells during human telencephalic myelinogenesis. Brain 93: 337-346

Norton WT (1981) Formation, structure and biochemistry of myelin. In: Siegel GJ, Wayne AR, Agranoff BW, Katzman R (eds) Basic neurochemistry. Little Brown , Boston, p. 63

Ono J. Harada K;, Sakurai K., Kodaka R., Shimidzu N., Tanaka J., Nagai T., Okada S. (1994). MR diffusion imaging in Pelizaeus-Merzbacher disease. Brain and Development 16: 219-223.

Paneth N., Rudelli R., Monte W., Rodriguez E. Pinto J. Kairam R., Kazam E. (1990). White matter necrosis in very low birth weight infants: neuropathologic and ultrasonographic findings in infants surviving six days or longer. J. Pediatr. 116: 975-984.

Peretti P, Raybaud C, Dravet C, Mancini J, Pinsard N (1989) Magnetic Resonance Imaging in partial epilepsy of childhood. J Neuroradiol 162: 308-316

Pidcok FS, Graziani LJ, Stanley C, Mitchell DG, Merton D (1990) Neurosonographic features of periventricular echodensities associated with cerebral palsy in preterm infants. J Pediatr 116: 417-422

Rakic P (1971) Mode of migration to the superficial layers of fetal monkey neocortex. Brain Res 33: 471-476

Rorke LB (1992) Anatomical features of the developing brain implicated in pathogenesis of hypoxic-ischemic injury. Brain Pathol 2: 211-221

Roth SC, Baudin J McCormick DC, Edwards AD, Townsend J, Stewart AL, Reynolds EOR (1993) Relation between ultrasound appearance of the brain of very preterm infants and neurodevelopment impairment at eight years. Dev Med Child Neurol 35: 755-768

Rutherford MA, Pennock JM, Dubowitz LM (1994) Cranial ultrasound and magnetic resonance imaging in hypoxic-ischaemic encephalopathy: a comparison with outcome. Dev Med Child Neurol 36: 813-825

Sarnat HB (1992) Cerebral plasticity in embryological development. In: Fukuyama Y, Suzuki Y, Kamoshita S, Casaer P (eds). Fetal and perinatal neurology. Karger, basel, p. 118

Sarnat HB, Sarnat M (1994) When is it the best to be born? A phylogenetic perspective. In: Amiel-Tison C, Stewart A (eds). The newborn infant: one brain for life. Les Editions INSERM, Paris, p. 47

Segal M (1995) Dendritic spines for neuroprotection: a hypothesis. Trans Int Neursci 11: 468-471

Shaywitz BA, Fletcher JM, Shaywitz SE (1995) Defining and classifying learning disabilities and attention-deficit/hyperactivity disorder. J Child Neurol S1: 50-57

Sheldon RA, Chuai J, Ferriero DM (1996) A rat model for hypoxic-ischemic brain damage in very premature infants. Biol Neonate 69: 327-341

Tanttu JI, Sepponen RE, Lipton MJ, Kuusela T (1992) Synergistic enhancement of MRI with Gd-DTPA and magnetization transfer. J Comput Assist Tomogr 16: 19-24

Thornberg E, Thiringer K, Hagberg H, Kjellmer I (1995) Neuron specific enolase in asphyxiated newborns: association with encephalopathy and cerebral monitor trace. Arch. Dis. Child 72: 39-42

Truwit CL, Barkovich AJ, Koch TK, Ferreiro DM (1992) Cerebral palsy: MR findings in 40 patients. An J Neurol Radiol 13: 67-78

van der Knaap MS, Valk J (1995) Magnetic resonance of myelin, myelination and myelin disorders. Springer-Verlag. Berlin (2nd edn).

Vannucci RC (1990) experimental biology of cerebral hypoxia-ischemia: relation to perinatal brain damage. Pediatr Res 27: 317-326

Volpe JJ (1992) Perinatal hypoxic-ischemic brain injury: overview. In: Fukuyama Y Suzuki Y, Kamoshita S, Casaer P (eds.) Fetal and perinatal neurology. Karger, Basel, p. 232

Volpe JJ (1995) Hypoxic-ischemic encephalopathy: biochemical and physiological aspects: In: Volpe J (ed.) Neurology of the newborn, (3rd ed) Saunders, Philadelphia, p. 211

Volpe JJ (1995) Neuronal proliferation, migration, organization and myelination. In: Volpe JJ (ed.) Neurology of the newborn, (3rd ed), Saunders, Philadelphia, p. 43

Wiklund LM, Uvebrant P, Flodmark O (1990a) Computed tomography as an adjunct in etiological analysis of hemiplegic cerebral palsy. I: Children born at term. Neuropediatrics 22: 50-56

Wiklund LM, Uvebrant P, Flodmark O (1990b) Computed tomography as an adjunct in etiological analysis of hemiplegic cerebral palsy. II: Children born before term. Neuropediatrics 22: 121-128

Wolff SD, Balaban RS (1989) Magnetization transfer contrast (MTC) and tissue water proton relaxation in vivo. Magn Reson Med 10: 135-144
Wolff SD, Balaban RS (1994) Magnetization transfer imaging: practical aspects and clinical applications. Radiology 192: 593-599
Young RSK, Petroff OAC, Novotny EJ, Wong M (1990) Neonatal excitotoxic brain injury. Physiologic, metabolic, and pathologic findings. Dev Neurosci 12: 210-230
Yoshioka K, Fujiwara K, Sawada T (1992) Perinatal hypoxic-ischemic brain injury. In: Fukuyama Y, Suzuki Y, Kamoshita S, Casaer P (eds) Fetal and perinatal neurology. Karger, Basel, p. 257

6. The ontogeny of cerebral metabolism

H.T. CHUGANI

The development of functional neuroimaging techniques has enabled energy metabolism in the developing human brain to be studied noninvasively. This can be accomplished using positron emission tomography (PET) and the principles underlying the ^{14}C-2-deoxyglucose autoradiographic method developed by Sokoloff et al. (1977). With PET and the tracer 2-deoxy-2(^{18}F)fluoro-D-glucose (FDG), measurements of regional cerebral glucose utilisation can be made during different stages of development and related to behavioural maturation, synaptogenesis, plasticity and other neuromaturational phenomena.

Developmental patterns of cerebral glucose metabolism

The pattern of glucose metabolism in the newborn brain is fairly consistent (Fig. 1), with the highest degree of activity in primary sensory and motor cortex, thalamus, brainstem and cerebellar vermis (Chugani and Phelps, 1986; Chugani et al., 1987; Chugani, 1994). The cingulate cortex, hippocampal region and occasionally the basal ganglia may also show relatively high glucose metabolism compared to most of the cerebral cortex in the newborn period (Chugani, 1996 in press). The relatively low functional activity of most of the cortex during the neonatal period is in keeping with the limited behavioural repertoire of newborns, characterised by the presence of intrinsic brain stem reflexes (Andre-Thomas and Saint-Anne Dargassies, 1960) and limited visuomotor integration (von Hofsten, 1982).

Increases in glucose utilisation are seen by two to three months in the parietal, temporal and primary visual cortex, basal ganglia, and cerebellar hemispheres (Fig. 2). These changes in glucose metabolism coincide with improved skills involving visuospatial and visuosensorimotor integration (Bronson, 1974), the disappearance or reorganisation of brain stem reflex neonatal behaviour (Andre-Thomas and Saint-Anne Dargassies, 1960; Parmelee and Sigman, 1983), and evidence of increasing cortical contribution to the electroencephalogram (Kellaway, 1979).

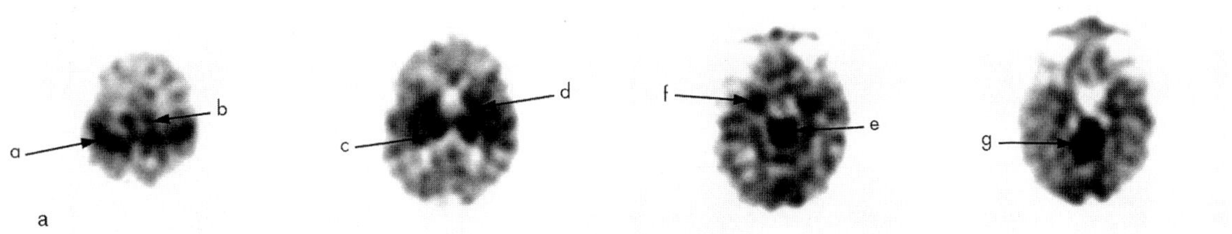

Fig. 1 - Newborn pattern of cerebral glucose metabolism. At this stage of development, glucose metabolism is most apparent in sensorimotor cortex (a), cingulate cortex (b), thalamus (c), basal ganglia (d), brain stem (e), mesial temporal region (f), and cerebellar vermis (g). Metabolic activity is low in most of the frontal, parietal, temporal and occipital cortex, and in the cerebellar cortex.

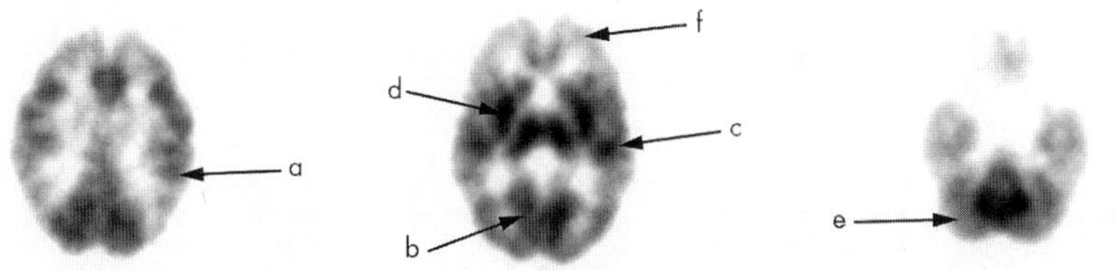

Fig. 2
Pattern of cerebral glucose metabolism in a 3-month-old infant. Glucose metabolism has increased in parietal (a), occipital (b), and temporal (c) cortex, basal ganglia (d), and cerebellar hemispheres (e). Metabolic activity in frontal cortex (f) remains low.

The frontal cortex is the last of the area brain to display an increase in glucose consumption during development. Starting between 6 and 8 months, lateral and inferior portions of frontal cortex become more functionally active (Fig. 3) and eventually, between 8 and 12 months, the dorsal and medial frontal regions also show increased glucose utilisation. These changes of frontal cortex metabolism come at a time when cognitively-related behaviours, such as the phenomenon of stranger anxiety (Kagan, 1972), and improved performance on the delayed response task (Fuster, 1984; Goldman-Rakic, 1984) begin to appear. Increased glucose requirement in frontal cortex also coincides with the expansion of dendritic fields (Schade and van Groenigen, 1961) and the increased capillary density (Diemer, 1968) observed in frontal cortex during the same period of development. By approximately one year of age, the infant's pattern of glucose utilisation resembles that of the adult, at least qualitatively.

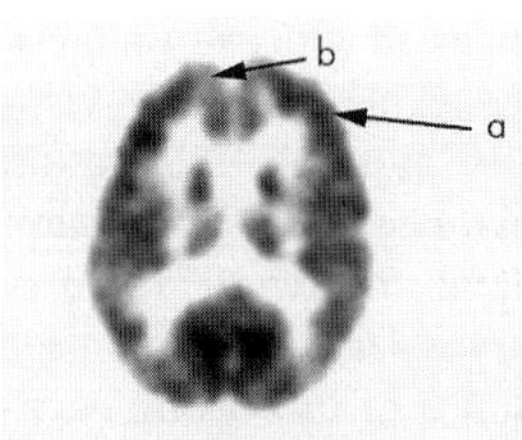

Fig. 3
Pattern of cerebral glucose metabolism in an 8-month-old infant. Glucose metabolism has increased in the lateral portion of the frontal cortex (a) but not in the medial portion (b).

From these observations, it appears that in the first year of life, the ontogeny of glucose metabolism follows a phylogenetic order, with functional maturation of older anatomical structures preceding that of newer areas (Chugani and Phelps, 1986;Chugani et al., 1987; Chugani, 1994). In addition, the suggestion by Kennedy et al. (1982) that "at any given developmental age, structures having metabolic rates equal to or exceeding their mature levels are those that dominate the behavior at that age" appears to be the case in human infant development since there is at least a general relationship between the maturational sequence of regional glucose metabolism and the behavioural maturation of the infant.

Glucose metabolic rates

An important aspect of the PET technique is that it allows for the *quantitative measurement* of biochemical and physiological processes. Thus, even though the brain of a one-year-old infant shows a similar distribution pattern of glucose utilisation similar to that of an adult, the *rate* at which glucose is being used by various brain regions is different. In fact, a dynamic, protracted and nonlinear process of "metabolic maturation" is apparent between birth and early adulthood (16-18 years).

Birth to 4 years

At birth, the regional or local cerebral metabolic rates of glucose utilisation (LCMRglc) are about 30% lower than those seen in normal healthy young adults (Fig. 4). Between birth and approximately 4 years, the cerebral cortex shows a dramatic increase in LCMRglc to reach levels that are more than twice adult rates (Fig. 4A,B). Such changes in LCMRglc are not observed in the brain stem (Fig. 4C), but a less dramatic increase is seen in the basal ganglia and thalamus (Fig. 4D).

Middle childhood

Between the ages of about 4 years and 9-10 years, the LCMRglc for cerebral cortex is essentially at a high plateau of over two-fold the glucose utilisation seen in adults (Chugani et al., 1987; Chugani et al., 1994) (Fig. 4A,B). This observation confirms the earlier results of Kennedy and Sokoloff (1957), who demonstrated that the average global cerebral blood flow (an indirect measure of energy demand in the brain) in 9 normal children (aged 3 to 11 years) was approximately 1.8 times that of normal young adults. Moreover, average global cerebral oxygen utilisation was approximately 1.3 times high in children as in adults.

Early and late adolescence

At about 9-10 years, LCMRglc for cerebral cortex begins to decline and gradually reaches adult values by 16-18 years (Fig. 4A,B) (Chugani et al., 1987; Chugani, 1994). It should be noted that all regions in cerebral cortex studied show the *same timing* of develop-

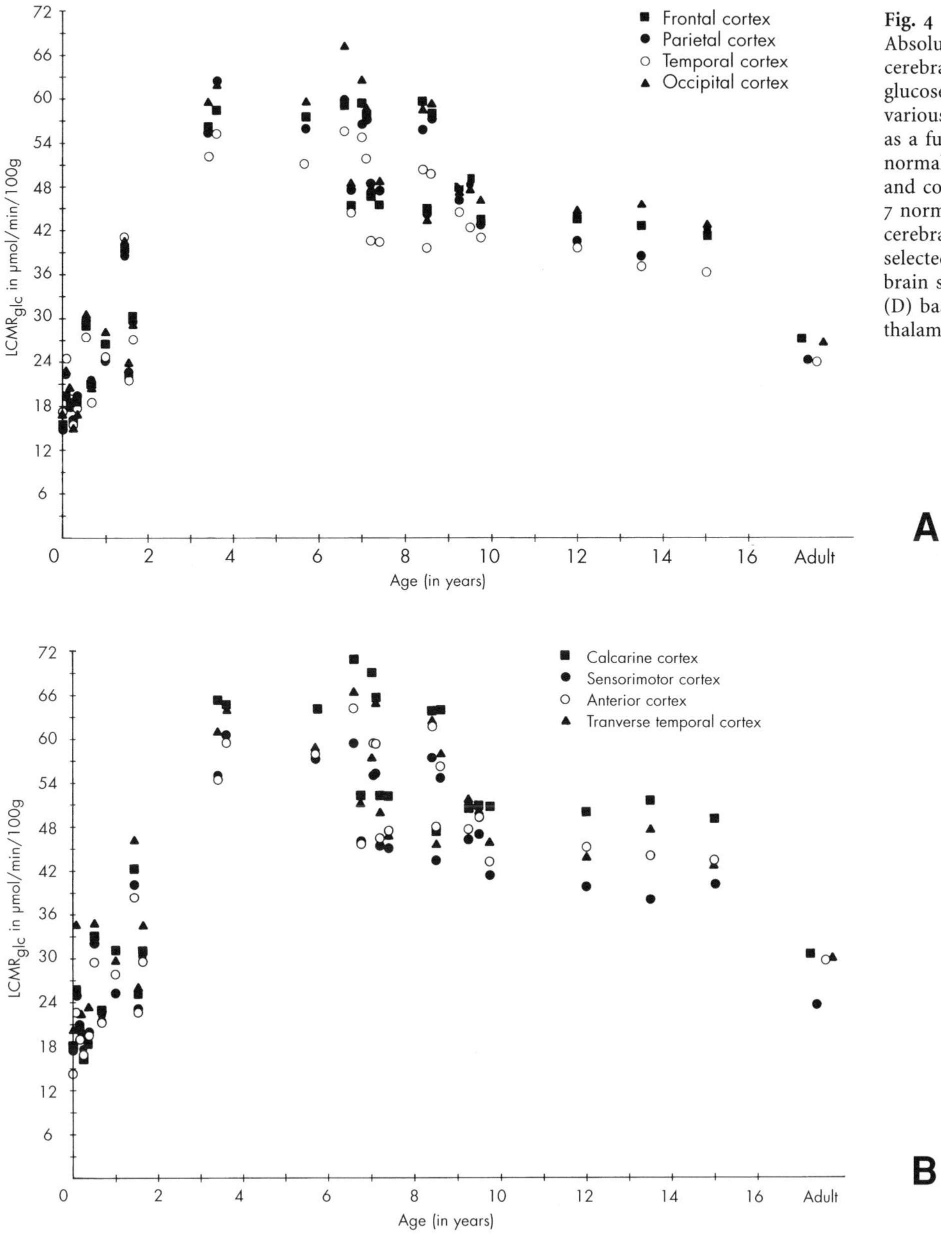

Fig. 4
Absolute values of local cerebral metabolic rates for glucose (LCMRglc) for various brain regions plotted as a function of age in normal infants and children, and corresponding values in 7 normal young adults. (A) cerebral cortex (lobes); (B) selected cortical regions; (C) brain stem and cerebellum; (D) basal ganglia and thalamus.

mental changes in LCMRglc. The time course is different only for basal ganglia and thalamus, whereas the brain stem does not show significant ontogenetic changes.

Regressive phenomena in development

Since the initial description of the ontogeny of cerebral glucose metabolism in children (Chugani et al., 1987), the relevance of these dynamic changes has been under active investigation. For over half a century, it has been recognised that the brain of an immature rat consumes more oxygen and glucose than that of an adult rat brain (Himwich and Fazekas, 1941; Tyler and van Harreveld, 1942). For example, the utilisation of both oxygen and glucose in excised rat cerebral cortex, striatum, cerebellum and brain stem was shown to be higher during the period between the fourth and seventh postnatal weeks and in the adult (Tyler and van Harreveld, 1942). Studies performed in other species using either in vivo autoradiography or PET have confirmed the presence of a developmental period during which local cerebral energy demand, as measured by local cerebral blood flow (LCBF) and, more directly LCMRglc, exceeds

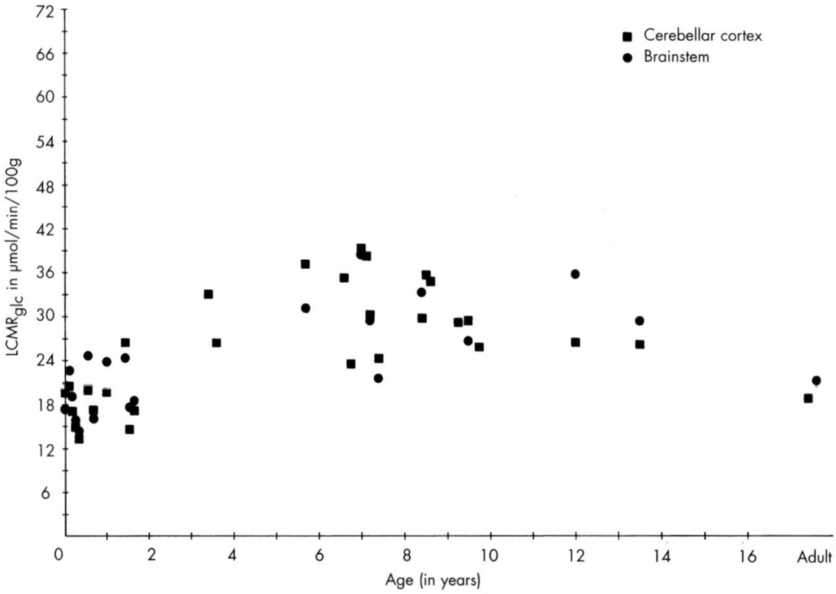

C

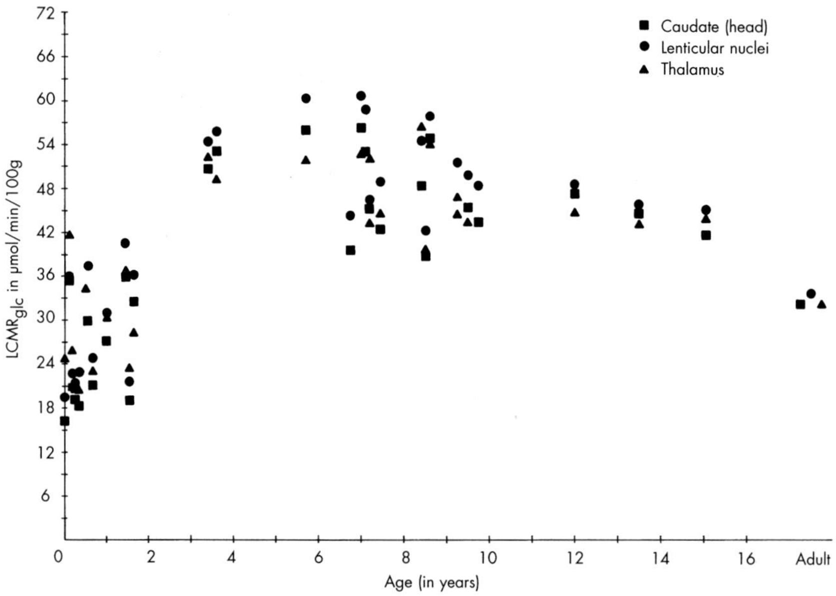

D

that of the adult (Kennedy et al., 1972; Chugani et al., 1991; Jacobs Chugani et al., 1995).

The ontogeny of cerebral glucose metabolism described in Fig. 4 is not surprising, considering the fact that regressive phenomena are not uncommonly seen during development of the nervous system (Changeux and Danchin, 1976; Jacobson, 1978; Cowan et al., 1984). Thus, there are periods during development when neurons, neuronal processes, synaptic contacts, various neurotransmitters and receptors are in excess of those seen in the adult. The proliferation and overproduction of neurons in humans occur prenatally, whereas programmed cell death begins prenatally and continues until about the second postnatal year (Rabinowicz, 1979). Surviving neurons undergo a similar phenomenon postnatally, characterised by overproduction of their arborisation and synaptic contacts, followed by an elimination or 'pruning' phase (Huttenlocher, 1979; Huttenlocher et al., 1982; Huttenlocher et al., 1987). Synaptic elimination in humans probably continues well into adolescence; for example, synaptic density in frontal cortex of children up to 11 years of age has been shown to exceed that in adults (Huttenlocher, 1979).

Synaptic pruning is not a random phenomenon, but rather, is based on activity-dependent stabilisation. In other words, repeated neuronal activity involving certain circuits during a critical period will result in stabilisation of those circuits rather than elimination during the pruning process (Rauschecker and Marler 1987). The advantage of activity-dependent stabilisation of neuronal pathways is that there will not be unnecessary expenditure of genes to code precisely for the large number of connections in the brain. Rather, repeated early environmental exposure will serve to guide the moulding of an optimum cortical cytoarchitecture for the individual's future needs. The molecular basis for the stabilisation and retention of some pathways, and vulnerability of others to be pruned or eliminated is an area of intense investigation. Recent studies have suggested that in the visual cortex of kittens, activity-dependent stabilisation may involve activation of the N-methyl-D-aspartate (NMDA) subclass of glutamate receptors (Rauschecker and Hahn, 1987; Bear et al., 1990), associated perhaps with the expression of specific neuronal proteins.

Neurobiological correlates of glucose metabolism ontogeny

Relationship to synaptogenesis

Under normal circumstances, the major portion of glucose used by the brain is for the maintenance of resting membrane potentials (Mata et al., 1980; Kadekaro et al., 1985; Nudo and Masterton, 1986). Therefore, there should be a direct relationship between the degree or density of 'connectivity' and the energy demand of the brain in the resting state. This is, in fact, the case when one compares the ontogeny of LCMRglc in cerebral cortex (Fig. 4A,B) with the developmental curve for synaptogenesis in humans (Huttenlocher, 1979; Huttenlocher et al., 1982; Huttenlocher and de Courten,1987). Similar comparisons performed in the developing kitten (Chugani et al., 1991) and rhesus monkey (Jacobs et al., 1995) have confirmed.

The ontogeny of LCMRglc in cerebral cortex may, therefore, provide an indirect measure of synaptogenesis in the brain. An analysis of the glucose metabolism curve (Fig. 4A,B) suggests that the ascending portion of the curve seen between birth and 4 years represents the period of synaptic proliferation in the cerebral cortex. The 'plateau' period of the curve seen during middle childhood represents the period of synaptic excess and exuberant connectivity associated with increased energy requirement by cortex compared to adults. This is also the critical period in development when the process of activity-dependent synaptic stabilization is at a maximum. With adolescence and the beginning of synaptic elimination, LCMRglc in cortex begins to decline gradually, as shown by the gradual downslope of the metabolism curve because of diminishing energy requirement (Chugani et al., 1989; Chugani, 1994).

Brain plasticity

There have been many studies relating synaptogenesis to a critical period of developmental brain plasticity. Since the ontogeny of LCMRglc appears to be related to synaptogenesis, it may indirectly provide a marker for a critical period of developmental brain plasticity in humans and, therefore, analyses correlating synaptogenesis, LCMRglc and brain plasticity may have important implications.

This relationship has been characterised in area 17 of the kitten's visual system. In the kitten, synapses are sparse in this region at birth (Voeller et al., 1963; Winfield, 1981), and LCMRglc values are correspondingly low (Chugani et al., 1991). During the second and third postnatal weeks, there is a well-documented rapid increase of synaptic density which reaches a peak at about 70 days (Winfield 1981; Winfield 1983); this phase of synaptogenesis coincides with the period when LCMRglc values rise dramatically in area 17. Moreover, this same time is characterised as a 'critical period' in the visual system of kittens. During this time, there considerable plasticity is manifest when the visual system is injured or manipulated experimentally (Morest, 1969; Hubel and Wiesel, 1970; Spinelli et al., 1972; Pettigrew, 1974; Timney, 1983). This 'critical period' of development in the kitten visual cortex extends from 4 weeks to about 3 months of life, during which LCMRglc values are high in this region of the brain. Subsequently, there is diminishing plasticity associated with regression of exuberant synapses and connections (Barlow 1975; Hirsch and Leventhal, 1978; Sherman and Spear, 1982), and a corresponding decline of LCMRglc presumably due to diminished energy requirements.

Interestingly, in the cat, the decline of LCMRglc in cerebral cortex is followed by a second, larger peak at about 180 days. Only after 180 days does LCMRglc decrease to reach final adult values. The period at about 180 days appears not to coincide with any known major neuroanatomical changes in the cat brain, but is the time when cats undergo sexual maturation (Kling, 1965). This timing of the gradual decline of LCMRglc in the cat roughly corresponds to that in humans (Fig. 4A,B). A similar relationship between synaptogenesis (Rakic et al., 1986) and LCMRglc (Jacobs et al., 1995) has been shown in the developing rhesus monkey.

Clinical implications of glucose metabolism ontogeny

The ontogeny of cerebral glucose metabolism appears to have profound implications for the study of human brain development, plasticity, and possibly childhood psychopathology. A central hypothesis in our laboratory is that at around 10 years, when LCMRglc in the cerebral cortex begins to decline (Fig. 4), developmental brain plasticity also begins to diminish in children. There is much support for this hypothesis in the clinical literature, only some of which will be reviewed.

Children who have been deprived of exposure to language since birth, for example, those raised in the wilderness (so-called 'feral' children), can still acquire reasonably normal language skills but only if intense speech and language therapy is introduced before the age of 10 years (Curtiss, 1981). Following damage to the language-dominant hemisphere, there is better recovery of language skills if the injury occurs before 8 - 10 years than if it occurs later (Basser, 1962; Curtiss, 1977). Based on an extensive review of this subject, Lenneberg (1967) postulated that there must be a "critical period for language acquisition" ending at about the age of 10 years, after which there is a more limited (but not absent) potential for acquiring language skills.

Analyses of the human visual system have also suggested a similar timing of diminished plasticity in children. A number of studies have looked at the upper age limit beyond which stimulus deprivation of one eye in young children, caused by monocular occlusion such as a cataract or certain kinds of strabismus, will induce irreversible reduction of visual acuity known as amblyopia (Marg, 1982). Two large clinical surveys have found that amblyopia can be prevented from occurring if the monocular occlusion is corrected prior to 8 — 10 years of age, but not after that(Awaya, 1978; Vaegan and Taylor, 1979). In addition, the compromise in visual depth perception induced by unilateral enucleation (e.g., for orbital tumours) can be minimised if enucleation is performed prior to about 8 years of age (Schwartz et al., 1987).

The notion of an extended period during childhood when activity-dependent synaptic stabilisation occurs has recently received considerable attention by groups dealing with early intervention to provide "environmental enrichment" and with optimal design of educational curricula. Thus, it is now believed by many (including the author) that the biological "window of opportunity" when learning is efficient and easily retained is perhaps not fully exploited by our educational system.

Finally, there are investigators who believe that the onset of some forms of psychopathology may be related to various segments of the synaptogenesis curve. For example, Feinberg et al. (1990) have noted that the maturational curves for LCMRglc, synaptogenesis, and delta wave amplitude during sleep in children are similar, and can be best described with a gamma distribution model. We suggested that, since the early symptoms of schizophrenia occur in early adolescence when the maturational curves begin their downslope, errors in synaptic pruning localised to certain areas of the brain (e.g., frontal cortex) may play an important role in the pathophysiology of this disorder.

In infantile autism, there is often a period of 'autistic regression' which occurs between 18 and 24 months of age. This is at a time of rapid synaptic proliferation and rapid rise in LCMRglc, and errors in this process may result in the formation of aberrant circuits. These interesting hypotheses merit further investigation.

References

Andre-Thomas CY, Saint-Anne Dargassies S. (1960) The neurological examination of the infant. Medical Advisory Committee of the National Spastics Society, London

Awaya S (1978) Stimulus vision deprivation amblyopia in humans. In: Reinecke RD (ed.) Strabismus. Grune and Stratton, New York, p 31-44

Barlow HB (1975) Visual experience and cortical development. Nature 258: 199-203

Basser LS (1962) Hemiplegia of early onset and the faculty of speech with special reference to the effects of hemispherectomy. Brain 85: 427-460

Bear MF, Kleinschmidt A, Gu Q.A, Singer W (1990) Disruption of experience-dependent synaptic modifications in striate cortex by infusion of an NMDA receptor antagonist. J. Neurosci 10: 909-925

Bronson G (1974) The postnatal growth of visual capacity. Child Dev 45: 873-890

Changeux JP, Danchin A (1976) Selective stabilization of developing synapses as a mechanism for the specification of neuronal networks. Nature 264: 705-712

Chugani, HT (1994) Development of regional brain glucose metabolism in relation to behavior and plasticity. In: Dawson G, Fischer W (eds.), Human behavior and the developing brain. Guilford Publications, New York, p 153-175

Chugani HT (in press) Neuroimaging of developmental non-linearity and developmental pathologies. In: Thatcher RW, Lyon RG, Rumsey J, Krasnegor N (eds.), Developmental neuroimaging: mapping the development of brain and behavior

Chugani HT, Hovda DA, Villablanca JR, Phelps ME, Xu WF (1991) Metabolic maturation of the brain: A study of local cerebral glucose utilization in the developing cat. J Cerebr Blood Flow Metab 11: 35-47

Chugani HT, Mazziotta JC, Phelps ME (1989) Sturge-Weber syndrome: a study of cerebral glucose utilization with positron emission tomography. J Pediatr 114: 244-253

Chugani HT, Phelps ME (1986) Maturational changes in cerebral function in infants determined by ^{18}FDG positron emission tomography. Science 231: 840-843

Chugani HT, Phelps ME, Mazziotta JC (1987) Positron emission tomography study of human brain functional development. Ann Neurol 22: 487-497

Chugani HT, Phelps ME, Mazziotta JC (1989) Metabolic assessment of functional maturation and neuronal plasticity in the human brain. In: von Euler C, Forssberg H, Lagercrantz H (eds.), Neurobiology of early infant behaviour. Stockton Press, New York, p 323-330

Cowan WM, Fawcett JW, O'Leary DDM, Stanfield BB (1984) Regressive events in neurogenesis. Science 225: 1258-1265

Curtiss S (1977) Genie: a psycholinguistic study of a modern-day "wild child". Academic Press, New York

Curtiss S (1981) Feral children. In: Wortis J (ed.) Mental retardation and developmental disabilities XII. Brunner-Mazel, New York, p 129-161

Diemer K (1968) Capillarisation and oxygen supply of the brain. In: Lubbers DW, Luft UC, Thews G, Witzleb E (eds.), Oxygen transport in blood and tissue Thieme, Stuttgart, p 118-123

Feinberg I, Thode HC, Chugani HT, March JD (1990) Gamma distribution model describes maturational curves for delta wave amplitude, cortical metabolic rate and synaptic density. J Theoret Biol 142: 149-161

Fuster JM (1984) Behavioral electrophysiology of the prefrontal cortex. Trends Neurosci 7: 408-414

Goldman-Rakic PS (1984) The frontal lobes: uncharted provinces of the brain. Trends Neurosci 7: 425-429

Himwich HE, Fazekas JF (1941) Comparative studies of the metabolism of the brain in infant and adult dogs. Am J Physiol 132: 454-459

Hirsch HVB, Leventhal AG (1978) Functional modification of the developing visual system. In: Jaconson M (ed), Handbook of sensory physiology, Vol.IX: Development of sensory systems. Springer-Verlag, Berlin Heidelberg, p 279-335

Hubel DH, Wiesel TN (1970) The period of susceptibility to the physiological effects of unilateral eye closure in kittens. J Physiol 206: 419-436

Huttenlocher PR(1979) Synaptic density in human frontal cortex-developmental changes and effects of aging. Brain Res 163: 195-205

Huttenlocher PR, de Corten C, Gary .LJ, Vanderloos H (1982) Synaptogenesis in human visual cortex: Evidence for synapse elimination during normal development. Neurosci Lett 33: 247-252

Huttenlocher PR, de Courten C (1987) The development of striate cortex in of man. Hum Neurobiol 6: 10-9

Huttenlocher PR, de Courten C, Gary LJ, van der Loos H (1982) Synaptogenesis in human visual cortex-evidence for synapse elimination during normal development. Neurosci Lett 33: 247-252

Jacobs B, Chugani HT, Allada V, Chen S, Phelps ME, Pollack DB, Raleigh MJ (1995) Developmental changes in brain metabolism in sedated rhesus macaques and vervet monkeys revealed by positron emission tomography. Cereb Cortex 3: 222-233

Jacobson M (1978) Developmental neurobiology. (2nd ed.). Plenum Press, New York

Kadekaro M, Crane AM, Sokoloff L (1985) Differential effects of electrical stimulation of sciatic nerve on metabolic activity in spinal cord and dorsal root ganglion in the rat. Proc Nat Acad Sci 82: 6010-6013

Kagan J (1972) Do infants think? Sci Am 226: 74-82

Kellaway P (1979) An orderly approach to visual analysis: parameters of the normal EEG in adults and children. In: Klass DW, Daly DD (eds.), Current practice of clinical electroencephalography. Raven Press, New York, p 69-147

Kennedy C, Grave GD, Jehle JW, Sokoloff L(1972) Changes in blood flow in the component structures of the dog brain during postnatal maturation. J Neurochem 19: 2423-2433

Kennedy C, Sakurada O, Shinohara M, Miyaoka M (1982) Local cerebral glucose utilization in the newborn macaque monkey. Ann Neurol 12: 333-340

Kennedy C, Sokoloff L (1957) An adaptation of the nitrous oxide method to the study of the cerebral circulation in children; normal values for cerebral blood flow and cerebral metabolic rate in childhood. J Clin Invest 36: 1130-1137

Kling A (1965) Behavioural and somatic development following lesions of the amygdala in the cat. J Psychiat Res 3: 263-273

Lenneberg E (1967) Biological foundations of language. Wiley, New York, p 125-187

Marg E (1982) Prentice Memorial Lecture: is the animal model for stimulus deprivation amblyopia in children valid or useful? Am J Optom Physiol Optics 59: 451-464

Mata M, Fink DJ, Gainer H, Smith CB, Davidsen L, Savaki H, Schwartz WJ, Sokoloff L (1980) Activity-dependent energy metabolism in rat posterior pituitary primarily reflects sodium pump activity. J Neurochem 34: 213-215

Morest DK (1969) The growth of dendrites in the mammalian brain. Z Anat Entwicklungsges 128: 290-317

Nudo RJ, Masterton RB (1986) Stimulation-induced {14C}2-deoxyglucose labeling of synaptic activity in the central auditory system. J Comp Neurol 245: 553-565

Parmelee AH, Sigman MD (1983) Perinatal brain development and behavior. In: Haith M, Campos J (eds.), Biology and Infancy, vol II. Wiley, New York, p 95-115

Pettigrew JD (1974). The effect of visual experience on the development of stimulus specificity by kitten cortical neurones. J Physiol 237: 49-74

Rabinowicz T (1979) The differentiated maturation of the human cerebral cortex. In: Falkner F, Tanner JM (eds), Human growth, Neurobiology and nutrition Vol 3. Plenum Press, New York, 97-123

Rakic P, Bourgeois JP, Eckenhoff MF, Zecevic N, Goldman-Rakic PS (1986) Concurrent overproduction of synapses in diverse regions of the primate cerebral Cortex. Science 232: 232-235

Rauschecker JP, Hahn S (1987) Ketamine-xylazine anaesthesia blocks consolidation of ocular dominance changes in kitten visual cortex. Nature. 326 (6109): 183-185

Rauschecker JP, Marler P (1987) What signals are responsible for synaptic changes in visual cortical plasticity? In: Rauschecker J, Marler P (eds.), Imprinting and Cortical Plasticity Wiley, New York, p 193-220

Schade JP, van Groenigen WB (1961) Structural organization of the human cerebral cortex. Acta Anat 47: 74-111

Schwartz TL, Linberg JV, Tillman W, Odom JV (1987) Monocular depth and vernier acuities: a comparison of binocular and uniocular subjects. Invest Ophthalmol Vis Sci 28(Suppl.): 304

Sherman SM, Spear PD (1982) Organization of visual pathways in normal and visually deprived cats. Physiol Rev 62: 738-855

Sokoloff L, Reivich M, Kennedy C, Des Rosiers MH, Patlak CS, Pettigrew KD, Sakurada O, Shinohara M (1977) The $[^{14}C]$ deoxyglucose method for the measurement of local cerebral glucose utilization: theory, procedure, and normal values in the conscious and anesthetized albino rat. J Neurochem 28: 897-916

Spinelli DN, Hirsch HVB, Phelps RW, Metzler J (1972) Visual experience as a determinant of the response characteristics of cortical receptive fields in cats. Exp Brain Res 15: 289-304

Timney B (1983) The effects of early and late monocular deprivation on binocular depth perception in cats. Dev Brain Res 7: 235-243

Tyler DB, van Harreveld A (1942) The respiration of the developing brain. Am J Physiol 136: 600-603

Vaegan E, Taylor D (1979) Critical period for deprivation amblyopia in children. Trans Ophthalmol Soc U K 99: 432-439

Voeller L, Pappas GD, Purpura DP (1963) Electron microscope study of development of cat superficial neocortex. Exp Neurol 7: 107-130

Von Hofsten C (1982) Eye-hand coordination in the newborn. Dev Psychol 18: 450-461

Winfield DA (1981) The postnatal development of synapses in the visual cortex of the cat and the effects of eyelid suture. Brain Res 206: 166-171

Winfield DA (1983) The postnatal development of synapses in different laminae of the visual cortex in the normal kitten and in kittens with eyelid suture. Dev Brain Res 9: 155-169

7. The ontogeny of the EEG during infancy and childhood: implications for cognitive development

M.A. BELL

Berger's initial publication (1929) on his recordings of electrical activity from the human scalp became the impetus for research describing the rhythmic nature of the EEG and its association with behavioural state and mental activity. It was not until Berger's (1932) report of EEG differences between children and adults, however, that interest in the normal developmental course of he electroencephalogram was generated. This work immediately spawned longitudinal studies of EEG development during infancy and childhood (Henry, 1944; Lindsley, 1939; Smith 1938a; b). The value of these initial developmental studies was their pictoral account of the appearance and changing nature of typical scalp electrical activity recorded during the first few years of life. As technology made EEG recording techniques more feasible, there was intensive research on visual analysis of the infant EEG during periods of sleep and alertness (Ellingson, 1958; Samson-Dollfus et al., 1964) and on the EEG in premature infants and neonates (Dreyfus-Brisac, 1964). These standards for visual analysis are still used by clinicians today in the assessment of diagnostic EEG recordings (Tharp, 1990).

The early intensive focus on the ontogeny of EEG during infancy and childhood was based on the assumption that EEG development reflects brain maturation. Efforts to examine this association have usually resulted in low to moderate correlations between EEG parameters and IQ (Henry, 1944; Beckwith and Parmelee, 1986). More contemporary efforts to relate EEG and cognitive function have shown moderate associations between electrophysiology and cognition within various special populations, including relations between EEG and psychosocial risk during infancy (Otero, 1994), Bayley test scores of alcohol-exposed infants (Ioffe and Chernick, 1990), learning disabilities in school-age children (Lukashevich et al., 1994), and attention deficit hyperactivity disorder in children (Crawford and Barabasz, 1996). What are missing from the literature, however, are studies looking at the ongoing relations between EEG maturation and cognitive development in a normal population.

Research concerning the ontogeny of the EEG has followed a "developmental pattern" that is directly correlated with technological advances. Limited by the science available to them, early EEG researchers relied solely on visual analysis and discussed development in terms of the appearance of EEG activity at certain scalp locations and in terms of the dominant frequency measured by manually counting wave activity (Smith, 1938a; Lindsley, 1939; Henry, 1944). Later, with the advent of frequency analysers, researchers began to pursue analogue broad band analysis of the dominant frequency and amplitude in EEG recordings (Gibbs and Knott, 1949; Hagne, 1968; Matousek and Petersen, 1973). With advances in computer technology, contemporary researchers have become sophisticated in digitally scrutinising the EEG via Fast Fourier transform (FFT); or discrete

Fourier transform, (DFT), using spectral analysis to obtain a wealth of information concerning the development of power and coherence at a specific EEG frequency (Hudspeth and Pribram, 1992; Thatcher, 1994a). Other researchers have examined the maturation of EEG power and coherence parameters in association with physical (Bell and Fox, 1996; Griesel et al. 1992), socio-emotional (Calkins et al., 1996; Davidson, 1992), and cognitive development (Bell, 1996; Bell and Fox, 1992).

Nunez (1981) speculated that EEG power reflects the excitability of groups of neurons, or neural networks. Power is expressed in terms of picowatt ohms or microvolts squared. It is measured over time and represents a sustained trend of activity at a specific frequency or frequency band. Power values have been found to be stable over a period of 1 year in children from 9 to 13 years of age (Fein et al, 1984; Gasser et al, 1985). During infancy, however, when the EEG signal is rapidly maturing, EEG power values are less stable over time, with only adjacent months showing moderate correlations (Bell and Fox, 1994).

With the advent of computer technology, EEG coherence has also been used to investigate brain maturation. Coherence is the frequency dependent squared cross correlation between two scalp electrode sites which reflects the degree of phase synchrony between them (Gevins, 1989; Nunez, 1981; Thatcher et al., 1986; Thatcher et al., 1987). Coherence values range from 0 to 1, may be related to the strength and number of synaptic connections (Thatcher, 1994a) and, thus, may reflect the level of connectivity between two EEG recording sites. Greater connectivity, however, does not indicate greater maturity. Higher coherence values mean that two specific brain regions are working together, the most effective use of cortex at each phase of life. EEG coherence, unlike EEG power, is not affected by arousal, opening or closing of the eyes or by state changes, because coherence varies with the connectivity of two particular brain regions and not with arousal (Thatcher, 1996).

The aim of this chapter is to consider the EEG correlates of cognitive development during infancy and childhood. Classic and contemporary works on the development of the EEG during infancy and reviewed first, with emphasis on the frontal EEG. Then EEG correlates of two specific cognitive behaviours between 6 and 12 months of age are described. Next, literature on the development of the EEG during childhood is reviewed. Finally, emphasis is placed on the contributions of environmental influences to EEG development.

Ontogeny of the EEG during infancy

In a previous review of the literature on the EEG during infancy (Bell and Fox 1994), we focussed on EEG development during the first year of life by chronologically detailing each longitudinal study which has focussed on the EEG in awake infants. In this chapter the focus will again be on the waking EEG. After a brief note about EEG development in premature infants, the classic infant EEG longitudinal studies will be highlighted. Also cited will be two of the more prominent cross-sectional studies of infant EEG development.

Premature infants

Brain development of premature infants has long been studied using EEG measures (Dreyfus-Brisac, 1964; Dreyfus-Brisac and Monod, 1975; Ellingson and Peters, 1980). Primarily descriptive in nature, this early literature traditionally used visual analysis of EEG recordings to show that EEG development of healthy premature infants paralleled the development that would have occurred during pregnancy. Thus, a healthy premature infant of 40 weeks conceptional age displayed an EEG pattern visually similar to that of a full-term infant (Dreyfus-Brisac, 1964; Parmelee, Wenner et al., 1967). Recently, however, researchers have focussed on a wider range of prematurity and have employed spectral analysis techniques to show that very low birthweight infants do not display the same course of EEG development as their full-term peers (Richards et al., 1986). Specifically, premature infants have been shown to display lower spectral power values across the entire frequency range than their full-term counterparts, in EEG recordings made at 40 weeks conceptional age (Scher et al., 1994).

In a report that looked at level of prematurity, early premature infants (born 26-32 weeks after conception) and later-born preterms (born 33-37 weeks after conception) appeared to be similar in the EEG spectra at 42 weeks after conception (Duffy et al., 1990). However, both groups' EEG data differed significantly from the EEG power data of the full-term infants (born 38-41 weeks after conception). She was speculated that the preterm infants may have received environmental stimulation at a time when their neural systems were not ontogenetically ready, thereby artifically triggering a "sensitive period" of brain development and that this forced exposure to environmental stimuli may have led to less than optimal subsequent neural development (Duffy et al., 1990).

Full-term infants

There have been four longitudinal samples of the waking EEG reported in the classic infant EEG literature. Two of these were accomplished in the 1930 s and appear to have been a result of Berger's (1932) publication examining EEG differences between children and adults. The EEG samples collected by Smith (1938a; b, 1939; 1941) and by Lindsley (1939; later republished by Henry, 1944) were examined by visual analysis and give us identical information on the ontogeny of the EEG. Both noted the emergence of a rhythm over the occipital area around 3 months of age and termed this rhythm "alpha" because its waveform is visually similar to the adult 8-13 Hz alpha oscillation. Measuring by hand, Smith and Lindsley both reported that this waveform oscillated at 3-5 Hz. Each speculated as to the significance of the appearance of this oscillation and agreed that it was associated with visual capacities of the occipital cortex (Lindsley, 1939; Smith, 1938b). The EEG data also showed that this occipital activity gradually increased to 6-7 Hz by 12 months of age. In addition to the occipital rhythm, Smith (1941) noted the emergence of a 7 Hz signal at central scalp locations around 3 months of age and hypothesised links between the appearance of this rhythm and the disappearance of primitive reflexes and the emergence of voluntary muscular control associated with reaching. This central activity remained stable for several months, not increasing in frequency until 10 months of age (Smith, 1941).

With the aid of advancing technology, the other two longitudinal samples of waking EEG were measured mechanically in terms of frequency and amplitude. The EEG data collected by Hagne (1968, 1972) and Mizuno et al.(1970) were accomplished via frequency analysers which divided the EEG into preselected frequency bands, but the researchers gave a consistent account of EEG frequency development during the first year of life. Hagne (1968, 1972) reported a decrease in amplitude at 1.5-3.5 Hz, with a corresponding increase in amplitude at 3.5-7.5 Hz during the first year of life at central, temporal, parietal, and occipital locations. The EEG at central sites was less stable than that recorded at the posterior locations. Reporting on the right occipital scalp EEG, Mizuno et al. (1970) showed a predominance of 2.0-4.15 Hz activity at 3 months and 3.5-8.6 Hz activity at 12 months. Interestingly, Hagne (1968) made note of individual differences in amplitude in same-age EEG recordings and stated that these persisted throughout the first year of life.

Mizuno et al. (1970) also made detailed observations of each infant's physical development, noting weight, height, head and chest circumference, and physical milestones (holding up head, sitting, standing, walking) at each EEG recording session. No attempt was made to relate physical development with EEG maturation, however.

Hagne (1972), on the other hand, did neurological and developmental assessments on each infant in association with each EEG recording. She reported correlations between peak frequency (frequency at which the infant displayed the greatest amplitude) at parietal/occipital and total score on the Griffiths scale of mental development at 4-months, and between peak frequency at central scalp locations and Griffiths score at 10 months of age. Hagne also reported a correlation between 4 month EEG activity at 1.5-7.5 Hz, temporal and central locations, and total score on the Griffiths scale. Given the large number of correlations tested, however, Hagne reported that "significant correlations were found only sporadically" (Hagne, 1972). She also went back to the original EEG recordings (Hagne, 1968, 1972) examined with frequency analysers and reanalysed them using spectral analysis via fast Fourier transform (Hagne, 1972; Hagne et al.,1973) and to confirm the original findings from the frequency analysers and to obtain a more detailed analysis of amplitude development (Hagne, 1972). Previous work with the frequency analysers was confirmed and noted that the development of peak frequency can be most clearly seen in the EEG from central scalp locations (Hagne et al., 1973).

There have been many cross-sectional studies of infant EEG development and two will be briefly noted here. One of the first cross-sectional studies was conducted by Gibbs and Knott (1949) and included a sample of 37 infants from birth to 12 months of age. (It also included EEG recordings from children and adults.) The infant sample confirmed the results of the longitudinal infant studies by Smith, Lindsley, and Henry. Using a frequency analyser, Gibbs et al.(1949) reported that the greatest amplitudes in the occipital EEG were associated with lower frequency values (< 6 Hz), but that by 12 months of age infants began to show greater amplitude at 9 Hz. Ohtahara (1964, 1981) also used a frequency analyser on parietal and occipital EEG samples of 585 infants and children to 14 years of age and reported that the amplitude in the lowest frequency band (1.5-3.5 Hz) decreased the first year of life. Amplitude from 3.5-8 Hz increased during the same time period, replicating with a cross-sectional sample the work of Hagne (1968, 1972; Hagne et al., 1973) and Mizuno et al. (1970).

Coherence

While there have been coherence studies on the newborn's sleeping EEG (Kuks et al., 1988), there has been no extensive work and on the development of coherence during infancy. In the large study of (1987) of 577 subjects from 2 months to 26 years of age, only 16 were less than one year of age and the data from these were treated as a group. Thatcher et al. (1987) reported that before 3 years of age coherence change with age was different for each electrode pairing. After that age, the coherence changes in each electrode pair become rhythmic. Coherence development in childhood will be discussed in the latter half of this chapter.

Development of frontal cortex during infancy

Despite many norming studies on EEG development, there has been no research on the ontogeny of the EEG from frontal scalp locations. As noted, previous work has focussed on EEG development from posterior scalp locations. Smith (1938a, b), Henry (1944), and Hagne (1968) all placed electrodes on the frontal scalp areas. None of them, however, reported on the frontal EEG recordings. Hagne (1968) and Hagne et al. (1972) stated that the frontal recordings were contaminated by eye movement and were not usable. In these norming studies, there may also have been an implicit assumption that the frontal lobes are not active during infancy. The frontal cortex always has been considered essential to complex cognitive functioning (Milner, 1982; Pribram, 1973), something many early researchers may have thought was beyond the realm of infancy.

Researchers from other disciplines, however, have recently shown that the frontal cortex is not undeveloped during infancy. Using PET data, Chugani and Phelps (1986) reported an increase in glucose metabolism in the frontal cortex during the last half of the first year of life. Specifically, Chugani and his colleagues noted that the lateral portion of the frontal cortex shows an increase in glucose metabolism at approximately 6 months of age (Chugani et al., 1987), while the medial frontal area (Chugani et al., 1987) and the dorsal prefrontal area (Chugani, 1994) show an increase from 8 months of age. By 1 year of age, the glucose metabolism pattern qualitatively resembles that of an adult (Chugani, 1994; Chugani et al., 1987).

Morphological studies have shown that a high rate of synaptogenesis occurs in the infant cortex during the first year of life. Through Huttenlocher's work, we now know a great deal about synaptic density and total synapse count in the visual cortex (Huttenlocher, 1990,1994). Depending on the specific layer of the visual cortex, the mean number of synapses per neuron peaks anywhere from 8 to 12 months of age (Huttenlocher, 1994). Neuronal development is much slower in the frontal cortex and much less information is available about synaptogenesis in this brain area (Huttenlocher, 1979, 1990). We do know, however, that maximum synaptic density in the frontal gyrus is achieved at 12 months of age and, with synaptic pruning, adult levels are reached by 16 years of age (Huttenlocher, 1979).

From the developmental neuropsychology literature, we know that specific EEG patterns at frontal sites are associated with mood state. Work by Fox and colleagues has shown a relation between frontal EEG asymmetry and expression of emotion during the first year of life (Bell and Fox, 1994; Davidson and Fox, 1982, 1989; Fox et al., 1992; Fox and Davidson, 1987, 1988). This asymmetry appears to be specific to frontal EEG recordings and not to those from posterior scalp locations. This work has been replicated by Dawson (1994) and Dawson et al. (1992) with infants in the second year of life.

EEG correlates of infant cognitive development

Longitudinal study of the frontal EEG and A-not-B performance

While the findings from the developmental neuropsychology literature confirm the PET and synaptic density data that the frontal cortex is "functional" during infancy, if not "mature", the EEG asymmetry research has been carried out without the benefit of norming studies on frontal EEG development. To fill this gap in the developmental literature, Nathan Fox and I (Bell and Fox, 1992, 1994; Fox and Bell, 1990) conducted a study on the ontogeny of the EEG from 7 to 12 months of age to observe both EEG power and coherence development. We sought to replicate, using modern technology, findings from the classic longitudinal EEG studies on the ontogeny of the EEG from posterior scalp locations. Of special interest was EEG development from frontal scalp locations. We were also concerned with the cognitive correlates of this frontal EEG maturation.

The participants in our longitudinal study were 13 healthy, full-term infants (7 girls) who had been carefully screened and found to have no medical conditions from the prenatal period through the first year of life. Infants were seen for monthly EEG recordings from frontal (F3, F4), parietal (P3, P4), and occipital (O1, O2) scalp locations. Using software developed by James Long Company, we computed EEG

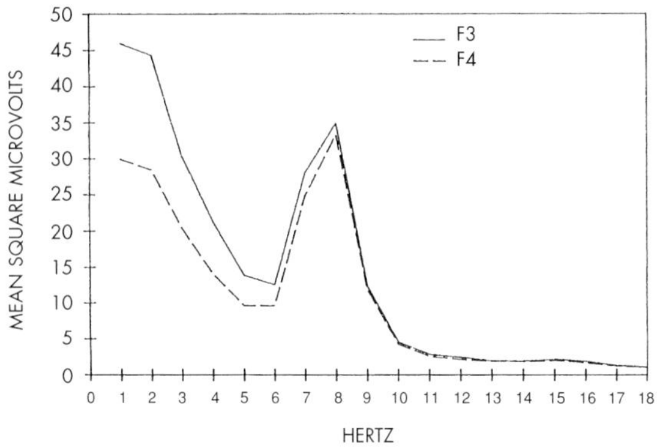

Fig. 1. Spectral plot for one 10-month-old girl for left and right medial frontal (F3, F4). Note the EEG power between 6 and 9 Hz.

power in single-Hertz bands between 1-18 Hz and plotted spectral power for each of the 6 scalp leads for each infant at each age.

Figure 1 shows the spectral plot for the frontal scalp locations for a girl at 10 months of age. This plot was typical of the spectral plots at each age. While little power was seen beyond 10 Hz, 2 dominant frequency bands were obvious from the individual spectral plots of the infants. One was between 1 and 4 or 1 and 5 Hz and the other between 6 and 9 Hz. To compare our findings with the classic infant EEG literature, we calculated relative power (6-9 Hz / 1-4 Hz) and found an increase in this ratio across age at frontal, parietal, and occipital scalp locations (Bell and Fox, 1994; Fox and Bell, 1990). Thus, we found that the developmental pattern reported for the posterior EEG for more than 50 years held true for the frontal EEG as well. Because relative power does not inform us whether the increase in this ratio was due to an increase in spectral power at 6-9 Hz or a decrease in spectral power at 1-4 Hz, we also examined developmental patterns of absolute power in the 6-9 Hz band and, likewise, found monthly changes in absolute power across age, the largest increase in spectral power at each scalp location occurring between 9 and 10 months of age (Bell and Fox, 1994).

Based on the classic infancy literature, we considered 6-9 Hz to be the most "mature" EEG frequency band and focussed on the EEG power and coherence in that band in our examination of the cognitive correlates of EEG development. The cognitive behaviour upon which we focussed was the A-not-B task, the classic marker of object permanence in Piaget's 4th substage of sensorimotor development. Briefly, this task involves hiding a desirable object in one of two possible adjacent locations in full view of the infant. The infant is allowed to search manually for the hidden object. Around 8 or 9 months of age, the typical infant will easily retrieve the object from multiple hidings at one location (side A), but upon seeing the object hidden in the other location (side B) will automatically reach back to the side of the original hidings (side A), hence the name of the task ("A not B").

Extensive work by Diamond and Goldman-Rakic (1983, 1986, 1989) and Diamond et al. (1989) demonstrated that the ability to succeed on the A-not-B task requires a mature or intact dorsolateral prefrontal cortex. Diamond (1988, 1990a, 1990b) proposed that the frontal functions of recall memory and inhibition are essential for successful reaching to side B during the A-not-B task, and shown that this task can appropriately be used with infants beyond the classic 8 or 9 month testing age by initiating a delay period between hiding the object and allowing the infant search (Diamond, 1985, 1990b).

In our longitudinal study (Bell and Fox, 1992, 1994) we replicated Diamond's (1985) report of the tolerance of increasing delay across age. What we were most impressed with, however, was the wide range of individual differences apparent at 12 months of age. Using K-means cluster analysis we placed the infants into 2 groups based on developmental progression on the A-not-B task. These was a group of 6 infants able to tolerate long delays and another of 7 who tolerated short delays at 12 months (Fig. 2).

We examined the EEG data of these two groups of infants using repeated-measures MANOVA and found a three-way interaction of group, hemisphere, and age for the frontal EEG power values. As seen in figure 3, the long delay group showed dramatic changes across age in frontal EEG power, the short delay group did not. The two groups did not differ in parietal EEG. In occipital EEG, the long-delay group displayed greater left than right occipital power across age. Thus, the only group-by-age effects were for the frontal EEG recordings.

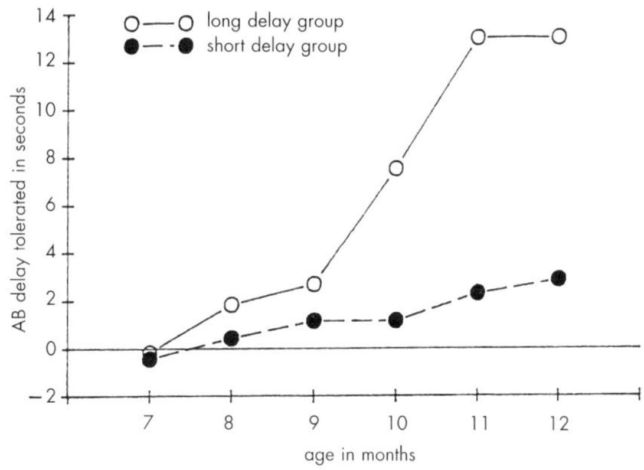

Fig. 2. Delay tolerated in seconds during the A-not-B task for the two performance groups across age. Failure to perform the A-not-B task was coded as -1. From Bell and Fox, 1994, by permission of Guilford Press.

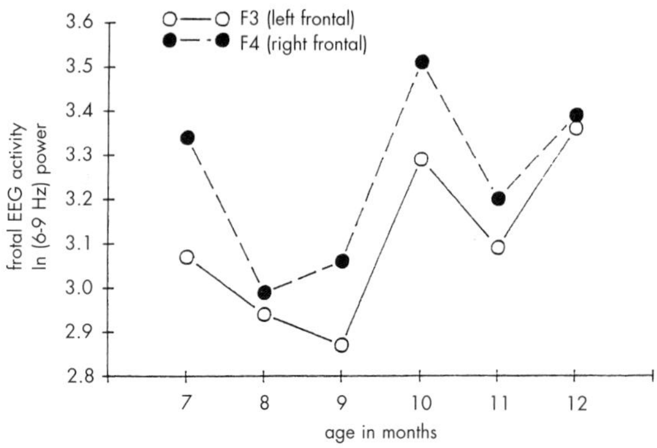

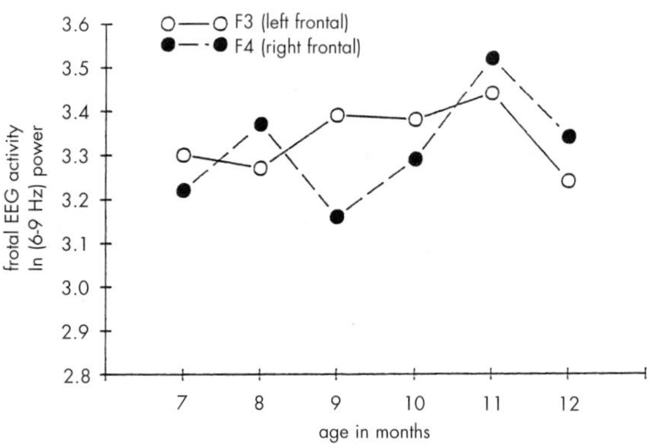

Fig. 3. Frontal EEG power across age for A-not-B performance group tolerating long delay (top) and short delay (bottom) at 12 months. From Bell and Fox, 1992, by permission of Society for Research in Child Development.

EEG coherence analyses revealed a similar group by age interaction, but only for the left hemisphere values. When collapsing across frontal/parietal and frontal/occipital coherence values, the long-delay group exhibited a change in EEG coherence across age that was cyclic (Fig. 4): a decrease in coherence between 7 and 9 months of age, stability from 9 to 10 months, and an increase from 10 to 12 months. The short delay group showed a more stable pattern (Fig. 4). Thus, for both EEG power and coherence in this data set, the change in frontal EEG across age distinguished between the long- and short-delay groups.

Case study of frontal EEG and language development

While our longitudinal study was the first to report systematically on changes in frontal EEG during infancy, we recorded from only two of the possible six left and right hemisphere frontal recording sites based on the 10/20 system. Information on frontal EEG development was thus still rather limited. To add to this growing knowledge base, René Schmauder and I (Bell and Schmauder, 1994, 1995; Schmauder and Bell, 1995) sought to carry out an intensive study of frontal EEG maturation during infancy by doing weekly EEG recording from one infant girl between 6 and 12 months of age (26-52 weeks). We recorded from all 6 frontal scalp locations: orbito (Fp1, Fp2), medial (F3, F4) and lateral (F7, F8) and from 4 temporal (T3, T4, T5, T6) locations. As in the previous longitudinal study, we focussed on the EEG at 6-9 Hz.

As seen in figure 5, the three pairs of frontal EEG leads showed different patterns of EEG maturation (at 6-9 Hz) from 6 to 10 months of age (Bell and Schmauder, 1995). The orbitofrontal (Fp1, Fp2) and lateral frontal (F7, F8) leads showed similar patterns of development. From 26 weeks (6 months) to 37 weeks (8.5 months), all four leads showed a gradual increase in EEG power. The left and right hemispheres showed similar patterns. A sharp increase in EEG power occurred in all four leads at 37 weeks. EEG power in the medial frontal (F3, F4) leads showed a very different pattern. These two recording sites showed greater variability in power from 6 to 10 months of age, with much less similarity between hemispheres than in the other four frontal leads. The medial frontal power was consistently greater than that at the other four frontal locations, except in weeks 40 and 41.

Figure 6 shows the frontal coherence data for these weekly EEG recordings. Orbitomedial coherence (Fp1/F3, Fp2/F4) exhibited a gradual increase between 29 and 39 weeks, while orbitolateral coher-

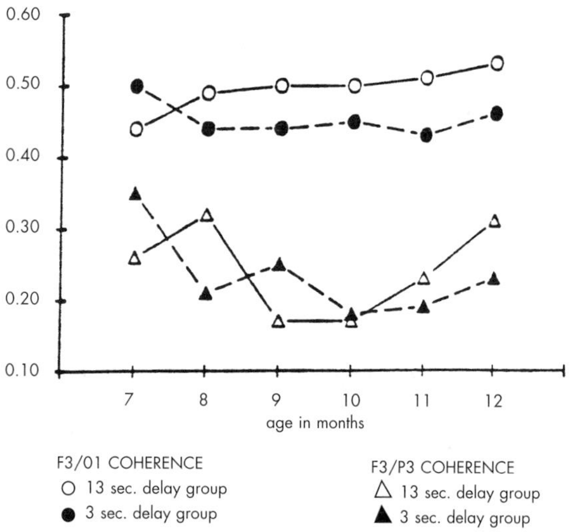

Fig. 4. Left hemisphere coherence across age for long delay and short delay groups. From Bell and Fox, 1992 by permission of Society for Research in Child Development.

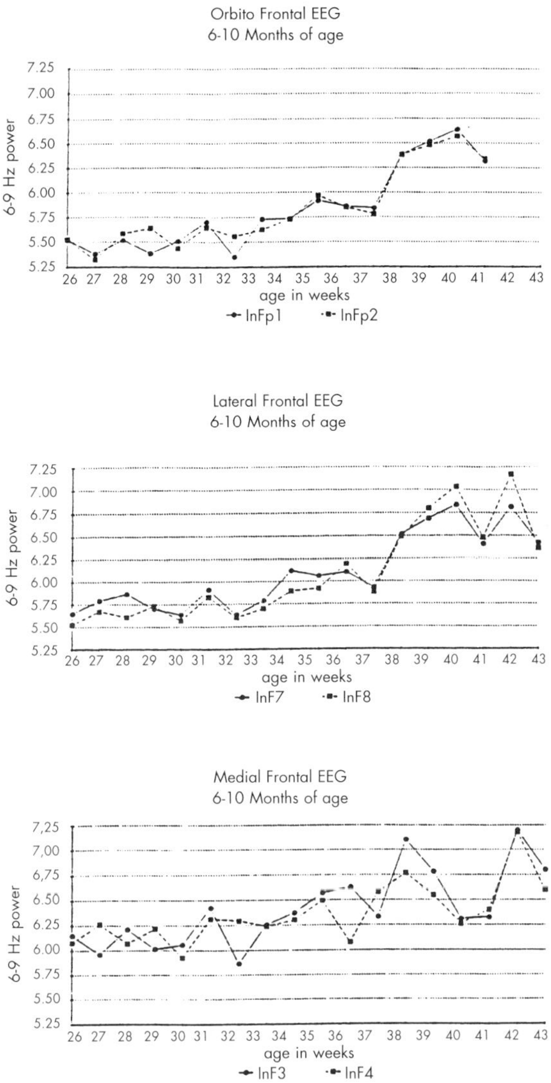

Fig. 5. Case study of weekly frontal EEG power from 26 to 43 weeks (6 to 10 months) for one girl.

ence (Fp1/F7, Fp2/F8) showed stability and a subsequent decrease after week 39. Medial-lateral coherence (F3/F7, F4/F8) displayed stability from 29 to 38 weeks and then showed a U-shaped pattern of coherence typical of cortical reorganisation (Thatcher, 1994a).

Because Dr. Schmauder is a psycholinguist, she had an interest in the language correlates of these monthly EEG recordings. We hypothesised that EEG maturation would be highly correlated with the onset of language production. After each weekly EEG recording session, there was a 15 minute play session involving the infant, mother, and research assistant during which audio recordings were made. The mother also made approximately 30 minutes of audio recordings each week. From these recordings the infant's rate of canonical syllable production was calculated and defined as the proportion of canonical to total syllables produced (Oller, 1986; Oller and Seibert, 1988). Canonical syllables are consonant-vowel or consonant-vowel-consonant combinations.

Weekly data from this infant girl from 27 to 52 weeks (6-12 months) showed that the rate of canonical syllable production increased with age, with canonical babbling reliably occurring from 30 weeks of age (Bell and Schmauder, 1994). We also examined medial frontal/anterior temporal coherence with age, hypothesising that the cortical area between these scalp locations may underlie the language areas of the left hemisphere. When we examined the coherence patterns with age we noted dissimilar patterns for left (F3/T3) and right hemispheres (F4/T4). More importantly, when we tested the relation between canonical syllable proportion and coherence for each hemisphere separately using a regression procedure, we found that left hemisphere coherence predicted language production, but right hemisphere coherence did not (Schmauder and Bell, 1995). As seen in figure 7, canonical syllable rate (CS/TS) paralleled left hemisphere coherence across age. While these data are from one infant, they do point to a need for more intensive study of relations between EEG maturation and cognitive development.

Individual differences in frontal EEG power and A-not-B performance

There appears to be a relation between frontal EEG maturation at 6-9 Hz and cognitive development, both object permanence and language production, at least when measured across time. In terms of individual variation in A-not-B performance, differences in cognitive task performance from 7 to 12 months of age appeared to be associated with different patterns of frontal EEG maturation. But can the frontal EEG differentiate among infants of the same age with differing levels of A-not-B object permanence development? That was the question we asked in a study of 80 infants 8 months of age. In addition to individual differences in frontal EEG maturation and A-not-B performance, we were also interested in the contribution of crawling experience to brain electrophysiology and cognitive performance. Many developmental psychologists have noted a relationship between the onset of hands-and-knees locomotion and the development of cognitive behaviour, especially associated with object search (Acredolo, 1990; Bai and Bertenthal, 1992, Kermoian and Campos, 1988). This locomotor experience may help the infant process information concerning the dynamic relations of objects within the environment more easily (Bertenthal et al., 1994).

The 80-8 month-old infants were recruited according to the amount of hands-and-knees locomotor experience each had and placed into one of four groups. These included infants with 1-4 weeks experience, 5-8 weeks experience, 9+ weeks and no experience. Each group consisted of 20 infants, half boys. Procedures were similar to the longitudinal study in that EEG recordings were achieved, and A-not-B performance was assessed. Spectral plots of the group EEG data verified what spectral plots of individual infant data from the longitudinal study had shown. Thus there we're 2 dominant frequency bands in the EEG data, one at 1-4 or 1-5 Hz and another at 6-9 Hz.

Results of repeated-measures MANOVA on the EEG revealed that infants successful at A-not-B at no imposed delay or a delay of 2 or more seconds exhibited greater medial frontal (F3, F4), and occipital EEG 6-9 Hz power than infants unsuccessful at the task (Fig. 8). In addition, infants with locomotor experience performed at a higher level on the A-not-B task than prelocomotor infants. There was no interelationship, however, of EEG, locomotor experience and object permanence performance. Thus, infants of the same age, both frontal and occipital EEG power values differentiated between infants successful or unsuccessful on the A-not-B task.

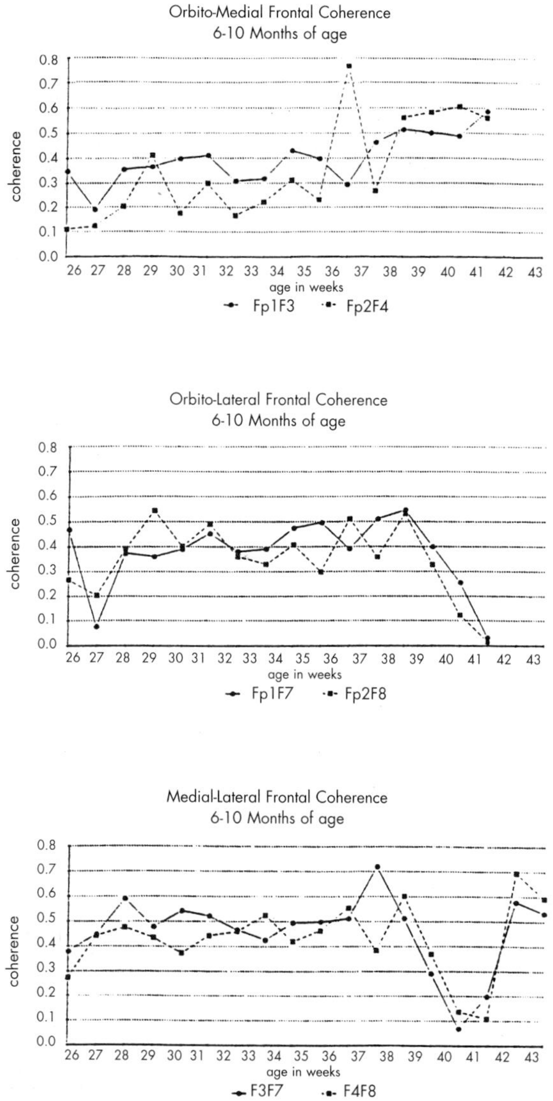

Fig. 6. Case study of weekly frontal EEG coherence from 26 to 43 weeks (6 to 10 months) for one girl.

Ontogeny of the EEG during childhood

The early infant longitudinal studies were remarkable in that they also contained longitudinal samples of children. Smith (1938a, b, 1939, 1941) continued to obtain EEG recordings from many his infant until they were 4.5 years of age. He is made single EEG recordings from 95 children aged 3-16 years (Smith, 1941). Using visual inspection, he noted that the occipital EEG had a frequency of almost 8 Hz and the central EEG of almost 9 Hz by 30 months of age. This period of rapid EEG development during infancy and early childhood was followed by a more gradual change in EEG (Smith, 1941). EEG frequency of 9 Hz at occipital locations was not obtained until 8 years of age (Smith, 1938b), while the adult occipital mean of 10 Hz was not seen until 16 years (Smith, 1941). Smith noted that Lindsley's data showed 10 Hz occipital EEG in some 12-year-old children (Smith, 1941), although Lindsley's (1939) data tables revealed that 10 Hz activity was displayed by some children from at 6 years of age.

The longitudinal data set begun by Lindsley (1939) and reanalyzed by Henry (1944) included 95 children ranging in age from 3 months to 19 years. Each contributed a minimum of 5 recordings, collected over a minimum of 5 years. Up to 1 year of age, recordings were made every 3 months. From 1 to 5 years, recordings were done every 6 months and then every year thereafter. Recordings were made from occipital and central sites and analysed using visual inspection. Lindsley (1939) reported that occipital amplitude began to decrease after 12 months of age, the sharpest decline occurring near the second birthday. He suggested that this was due to the closing of the fontanelle, because the drop in amplitude was not accompanied by a change in frequency, and that the continued drop in amplitude evident throughout childhood was associated with increase in skull thickness.

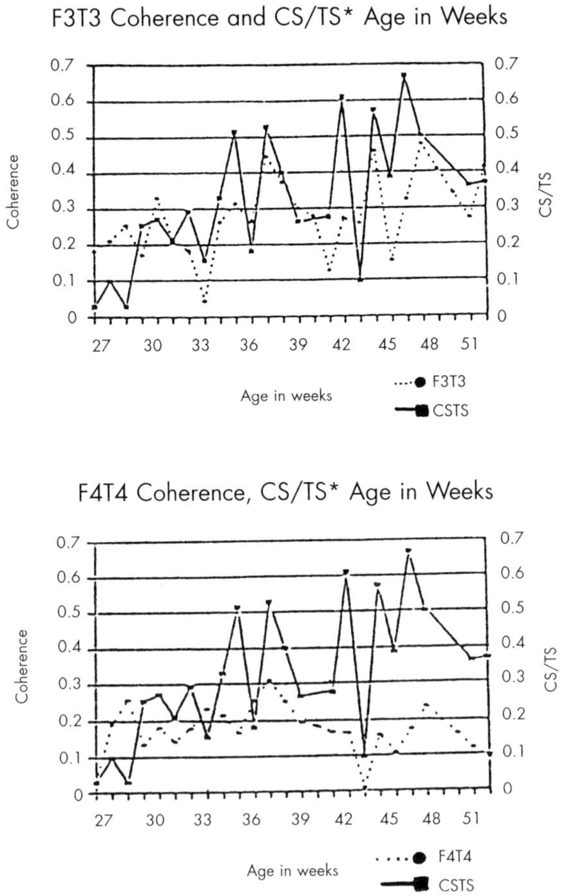

Fig. 7. Proportion of canonical syllables to total syllables plotted against left (top) and right (bottom) hemisphere frontal/temporal coherence for one case study infant from 27 to 52 weeks of age. From Schmauder and Bell, 1995, by permission of Cascadilla Press.

Henry (1944) reported sudden frequency changes in occipital recording sites prior to the age of 4, but that after 6 years most children exhibited an occipital EEG in the 9-11 Hz range, and that individual differences in maturation of the adult-like EEG frequency were evident in his visual analysis of the EEG data. Some children appeared to reach this mature frequency early, while others showed slow increases throughout childhood. Individual differences in dominant frequency tended to be stable, however. Children with faster (> 11 Hz) and slower (< 9 Hz) dominant frequencies tended to be at the maximum and minimum levels of the group mean respecting throughout the longitudinal study (Henry, 1944).

Two cross-sectional studies often cited in the classic EEG development literature examined EEG with frequency analysers. Gibbs and Knott (1949) studied 930 premature infants, full-term infants, children, and younger adults to age 29, recording whole head EEG, but only report only occipital EEG findings. Corbin and Bickford (1955) included 64 children ages 1 to 10 and also recorded from the entire scalp, but reported only on occipital recordings. Gibbs and Knott (1949) reported that 4-6 Hz EEG activity increases until 2 years and then declines, while Corbin and Bickford (1955) reported that the greatest levels of EEG activity in this frequency band are evident at 3 years. The latter suggested that EEG activity gradually shifts upwards to the adult frequency range of 8-12 Hz from this lower frequency band. This probably explains the Gibbs and Knott finding by of an increase and then a decline in 4-6 Hz activity after 2 years. Both pairs of researchers reported that adult-like frequencies (10-12 Hz) exhibited gradually increasing amounts of activity during childhood, but as opposite findings regards activity in the lowest frequency band. Gibbs and Knott (1949) found that 1-3 Hz activity steadily decreased across age, while Corbin and Bickford (1955) reported that 1-3 Hz activity increased until 4 years before decreasing. Ohtahara (1964, 1981) reported on a data set of occipital EEG recordings from 576 children from newborn to 14 years of age. Results using a frequency analyser corroborated the report of Gibbs and Knott (1949) that 1-3 Hz activity decreased steadily with age.

Petersen and Eeg-Olofsson (1971) used visual analysis to assess development of the EEG in children from 1 to 15 years of age and in adolescents from 16 to 21 years (Eeg-Olofsson, 1971). Recordings were made from frontal, central, temporal, parietal and occipital locations. From these original data sets, 561 EEG sessions had been recorded on tape and were submitted to broad-band frequency analysis by Matousek and Petersen (1973). This confirmed earlier cross-sectional work, showing decreases in 1.5-3.5 Hz activity and increases in 9.5-12.5 Hz activity with age. EEG development occurred more quickly at posterior than central scalp locations; age-related EEG changes were linear during childhood and logarithmic during adolescence.

John et al. (1980) compared 306 children aged 6 to 16 years of age with the 324 children 6-16 year examined by Matousek and Petersen (1973) and confirmed the notion of linear changes in the EEG with increasing age. Again, EEG activity in the 1.5-7.5 Hz frequency band decreased with age, while EEG activity over 7.5 Hz increased with age.

These earlier notions of linear changes in EEG development were questioned with a graphical display of the EEG data by Epstein (1980). Examining EEG activity reported longitudinally by Smith (1938b), Lindsley (1939), and Henry (1944), and cross-sectionally by Matousek and Petersen (1973), Epstein recalculated the EEG changes with age to reflect biennial increments in 8-13 Hz activity. This reconfiguration of the data revealed 5 stages of EEG development which correlated with the stages of brain growth in

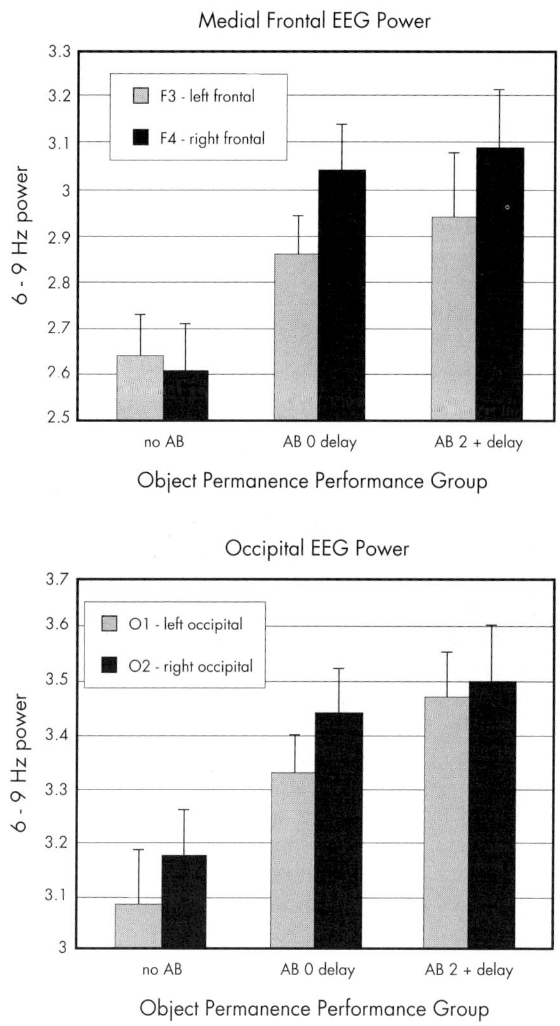

Fig. 8. Frontal and occipital EEG power values for the A-not-B performance groups at 8 months of age. From Bell and Fox, under review.

terms of gross weight reported earlier (Epstein, 1974).

Hudspeth and Pribram (1990, 1992) reanalysed the Matousek and Petersen (1973) data and reported evidence stages or "growth spurts" in EEG development. Estimating age dependent changes in the total EEG spectra (1-25 Hz), as opposed to changes in individual frequency bands, they examined the data for each scalp location separately to account for regional differences in cerebral maturation. The first stage of brain maturation was from 1 to 6 years of age. EEG activity from all recording sites reached peak levels of change at about the same age. The second stage was from 6 to 10.5 years, with peak change occurring at 7.5 years. Maturation patterns across each brain region appeared synchronised during the first 10 years of life. The third stage was from 10.5 to 13 years of age and involved mostly parietal-occipital change. The fourth spanned 13 to 17 years and showed major changes in the temporal and frontal EEG. The last stage, from 17 to 21 years involved only frontal recording sites.

Using EEG recordings from 142 children aged 5 to 12 years, Somsen and van 't Klooster (1994) attempted to replicate these findings of stages, or "growth spurts", in the EEG during childhood. Using the same calculations, they replicated the stages of EEG development; they went further, however, and demonstrated that the apparent stages of EEG maturation could be manipulated by using monopolar, as opposed to bipolar, recordings, and by calculating relative, as opposed to absolute, EEG power.

The stages of EEG maturation reported by Hudspeth and Pribram (1990) coincide with data on regional brain development (Chugani, 1994; Huttenlocher, 1994). In addition, Hudspeth and Pribram (1990) argumed that they also coincide with the basic tenets of Piaget's theory. A correspondence between Piaget's stages of cognitive development and stage-like patterns of brain development also has been posited by Fischer (1987; Fischer and Rose, 1994) and Case (1992). The EEG data of Matousek and Petersen (1973) EEG data were collected without cognitive or behavioural complements, however. Fischer and Rose (1994) has noted the need for more precise and simultaneous brain-behaviour assessments to detect discontinuities in brain maturation and cognitive development during childhood.

Coherence

As noted previously, coherence values may be related to the strength and number of synaptic connections (Thatcher, 1994a) and, may thus reflect the level of connectivity between two EEG recording sites. Using 577 EEG recordings on infants, children, and young adults aged 2 months to 26 years, Thatcher et al. (1987) showed that EEG coherence values also follow a cyclical pattern of increases and decreases which appear to occur at ages corresponding to Piaget's stages of cognitive development. The "growth spurts" appeared very similar to those demonstrated by Hudspeth and Pribram (1990) in the data of Matousek and Petersen (1973).

Recording EEG from 19 scalp locations, Thatcher et al. (1986) divided the EEG into 4 frequency bands, but later publications appear to present data for the 7-13 Hz band only. Initially, they noted 5 growth periods in the coherence data. Period one, from birth to 3 years was characterised as "topographically scattered developmental change", with coherence values from each electrode pair displaying no obvious developmental pattern. After this first period, coherence values from different electrode pairs became more synchronised. Period two, from 4 to 6 years involved changes in left hemisphere frontal-occipital and frontal-temporal coherence and right hemisphere frontal-frontal pole coherence. Growth period three included ages 8 to 10 years and involved right hemisphere frontal-temporal coherence. Both period four, ages 11 to 14 years, and period five, ages 15 years to adult, involved changes in frontal scalp locations.

Later publications focussed on the 436 recordings made from the children 1 to 16 years of age (Thatcher, 1994a, 1991) and highlighted the notion that "growth spurts" are nested within continuous developmental trajectories. Most recently, Thatcher has discussed these growth spurts in terms of three cycles of EEG coherence development. Cycle one is from 1.5 to 5, cycle two from 5 to 10, and cycle three from 10 to 16 years. The major difference between this new configuration of development and the original one (Thatcher et al., 1987) appears to be the combination of the original first two periods of growth (ages birth to 3 years and ages 4 to 6 years) into one cycle of development. Between these three cycles of growth there are major phase transitions or bifurcations occurring around ages 5-7 and 9-11 years.

Thatcher (1991) noted that EEG coherence from frontal recording sites figures prominently in developmental cycles. Most of the growth spurts in coherence involve frontal lobe connections (Thatcher et al, 1987). Thatcher has often used the predator-prey analogy to describe this phenomenon , reasoning that the frontal lobes are responsible for the synaptic organisation and reorganisation of the posterior regions (Thatcher, 1994b).

Effects of experience on EEG development

Thatcher (1994b) also noted the dual influences of genetics and environmental experience on the growth spurts in EEG coherence development. He suggested that genetics are involved in the increased synaptic production and the accompanying increases in coherence and that experience is involved in the pruning of unneeded synapses and decreases in coherence. Greenough and his coworkers proposed a model of the role of experience on brain structure and function during maturation of the brain and on the further refinement of brain structure after maturation (Black and Greenough, 1986; Greenough and Black, 1992; Greenough et al., 1987). Drawing upon Piaget, Black and Greenough (1986) proposed that two types of information can be gleaned from the environment. Expected information is common to all members of a species and, is thus, developmental or maturational. Unexpected or situation-dependent information is specific to the individual and therefore has a learning component.

Greenough had labelled experience-expectant processes as those which have been widely available throughout evolutionary history (Greenough and Black, 1992). The events occur early in life and are invariant across individuals. The timing of the event is relatively critical. Physiologically, synaptic overproduction in critical areas of the cortex anticipates an expected experience. Greenough's model also accounts for the later pruning of inappropriate synapses, while retaining a subset of synapses as a result of the experience (Fig. 9).

Given Greenough's model, one could hypothesise that the experience-expectant event of crawling in human infants would result in anticipatory modifications in brain structure during maturation and that the actual experience of crawling could further refine that structure. Hands-and-knees crawling may be functionally related to the development of cognitive and socio-emotional behaviour during infancy and has thus received a considerable amount of attention in the developmental literature (Bertenthal and Campos, 1990; Bertenthal et al., 1994; Campos et al., 1992). We used Greenough's model to examine EEG coherence among four groups of 8-month-old infants who had various amounts of hands-and-knees crawling experience (Bell and Fox, 1996). These groups were detailed in the section of this chapter concerning individual differences in frontal EEG and A-not-B performance. Briefly, novice crawlers had 1-4 weeks, moderate crawlers 5-8 weeks, and proficient crawlers 9 or more weeks crawling experience. The fourth group included prelocomotor infants. The resting, awake EEG was recorded from frontal, parietal, and occipital scalp locations. Coherence was computed for the 6-9 Hz frequency band.

We found that novice crawlers (1-4 weeks) displayed greater levels of coherence between medial

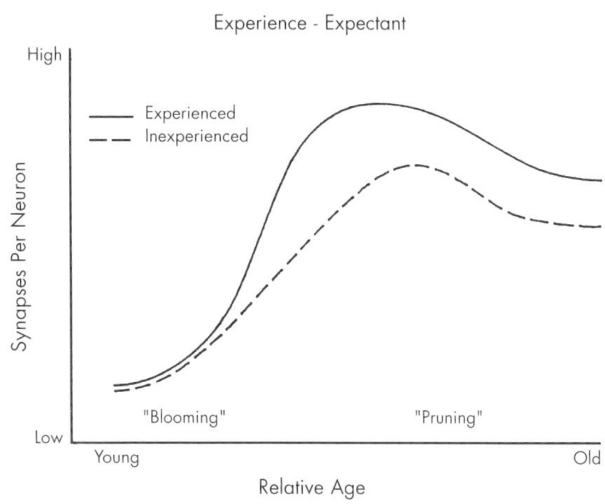

Fig. 9. Greenough's model of synaptic overproduction ("blooming") and deletion ("pruning") associated with an experience-expectant process. From Black and Greenough, 1986, by permission of Erlbaum.

frontal/occipital, medial frontal/lateral frontal, and parietal/occipital scalp locations than either the prelocomotor infants or those with long-term (9+ weeks) crawling experience (Fig. 10). Infants with 5-8 weeks experience had greater medial frontal/occipital coherence than prelocomotor or infants with 9 or more weeks experience. Group differences were limited to right-hemisphere EEG coherence values.

Thus, the onset of locomotion may have been associated with changes in cortical organisation. The specific pattern of pruning (gradual or quick) appears to have depended on the particular cortical connection. For example, the gradual decrease in medial frontal/occipital coherence may be related to long-term connections between visual cortex and motor planning areas of the frontal cortex. The visual cortex and prefrontal cortex both have areas serving object and spatial vision (Wilson et al., 1993). Competence at both spatial and object vision may be essential to crawling. The rather quick decline in parietal/occipital coherence may suggest that these connections are not needed after some crawling experience, even though they were essential to locomotor onset (Bell and Fox, 1996). These data provide a neural model for motor experience during infancy and perhaps set the stage for a neural model of the effects of experience on cognitive functioning.

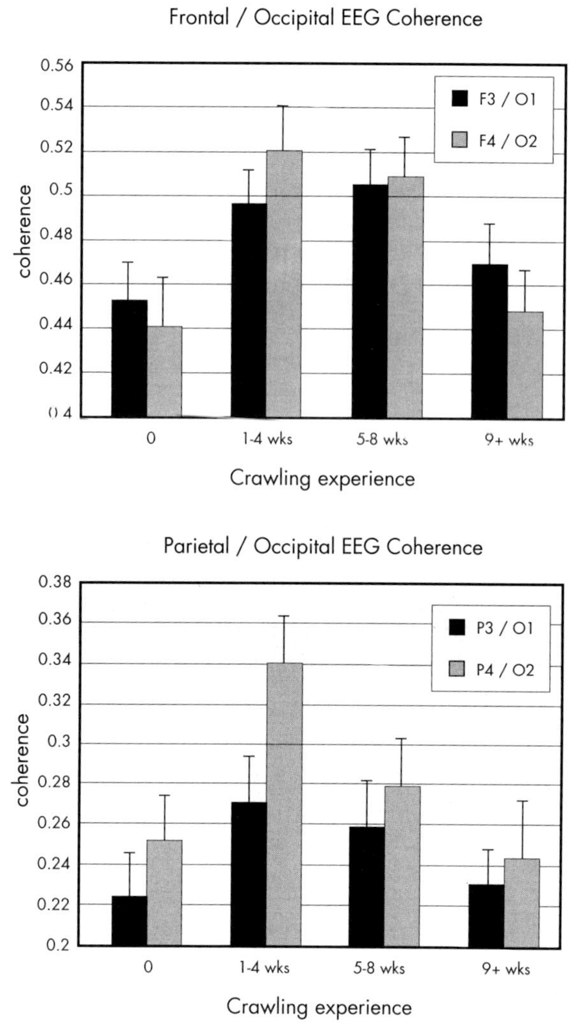

Fig. 10. Medial frontal/occipital (top) and parietal/occipital (bottom) EEG coherence (bottom) for 4 locomotor experience groups. From Bell and Fox, 1996, by permission of Wiley.

Conclusions

As noted at the beginning of this chapter, our ability to examine the ontogeny of the EEG has changed with advances in technology. Despite our accomplishments, however, it is those classic studies of EEG development from the 1930 s to the 1960 s which are the foundation for clinical assessment of EEG today. Present day research on the EEG maturation continues to be intent on describing normal developmental patterns of EEG power and coherence change with age. The addition of cognitive measures to infancy EEG research has given us much more information as to the value of these maturational patterns of change in the EEG. Perhaps one of the most exciting areas of EEG research during infancy is the confirmation of frontal functioning. There is indeed brain wave activity from frontal scalp leads prior to the first birthday and the pattern of maturation appears to be related not only to the development of A-not-B object permanence skills and language production, but to the effects of locomotor experience as well. These types of studies are adding greatly to our knowledge of brain behaviour relations during infancy.

We have a great deal of information concerning the ontogeny of the EEG during childhood and adolescence. With the large cross-sectional data sets reviewed in this chapter, we can now make statements concerning the gradual increase in EEG activity with age and the corresponding "growth spurts" or maturational cycles in EEG power and coherence. It is interesting to note that these large cross-sectional studies are in agreement as to the cycles of EEG maturation. It is also fascinating that the EEG experts, as well as other researchers, have noticed the agreement of these cycles of development with Piaget's stages of cognitive development. The coincidence is very enticing, but what is really essential is the intensive work needed to do more than just speculate about a relation between EEG ontogeny and cognitive development. We need to incorporate cognitive measures into this type of research to show that this is indeed a true relationship and not a mere coincidence. Measures of IQ will not satisfy this requirement. Only measures which account for qualitative change in cognitive complexity or that have similar complexity levels but cover many different domains of processing can meet this demand (Fischer and Rose, 1994).

Finally, the value of EEG coherence as a measure of brain maturation has been highlighted. Because coherence values may reflect the connectivity of two EEG recording sites (Thatcher, 1994a), this brain measure gives us a way of examining the dynamic inter-relations of various brain regions. This may, indeed, prove to be a more informative measure of developing brain function than traditional amplitude and power measures. In either event, it is the combination of brain and behavioural measures that gives us the most accurate account of the dynamics of cognitive development.

References

Acredolo L (1990) Individual differences in infant spatial cognition. In: Colombo J, Fagen J (eds) Individual differences in infancy: Reliability, stability, prediction.Erlbaum, Hillsdale, NJ, p 321

Bai DL, Bertenthal BI (1992) Locomotor experience and the development of spatial search skills. Child Dev 63: 215-226

Beckwith L, Parmelee AH (1986) EEG patterns of preterm infants, home environment, and later IQ. Child Dev 57: 777-789

Bell MA (1996) Frontal EEG activation in 8-month-old infants during a looking version of the classic A-not-B object permanence task. Paper presented at the annual meeting of the Society for Psychophysiological Research, Vancouver, BC

Bell MA, Fox NA (1992) The relations between frontal brain electrical activity and cognitive development during infancy. Child Dev 63: 1142-1163

Bell MA, Fox NA (1994) Brain development over the first year of life: Relations between electroencephalographic frequency and coherence and cognitive and affective behaviors. In: Dawson G, Fischer KW (eds) Human behavior and the developing brain. Guilford, New York, p. 314

Bell MA, Fox NA (1996) Crawling experience is related to changes in cortical organization during infancy: Evidence from EEG coherence. Dev Psychobiol 29: 551-561

Bell MA, Fox NA (under review) Individual differences in object permanence performance at 8 months: Locomotor experience and brain electrical activity. Manuscript under review

Bell MA, Schmauder AR (1994) Electrophysiological correlates of language development during infancy: a case study [Abstract]. Psychophysiology 31: s25

Bell MA, Schmauder AR (1995). Frontal lobe development from 6 to10 months of age: An EEG case study. Paper presented at the Society for Research in Child Development, Indianapolis

Berger H (1929) Über das Elektroenkephalogramm des menshen. Arch Psychiat Nervenkr 87: 527-570

Berger H (1932) Über das Elektroenkephalogramm des menshen. V., Arch Psychiat Nervenk 98: 231-254

Bertenthal BI, Campos JJ (1990) A system approach to the organizing effects of self-produced locomotion during infancy. In: Rovee-Collier C, Lipsitt LP (eds)Advances in infancy research Vol. 6. ABLEX, Norwood, NJ, p 1

Bertenthal BI, Campos JJ, Kermoian R (1994) An epigenetic perspective on the development of self-produced locomotion and its consequences. Curr Dir Psychol Sci 5: 140-145

Black JE, Greenough WT (1986) Induction of pattern in neural structure by experience: Implications for cognitive development. In: Lamb ME, Brown AL, Rogoff B (eds) Advances in developmental psychology Vol. 4. Erlbaum: Hillsdale NJ, p 1

Calkins SD, Fox NA, Marshall TR (1996) Behavioral and physiological antecedents of inhibited and uninhibited behavior. Child Dev 67: 523-540

Campos JJ, Kermoian R, Zumbahlen MR (1992) Socioemotional transformations in the family system following infant crawling onset. In: Eisenberg N, Fabes RA (eds) New directions for child development. No. 55. Fossey-Bass, San Francisco, p 25

Case R (1992) The role of the frontal lobes in the regulation of cognitive development. Brain Cognition 20: 51-73

Chugani HT (1994) Development of regional brain glucose metabolism in relation to behavior and plasticity. In: Dawson G, Fischer KW (eds) Human behavior and the developing brain. Guilford, New York, p.153

Chugani HT, Phelps ME (1986) Maturational changes in cerebral function in infants determined by FDG Positron Emission Tomography. Science 231: 840-843

Chugani HT, Phelps ME, Mazziotta JC (1987) Positron emission tomography study of human brain functional development. Ann Neurol 27: 1178-1188

Corbin HPF, Bickford RG (1955) Studies of the electroencephalogram of normal children: Comparison of visual and automatic frequency analyses. Electroencephalogr Clin Neurophysiol 7: 15-28

Crawford HJ, Barabasz M (1996) Quantitative EEG magnitudes in children with and without attention deficit disorder during neurological screening and cognitive tasks. Child Study J 26: 71-86

Davidson RJ (1992) Anterior cerebral asymmetry and the nature of emotion. Brain Cognition 20: 125-151

Davidson RJ, Fox NA (1982) Asymmetrical brain activity discriminates between positive versus negative affective stimuli in human infants. Science 218: 1235-1237

Davidson RJ, Fox NA (1989) Frontal brain asymmetry predicts infants' response to maternal separation. J Abn Psychol 98: 127-131

Dawson G (1994) Development of emotional expression and emotion regulation in infancy: Contributions of the frontal lobe. In: Dawson G, Fischer KW (eds), Human behavior and the developing brain. Guilford, New York, p 346

Dawson G, Panagiotides H, Grofer Klinger L, Hill D (1992) The role of frontal lobe functioning in the development of self-regulatory behavior in infancy. Brain Cognition 20: 152-175

Diamond A (1985) Development of the ability to use recall to guide action, as indicated by infants' performance on AB. Child Dev 56: 868-883

Diamond A (1988) Abilities and neural mechanisms underlying AB performance. Child Dev 59: 523-527

Diamond A (1990a) Developmental time course in human infants and infant monkeys, and the neural bases, of inhibitory control in reaching. In: Diamond A (ed) The development and neural bases of higher cognitive functions. New York Academy of Sciences Press, New York, p 637
Diamond A (1990b) The development and neural bases of memory functions as indexed by the AB and Delayed Response tasks in human infants and infant monkeys. In: Diamond A (ed) The development and neural bases of higher cognitive functions. New York Academy of Sciences Press, New York, p 267
Diamond A, Goldman-Rakic PS (1983) Comparison of performance on a Piagetian object permanence task in human infants and rhesus monkeys" Evidence for involvement of prefrontal cortex. Society for Neuroscience Abstracts 9: 641
Diamond A, Goldman-Rakic PS (1986) Comparative development in human infants and infant rhesus monkeys of cognitive functions that depend on prefrontal cortex. Society for Neuroscience Abstracts 12: 742
Diamond A, Goldman-Rakic PS (1989) Comparison of human infants and rhesus monkeys on Piaget's AB task: Evidence for dependence on dorsolateral prefrontal cortex. Exp Brain Res 74: 24-40
Diamond A, Zola-Morgan S, Squire LR (1989) Successful performance by monkeys with lesions of the hippocampal formation on AB and Object Retrieval, two tasks that mark developmental changes in human infants. Behav Neurosci 103: 526-537
Dreyfus-Brisac C (1964) The electroencephalogram of the premature infant and full-term newborn. In: Kellaway P, Petersen I (eds) Neurological and electroencephalographic correlative studies in infancy. Grune and Stratton, New York, p 186
Dreyfus-Brisac C, Monod N (1975) The electroencephalogram of full-term new borns and premature infants. In: Lairy GC (ed) Handbook of electroencephalography and clinical neurophysiology: Volume 6. The normal EEG throughout life. Elsevier, Amsterdam, p 6B-6.
Duffy FH, Als H, McAnualty GB (1990) Behavioral and electrophysiological evidence for gestational age effects in healthy preterm and fullterm infants studies two weeks after expected due dates. Child Dev 61: 1271-1286
Eeg-Olofsson O (1971) The development of the EEG in normal young persons from the age of 16 through 21 years. Neuropadiatrie 2
Ellingson RJ (1958) Electroencephalograms of normal, full-term newborns immediately after birth with observations on arousal and visual evoked responses. Electroencephalogr Clin Neurophysiol 10: 31-50
Ellingson RJ, Peters JF (1980) Development of EEG and daytime sleep patterns in low risk premature infants during the first year of life: Longitudinal observations. Electroencephalogr Clin Neurophysiol 50: 165-171
Epstein HT (1980) EEG developmental stages. Dev Psychobiol 13: 629-631
FeinG et al (1984) EEG spectra in 9-13 year old boys are stable 103 years. Electroencephalogr Clin Neurophysiol 58: 517-518
Fischer KW (1987) Relations between brain and cognitive development. Child Dev 58: 623-632
Fischer KW, Rose SP (1994) Dynamic development of coordination of components in brain and behavior: A framework for theory and research. In: Dawson G, Fischer KW (eds) Human behavior and the developing brain. Guilford, New York, p 3
Fox NA, Bell MA (1990) Electrophysiological indices of frontal lobe development: relations to cognitive and affective behavior in human infants over the first year of life. In: Diamond A (ed) The development and neural bases of higher cognitive functions. New York Academy of Sciences, New York, p 677
Fox NA, Bell MA, Jones NA (1992) Individual differences in response to stress and cerebral asymmetry. Dev Neuropsychol 7: 161-184
Fox NA, Davidson RJ (1987) EEG asymmetry in ten month old infants in response to approach of a stranger and maternal separation. Dev Psychol 23: 233-240
Fox NA, Davidson RJ (1988) Patterns of brain electrical activity during the expression of discrete emotions in ten month old infants. Dev Psychol 24: 230-236
Gasser T, et al (1985) Test-retest reliability of spectral parameters of EEG. Electroencephalogr Clin Neurophysiol 60: 312-319
Gevins AS (1989) Dynamic functional typography of cognitive tasks. BrainTopogr 2: 37-56
Gibbs FA, Knott JR (1949) Growth of the electrical activity of the cortex. Electroencephalogr Clin Neurophysiol 1: 223-229
Greenough WT, Black JE (1992) Induction of brain structure by experience: Substrates for cognitive development. In: Gunnar MR, Nelson CA (eds) Developmental behavioral neuroscience: The Minnesota Symposia on Child Psychology. Vol. 24. Erlbaum, Hillsdale, NJ, p 155
Greenough WT, Black JE, Wallace C (1987) Effects of experience on brain development. Child Dev 58: 540-559
Griesel RD, Belciug M, Richter LM (1992) Changes in brain function accompanying behavioural maturation. S A Tydsk Wetenskap 88:147-153
Hagne I (1968) Development of the waking EEG in normal infants during the first year of life. In: Kellaway P, Petersen I (eds) Clinical electroencephalography of children. Grune & Stratton, New York, p 97
Hagne I (1972) Development of the EEG in normal infants during the first year of life. Acta Ped Scand, (Suppl) 232: 25-53
Hagne I, Persson J, Magnusson R, Petersen I. (1973) Spectral analysis via fast fourier transform of waking EEG in normal infants. In: Kellaway P, Petersen I (eds) Automation of clinical EEG. Raven Press, New York
Henry JR (1944) Electroencephalograms of normal children. Monographs of the Society for Research in Child Development 9 (3 Serial No 39)
Hudspeth WJ, Pribram KH (1990) Stages of brain and cognitive maturation. J Educa Psychol 82: 881-884
Hudspeth WJ, Pribram KH (1992) Psychophysiological indices of cerebral maturation. Int J Psychophysiol 12: 19-29
Huttenlocher PR (1979) Synaptic density of human frontal cortex: Developmental changes and effects of aging. Brain Res 163: 195-205
Huttenlocher PR (1990) Morphometric study of human cerebral cortex development. Neuropsychologia 28: 517-527
Huttenlocher PR (1994) Synaptogenesis in human cerebral cortex. In: Dawson G, Fischer KW (eds) Human behavior and the developing brain. Guilford, New York, p 137
Ioffe S, Chernick V (1990) Prediction of subsequent motor and mental retardation in newborn infants exposed to alcohol in utero by computerized EEG analysis. Neuropediatrics 21: 11-17
John ER, Ahn H, Prichep L, Trepetin M, Brown D, Kaye H (1980) Developmental equations for the electroencephalogram. Science 210: 1255-1258

Kermoian R, Campos JJ (1988) Locomotor experience: A facilitator of spatial cognitive development. Child Dev 59: 908-917

Kuks JBM, Vos JE, O'Brien MJ (1988) EEG coherence functions for normal newborns in relation to their sleep state. Neurophysiology 69: 295-302

Lindsley DB (1939) A longitudinal study of the occipital alpha rhythm in normal children: Frequency and amplitude standards. J Gen Psychol 55: 197-213

Lukashevich IP, Machinskaya RI, Fishman MN (1994) Determination of brain function in young school children with learning problems. Hum Physiol 20: 353-358

Matousek M, Petersen I (1973) Frequency analysis of the EEG in normal children and adolescents. In: Kellaway P, Petersen I (eds) Automation of clinical electroencephalography. Raven Press, New York, p 75.

Milner B (1982) Some cognitive effects of frontal-lobe lesions in man. Phil Trans Roy Soc Lond 298: 211-226

Mizuno T, Yamaguchi N, Iinuma K, Arakawa T (1970) Maturation of patterns of EEG: Basic waves of healthy infants under 12 months of age. Tohoku J Exp Med 102: 91-98

Nunez P (1981) Electrical fields of the brain. Oxford, New York

Ohtahara S (1964) Development of electroencephalogram during infancy and childhood. Proc Jap EEG Soc 18-23

Ohtahara S (1981) Neurophysiological development during infancy and childhood. In: Yamaguchi N, Fujisawa F (eds) Recent advances in EEG and EMG data processing. Elsevier, Amsterdam, p. 369

Oller DK (1986) Metaphonology and infant vocalizations. In: Lindblom B, Zetterstrom R (eds) Precursors of early speech. Macmillan, Basingstroke, Hampshire, p 21

Oller DK, Seibert JM (1988) Babbling of prelinguistic mentally retarded children. Am J Mental Retard 92: 369-375

Otero GA (1994) EEG spectral analysis in children with sociocultural handicaps. Int J Neurosci 79: 213-220

Parmelee AH, Wenner WH, Akiyama Y, Stern E, Flescher J (1967) Electroencephalography and brain maturation. In: Minkowski A (ed) Regional development of the brain in early life. Davis, Philadelphia, p 459

Petersen I, Eeg-Olofsson O (1971) The development of the electroencephalogram in normal children from the age of 1 through 15 years: Non-paroxysmal activity. Neuropadiatrie 2: 247-301

Pribram KH (1973) The primate frontal cortex: Executive of the brain. In: Pribram KH, Luria AR (eds) Psychophysiology of the frontal lobes. Academic, New York, p 293

Richards JE, Parmelee AH, Beckwith L (1986) Spectral analysis of infant EEG and behavioral outcome at age five. Electroencephalogr Clin Neurophysiol 64: 1-11

Samson-Dollfus D, Forthomme J, Capron E (1964) EEG of the human infant during sleep and wakefulness during the first year of life. In: Kellaway P, Petersen I(eds) Neurological and electroencephalographic correlative studies in infancy. Grune and Stratton, New York, p 208

Scher MS, Sun M, Steppe DA, Banks DL, Guthrie RD, Sclabassi RJ (1994) Comparisons of EEG sleep state-specific spectral values between healthy full-terms and perterm infants at comparable postconceptional ages. Sleep 17: 47-51

Schmauder AR, Bell MA (1995) EEG, brain and language development: A case study. In: MacLaughlin D, McEwen S (eds) Proceedings of the 19th annual Boston University conference on language development. Casacadilla, Somerville, MA, p 533

Smith JR (1938a) The electroencephalogram during normal infancy and childhood: I. Rhythmic activities present in the neonate and their subsequent development. J Gen Psychol 53: 431-453

Smith JR (1938b) The electroencephalogram during normal infancy and childhood: II. The nature and growth of the alpha waves. J Gen Psychol 53: 455-469

Smith JR (1939) The "occipital" and "pre-central" alpha rhythms during the first two years. The J Psychol 7: 223-226

Smith JR (1941) The frequency growth of the human alpha rhythms during normal infancy and childhood. J Psychol 11: 177-198

Somsen RJM, van 't Klooster BJ (1994) Growth spurts in the EEG? Paper presented at the annual meeting of the Society for Psychophysiological Research, Atlanta, GA

Tharp BR (1986) Neonatal and pediatric electroencephalography. In: Aminoff MJ (ed) Electrodiagnosis in clinical neurology,2nd ed. Churchill Livingstone, New York, p 77

Tharp BR (1990) Electrophysiological brain maturation in premature infants: An historical perspective. J Clin Neurophysiol 7: 302-314

Thatcher RW (1991) Maturation of the human frontal lobes: Physiological evidence for staging. Dev Neuropsychol 7: 397-419

Thatcher RW (1994a) Cyclic cortical reorganization: Origins of human cognitive development. In: Dawson G, Fischer KW (eds) Human behavior and the developing brain. Guilford, New York, p 232

Thatcher RW (1994b) Psychopathology of early frontal lobe damage: Dependence on cycles of development. Dev Psychopathol 6: 565-596

Thatcher RW, Krause PJ, Hrybyk M (1986) Cortico-cortical associtions and EEG coherence: A two-compartmental model. Electroencephalogr Clin Neurophysiol 64: 123-143

Thatcher RW, Walker RA, Giudice S (1987) Human cerebral hemspheres develop at different rates and ages. Science 236: 1110-1113

Wilson FAW, O-Scalaidhe SP, Goldman-Rakic PS (1993) Dissociation of object and spatial processing domains in primate prefrontal cortex. Science 260: 1955-1958

8. Auditory evoked potentials (N1 wave) as indices of cortical development

N. BRUNEAU, M. GOMOT

The neurophysiology of sensory and cognitive processing can be studied with a high degree of temporal resolution by recording evoked potentials (EPs) on the scalp. These potentials are extracted from the EEG by averaging a number of EEG samples time-locked to the event. They offer the possibility of measuring the function of numerous neural systems in a completely noninvasive fashion. Moreover, evoked potentials can be assessed in paradigms which do not require the active participation of the subject. These advantages make them easily applicable to children and therefore particularly suitable for the study of normal and abnormal brain development. One of the most important uses of EPs is assessment of auditory function. Applications are quite extensive, particularly in developmental disorders. Indeed, in disorders such as those including language and communicative impairment, it is important to identify the possible disturbances which can affect various levels of the central auditory system.

A series of EP measurements is available for assessment of neural activity elicited by auditory stimuli. The most commonly used classification of auditory evoked potentials (AEPs) is based upon the latency of the responses and their sensitivity to auditory stimulus parameters (Regan, 1989; Picton, 1990) and can be summarised as follows. Brainstem AEPs, present during the first 15 ms following an auditory stimulus, provide a measurement of the functional integrity of the peripheral and brainstem auditory pathways. Middle-latency AEPs, present between 15 to 80 ms, represent the initial activation of the auditory cortex. Slow AEPs are several hundred ms in duration and represent continued cortical processing mainly related to the physical properties of the stimulus. They include a negative phase (N1) followed by a positive one (P2) that peak at about 100 and 200 ms respectively in adults. Late AEPs comprise cerebral activity associated with perceptual and cognitive operations. These potentials include several negative and positive deflections which overlap or follow the slow auditory evoked potentials (Picton and Hillyard, 1988). Their application to developmental studies of both normal and abnormal cognitive processes is reviewed in Courchesne (1990), Steinschneider et al (1992) and Taylor (1995).

This chapter will focus on slow AEPs and particularly on the N1 wave which reflects the initial sensory registration of the auditory stimuli.

After comments on some methodological aspects of AEP recordings, we review the literature on the N1 wave in adults and in children; thereafter, we present our recent data demonstrating the usefulness of this electrophysiological response as a tool for studying normal brain maturation. We then finish with a review of applications of the N1 wave in the study of developmental disorders with particular focus on language impairment and autism.

Methodological issues

The study of evoked potentials was previously limited to analysis of waveforms (peak latency, amplitude) recorded at a few electrode locations. By recording AEP simultaneously from multiple scalp electrodes, the scalp distribution of the potential field can be obtained at different selected time.

Despite the value of scalp potential topography in developmental studies — as will be shown later in this chapter — these studies are not always possible, particularly in child psychiatry. Indeed these patients, particularly the very disturbed, do not accept long electrode placement procedures or reject the cap used for multielectrode recordings. In these cases, recordings using a few electrodes are the only possibility. Normative topographical data can thus provide information guiding the choice of optimal electrode location for picking up the expected responses according to age.

Another important consideration in electrode positioning is the location of the reference electrode. Indeed, evoked potentials are obtained using a monopolar montage which allows recording of the potential difference between the active electrode placed on the scalp — i.e., over active neural tissue — and the "inactive" reference electrode, placed over an area of minimal electrical activity. However, no electrode location is completely inactive. The results must therefore be interpreted according to the location of the reference chosen.

Evoked potential brain mapping is based on averaged EPs recorded simultaneously from multiple electrodes. Mapping is achieved by interpolating values obtained at each electrode site. Different interpolating algorithms can be used. The 4-nearest neighbours method (Shepard, 1968) is easy to calculate but it implies that extreme values are always located at electrode sites, leading to discontinuities in isovoltage surface representation. These problems are not found when using spline interpolation algorithms (Perrin et al., 1987, 1989).

At a selected time, scalp potential distribution constitutes a surface field which results from overlapping activities from multiple sources in the brain. This is therefore a limitation to the interpretation of the maps in terms of the origins of the features observed. The resolution of scalp topography is considerably improved by using scalp current density (SCD) mapping. These maps are obtained by computing the second spatial (Laplacian) derivative (Perrin et al., 1987, 1989) of the interpolated potential distribution. SCDs have the property of being reference-free, and of having sharper peaks and valleys than scalp potential distributions. This facilitates interpretation in cases in which there are multiple overlapping components.

Other methods have been developed to increase the localising power of noninvasive electrophysiological methods. The most widely used is searching for a current source location and time course that could plausibly account for EP fields on the scalp. In these spatio temporal modelling procedures (Scherg and von Cramon 1985, 1986), the source distribution is modelled by several equivalent current dipole (ECD) and a nonlinear least squares minimisation is used to estimate ECD parameters. The method determines both the best fitting location and orientation for the different ECD, and computes the strength of each ECD over the time course considered. Neuroanatomical locations of the generators can then be defined by superimposing the ECD on brain imaging provided by MRI.

N1 wave in normal development

The N1 wave in adults

Description of components

The N1 wave is the most prominent deflection of the AEP in human adults. It was classically described as a broad negative deflection maximally recorded at frontocentral sites and culminating approximately 100 msec after stimulus onset. There are now several lines of evidence indicating that a number of components representing different cerebral processes occur in the latency range of the N1 wave (Näätänen and Picton, 1987; Woods, 1995). Wolpaw and Penry (1975) first suggested that the N1 wave consisted of midline and temporal components. They described a positive-negative response negative (Ta-Tb) response named the "T complex" with peaks occurring at about 100 and 150 msec respectively, distributed around the midtemporal areas. The terminology introduced by McCallum and Curry (1980) is commonly used to describe the deflections recorded in the N1 latency range and is adopted in this chapter (Fig. 1). N1b refers to the negative frontocentral wave peaking around 100 ms, N1a and N1c refer to the successive negative waves recorded from temporal electrodes, peaking at approximately 80 and 150 ms respectively and separated by a positive deflection peaking around 100 msec. According to Wolpaw and Penry's nomenclature, this positive deflection corresponds to Ta and the subsequent negative deflection N1c to Tb.

Therefore, the terminology "N1 wave" does not correspond to a specific deflection but to the three deflections previously described (N1a, N1b, N1c) which occurred in the 80-200 ms latency period.

Brain structures involved in the generation of the different components recorded in the N1 latency range.

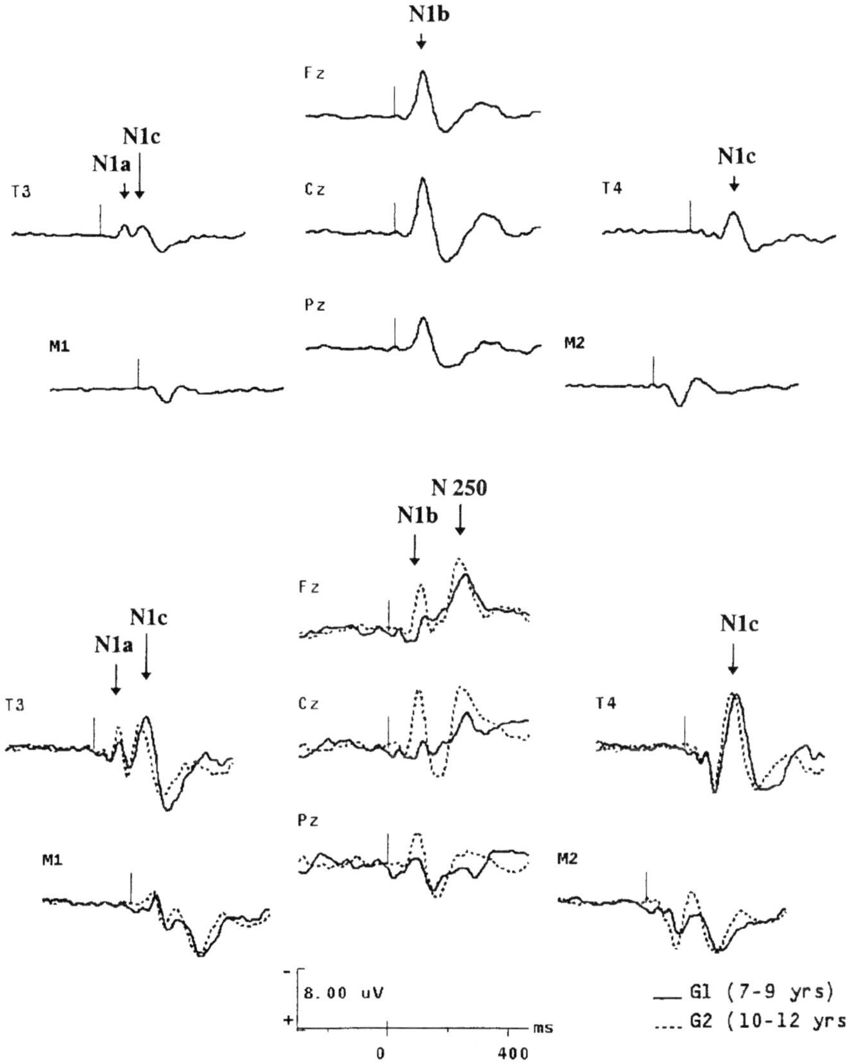

Fig. 1
Grand average AEPs across subjects for left ear tone stimuli (750 Hz, 200 ms, 70 dB SPL) (N= 8 adults , 8 children aged 7- 9-years and 8 children aged 10- 12 years).
At midline electrodes: 1) N1b clearly emerges up to 10 years 2) N 250 is mainly recorded in children.
At temporal electrodes: 1) N1a is recorded on left side at all ages 2) N1c is of larger amplitude in children than in adults.
At mastoïde electrodes: Positive deflections are recorded at the latency peak of N1b and N 250.

Although until recently the subject of debate, localisation of the generators responsible for the different components elicited in the N1 latency range has been clarified in adults (Näätänen and Picton, 1987; Woods, 1995). Electrical and magnetic studies have provided evidence that the N1b component originates, at least in part, from generators in the supratemporal plane of the auditory cortex (Vaughan and Ritter, 1970; Peronnet et al., 1974; Hari et al., 1980; Scherg and Von Cramon, 1985, 1986). Nonspecific brain regions (Hari et al., 1982; Velasco and Velasco, 1986) and particularly frontal areas (Alcaini et al., 1994, Giard et al., 1994) are also involved. Data from lesioned patients also indicate that N1b generation involves the postero superior temporal plane near the temporo parietal junction (Woods et al., 1993). The generation of the N1c component recorded at temporal sites involves sources in the secondary auditory cortex on the lateral part of the temporal lobe. This conclusion derives from results of the intracerebral recordings (Celesia 1976), the scalp distribution analysis (Wood and Wolpaw, 1982) and cortical recordings in lesioned patients (Woods et al., 1993).

Scherg and Von Cramon (1985, 1986), using a spatio-temporal dipole model, suggested that scalp-recorded AEP activity in the N1 latency range could be modelled by two bilateral superotemporal lobe sources, one source oriented vertically (tangentially to the lateral surface of the skull) and the other horizontally (radially). The first should correspond to the activation of the supratemporal area which generates the frontocentral N1b, the second corresponds to the activation of the lateral surface of the temporal lobe and generates a somewhat later negative wave with maximal amplitude over the temporal scalp, i.e., N1c.

Several groups (Mc Callum and Curry, 1980; Knight et al., 1988; Woods et al., 1993) interpret the hemisphere asymmetry of the N1a component (L>R) as suggesting possible generation in the planum temporale, which is larger in the left hemisphere (Steinmetz et al., 1989).

The N1 wave in normal children

Review of N1 wave studies in children

The influence of maturation on the different cortical responses evoked in the N1 latency range has not yet been elucidated. Topographical studies of auditory evoked responses to speech sounds by Kurtzberg et al., (1984) through the first 2 years of life demonstrate two distinct but spatiotemporally overlapping waveforms. One is maximal frontocentrally maximum and extends over most of the frontal portion of the head; the other is similar in general waveform but longer in latency and largest over the lateral portions of the head, overlying the superior temporal gyrus. Studying responses to click stimulation in preterm infants, Weitzman and Graziani (1968) also reported such lateral/midline dissociation of the waveforms. Relatively few developmental data have been reported on the different components of the auditory evoked responses throughout childhood. Most of the information has been obtained from electrodes positioned on midline or near-midline sites and has emphasised the lack of reliability of midline auditory responses in the 80-250 ms latency range (Allison et al., 1984; Callaway and Halliday, 1973; Courchesne, 1977, 1978; Goodin et al., 1978; Johnson, 1989; Martin et al., 1988; Polich et al., 1990); all of these studies indicate that there are longer peak latencies in children than in adults. In one study, responses were recorded from a coronal chain of electrodes (De Crévoisier et al., 1975); the N1 wave was of greater amplitude and longer latency at temporal sites than at the vertex in 2- 12-year-old children.

In a recent study (Bruneau et al., 1997), we therefore focussed on the 4- 8-year-old period to clarify frontocentral and temporal components of the N1 wave at this age. The effect of stimulus intensity was used in order to facilitate the dissociation of the different components. Indeed in adults, the different components of the N1 wave are differentially affected by stimulus intensity. N1b displays an increase in amplitude and a decrease in latency with increasing stimulus intensity, but these effects decline as higher levels of intensity are reached (Picton et al., 1970, 1977; Prescott et al., 1984; Bruneau et al., 1985) whereas temporal responses were reported to be minimally affected by stimulus intensity (Cacace et al., 1988; Connolly, 1993; Wolpaw and Cacace, 1994). Therefore, the use of stimuli of different intensities may be a means of ascertaining the different components of the N1 wave and their maturation.

Comparison between 4- 8-year-old children and adults indicated strong differences at both frontocentral and temporal sites. In adults, the predominant response is the frontocentral N1b component, whereas in children the predominant response is the temporal N1c. Indeed, at this age, N1c is very reliable, culminates at around 170 ms in children (i.e. later than in adults in whom it is 140 ms), and is modified with increasing stimulus intensity (decreased latency and increased amplitude). Frontocentral N1b in children is of smaller amplitude and less variable than temporal N1c. Significant amplitude differences are found at frontocentral sites according to age: N1b culminates at the frontal site at ages 4-6 years and at ages 6-8 years tends to culminate at the vertex. It would be hypothesised that these age-related differences in frontocentral amplitude to reflect development in scalp potential distribution of N1b, with negativity shifting from frontal to central sites with increasing age. Scalp potential distributions are needed to clarify this hypothesis.

The effect of stimulus intensity on frontocentral N1b was strong in adults. In children this effect was very slight and preferentially recorded at the frontal site, supporting the hypothesis that the frontal negative wave recorded in young children might correspond to N1b.

In summary, the N1 wave in 4- 8-year-old children ("children pattern") mainly comprises predominant temporal N1c components and a small amplitude N1b component which culminates at the frontal sites in young children.

Few data are available on scalp potential topography of the N1 wave in children. The distribution of the frontocentral N1 wave (N1b) in 8- 16-year-old children was reported to be similar to that of adults (Borg et al., 1988; Tonnquist-Uhlén et al., 1995). Therefore we studied scalp potential distribution of the different components of the N1 wave between 7 and 12 years in order to assess the transition from the "children's pattern" to the adult-like pattern previously reported as beginning from 8 years onwards.

Scalp potential distribution of N1b and N1c in 7-12-year-old children

This on-going study includes to date 16 children ranging from 7 to 12 years of age and 8 young adults. All subjects were right-handed.

The stimuli were 750 Hz tone bursts of 200 ms duration (5 ms rise/fall time) delivered monaurally (left and right ears) with a random interstimulus interval varying from 1 to 2 s. Intensities were 50 and 70 dB SPL. Each subject received a run of 400 randomised stimuli, 100 for each intensity and each ear. Maps were obtained using linear interpolations. Evoked potentials were recorded from 28 Ag-AgCl scalp electrodes referenced to the nose, 19 placed according to the 10-20 International System, the other 9 at additional intermediate locations. Horizontal and vertical ocular movements were also recorded. Only data obtained at 70 dB SPL are reported in this preliminary presentation.

We will successively describe evolution of AEP waveforms and topographic changes of the different waves according to age.

The Top of the Fig. 1 shows grand mean AEPs in adults. Responses are similar to those classically described. At temporal sites two negative waves, N1a and N1c, occurred with peak latencies around 70 and 140 ms respectively which precede and follow the latency of the prominent vertex N1b which culminates at 95 ms. A positive deflection occurs at mastoid sites at around the same peak latency as N1b.

The lower part of the Fig. 1 shows superimposition of AEPs recorded on children aged 7-9 years and 10-12 years. Waveforms differed according to age at frontocentral sites. Up to 10 years, children displayed a large frontocentral N1b component, culminating at the vertex, similar to that recorded in adults in both amplitude and peak latency (95 ms). In younger children aged 7-9 this response displayed smaller amplitude and longer peak latency (110 ms) than in older children. Following N1b, both groups of children displayed a large frontocentral negative wave peaking at around 250-260 ms. A late negative wave was also recorded after N1b in adults, but was of smaller amplitude and longer latency than that of children. This late fronto-central negative response will be described in detail in paragraph III.3. Waveforms at temporal sites did not vary wit age in children. A first negative component (N1a) was specifically recorded on the left side, followed by a second negative component (N1c) on both sides. Their peak latencies decreased from ages 7-9 to ages 10-12 (approximately from 75 ms to 70 ms for N1a and from 170 ms to 150 ms for N1c). However, in contrast to N1b, adult values (145 ms) were not reached for N1c at 10-12 years. Peak amplitudes in children did not vary with age. Although similar in waveform, the temporal responses in children were much greater than in adults.

Figure 2 (left part) shows the mean scalp potential distribution of N1b according to age. Maps were plotted of the latency of the peak at Cz. N1b topography presents similar characteristics in both children and adults, with the highest negative amplitude over the frontocentral regions and positive potentials over the temporomastoid sites. The maps disclosed topographical changes from childhood to adulthood. The negative potential fields over the frontocentral regions became broader with increasing age whereas the broad positive potential fields over the temporomastoid electrodes narrowed to mastoid site localisation with increasing age.

The temporomastoid positive wave was of higher amplitude on the right than on the left, consistent with preferential right sided activation in children whatever the ear stimulated. In adults, the positivity was of greater amplitude on the contralateral side for left ear stimulation and similar on both sides for right ear stimulation, indicating that the right hemisphere is always activated regardless of which the is ear stimulated.

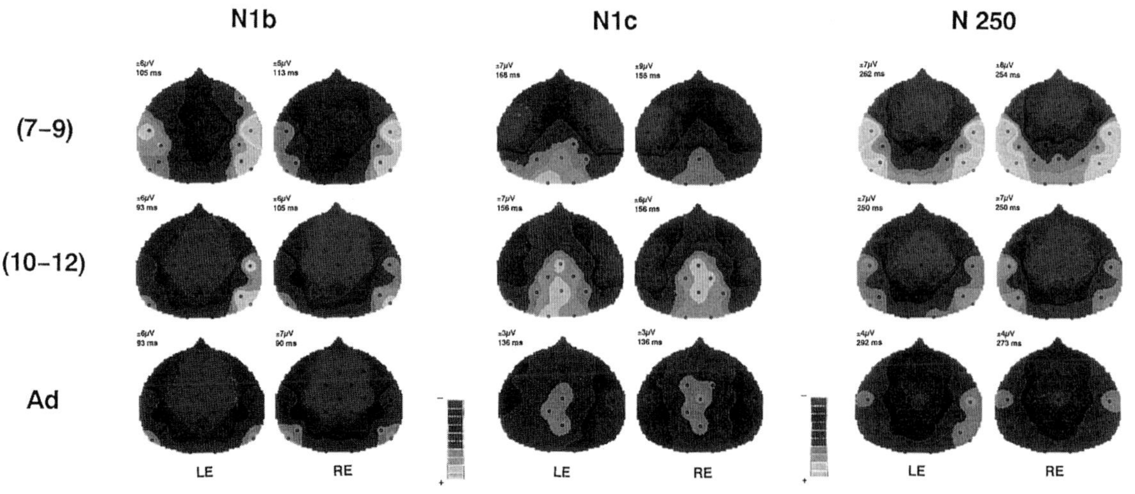

Fig. 2. Mean scalp potential distribution of N1b, N1c and N 250 to left ear (LE) and right ear (RE) tone stimuli in 8 children aged 7- 9-years, 8 children aged 10- 12 years and 8 adults.
Maps are plotted at the peak latency at the vertex for N1b and at the peak latency at the temporal site (T3, T4) contralateral to the ear stimulated for N1c.
For N 250, maps are plotted at the peak latency at Fz in children aged 7-9 and at the peak latency at Cz in children aged 10-12 and in adults. *See colour illustrations appendix.*

Figure 2 (middle part) shows the mean scalp potential distribution of N1c according to age. Maps were plotted of the peak latency of N1c at the temporal electrode contralateral to the stimulated ear.

The maps were characterised by lateral negative wave associated with positivity at posterior midline sites. They disclosed topographical changes with to age. The lateral negative wave shifted from temporofrontal sites at 7-9 years to temporal sites at 10-12 years to reach temporal posterior sites in adults. In parallel, positivity shifted from occipital sites at 7-9 years to parietocentral sites at 10-12 years to reach central sites in adults.

Hemisphere differences varied according to age. N1c showed an asymmetrical scalp distribution, with the largest potential amplitudes over the hemiscalp contralateral to the stimulated ear in 7- 9-year old children. Up to this age, N1c showed a greater distribution on the contralateral side for left ear stimulation whereas a bilateral distribution was obtained after stimulating the right ear.

Discussion

Our findings in adults are in agreement with those classically described. The auditory response mainly involved the N1b deflection around 100 ms after stimulus onset, with the largest negative amplitude at frontocentral electrodes and positive peaks at mastoid sites. The polarity reversal of potential at inferotemporal levels (with the reference electrode at the nose) is consistent with an origin in or near the supratemporal plane of the auditory cortex, as previously reported (Näätänen and Picton, 1987; Woods, 1995 for reviews).

This N1b wave is quite different in children. It is clearly obtained at frontocentral sites up to 10 years with similar characteristics (maximal peak latency, amplitude) to adult N1b. However scalp potential distribution of N1b in children aged 10-12 years is different from that of adults. The distribution of the frontocentral negative wave is similar in both groups, in agreement with data reported by Tonnquist-Uhlèn et al. (1995). However, we found between-group differences in the distribution of temporomastoid positive deflections, which is much more broader in children than in adults. This might indicate differences in the location and/or orientation of the generators of N1b which are thus presumably not completely mature at age 10-12.

The lack of N1b at frontocentral sites in 7- 9-year-old children was also previously reported in younger children aged 4-8 years (Bruneau et al., 1997) and was interpreted as reflecting possible differences in the orientation of the generators of N1b at this age, impeding scalp recording at frontocentral sites. The data presented here from scalp topography provides support for this hypothesis. Indeed, the slight frontocentral negative deflection is associated with a broad positive wave at temporomastoid electrodes which suggest different orientation of generators in the supratemporal plane of the auditory cortex at this age.

Although scalp distribution of N1b in 4- 6-year-old children has not been documented, our previous data (Bruneau et al., 1997) showed larger N1b amplitude at the frontal than at the central site. This allows to suppose an earlier step in the orientation of these temporal generators with a more anteroposterior orientation of the tangential dipole responsible for N1b.

This frontal component could also be interpreted as resulting from activation of generators in the frontal cortex. Indeed, the involvement of such frontal generators in the N1 response of adults was recently demonstrated (Alcaini et al., 1994; Giard et al., 1994) using combined scalp current density and dipole model analyses. The development of the frontocentral negativity with age in children might also be thought to reflect a possible development in these frontal generators. The behavioural evolution observed from 6 years of age could be dependent on the same underlying set of frontally mediated changes which influence the evolution of frontal electrical activity. Cognitive development studies have shown that up to 6 years, substantial improvements are evident in functions controlled by the frontal system such as executive and self-reflexive capabilities which are essential for high level cognitive activity in humans (Stuss, 1992; Chelune and Baer, 1986; Griffin, 1992; Passler et al., 1985; Case, 1992). The frontal prominence of the N1 wave in young children could also be interpreted in the light of the frontal response enhancement observed by Knight et al. (1980) in adults with frontal lesions. This enhancement has been interpreted as reflecting suppression of frontal inhibitory influences on the generation of the N1 auditory response. The pattern obtained in 4- 6-year-old children (Fz>Cz) is compatible with a hypothesis of immature inhibitory frontal functioning which develops subsequently. It has been shown that myelination of the frontal lobes (Yakovlev and Lecours 1967) and synaptic density counts of the frontal cortex (Huttenlocher, 1979; Huttenlocher, 1990) do not appear to be completely mature until adolescence.

Scalp potential distribution of N1c is clearly different from that of N1b. Moreover, like N1b, it evolves with age. Our findings in adults are in accord with those previously reported (Wood and Wolpaw, 1982). The negative potentials over the temporal areas with positive potentials over central sites suggest a more radial distribution for the generators of N1c than for those of N1b. This is consistent with a previous hypothesis suggesting generation of N1c in the lateral surface of the superior temporal plane (Näätänen and Picton, 1987; Woods, 1995) as supported by data from intracerebral recordings (Celesia, 1976) and cortical recordings in lesioned patients (Woods et al., 1993).

Our data clearly show changes in scalp potential distribution of N1c with age: the lateral negative deflection shifts an anteroposterior direction, whereas the midline positive wave shifts from occipital to central, consistent with evolution of the location and/or orientation of the generators with age. As for N1b, generators underlying N1c are thus not completely mature at 10-12 years.

Scalp potential distribution of N1a was not considered in this study. At the peak latency of N1a (70 ms), there is overlapping of N1a with the ascending part of N1b. Studies of waveforms have indicated that in both children and adults, N1a predominates on the left which ear is stimulated. This was previously found in adults (Knight et al., 1988; Woods et al., 1993) and proposed as consistent with possible generation in the planum temporale which is larger in the left hemisphere (Steinmetz et al, 1989).

All of these findings suggest age-related differences in location and/or orientation of neural generators contributing to scalp recorded potentials N1b and N1c. This could be linked to changes in the relative geometry of the brain and skull during development (Dekaban, 1970; Giedd et al., 1996) and/or to differences in cortical myelination between the 8 years of age and adulthood, as described by Jernigan and Tallal (1990). Moreover, the recording of responses from the temporal association cortex is perhaps easier in children whose temporal bone window is thinner than in adults. This characteristic also facilitates recording of other physiological parameters such as cerebral blood flow velocity in the middle cerebral artery by transcranial Doppler ultrasonography in children (Bruneau et al., 1992).

A final aspect worthy of comment is the age-related hemisphere differences according to which ear is stimulated. Although not detailed in this chapter, preliminary results indicate that differences exist according to age. Detailed measurement will be very valuable to assess maturation of lateralisation.

N 250: a component of AEP specific of children

Following the components evoked in the N1 latency range, waveforms of children clearly show a late negative wave which culminates at frontocentral sites at approximately 250 ms (Fig. 1). This might correspond to the small negative wave recorded at the frontocentral site in adults which culminates later (around 280 ms) than in children. It was recorded on both groups of children but culminated at frontal sites in younger children and at the vertex up to 10 years. Figure 2 (right part) shows the scalp potential distribution of the grand average N 250 elicited by left and right ear tones on both groups of children, at the peak latency at Fz for 7- 9-year-old children and at the peak latency at Cz for 10- 12-year-old children.

The maps are characterised by broad negative potential fields over the frontocentral regions and positive potentials at mastoid sites. Moreover, the scalp distribution of N250 is symmetrical. The amplitude of the positive wave and its distribution are similar on both sides, which ever ear is stimulated.

The distribution of N 250 is therefore similar to that of N1b. Both showed polarity reversals of potential at inferotemporal levels, consistent with an origin in the supratemporal plane of the auditory cortex. The functional significance of such prominent N 250 elicited in passive conditions in children remains to be elucidated. Either this step in the auditory processing is specific to children or it also exists in adults but the orientation of the generators involved in such processing does not allow recordings on the scalp. As previously discussed for the N1 wave, the analysis of N 250 using Laplacian methods and dipole localisation analysis will lead to better understanding of the cerebral processes underlying this response recorded in children.

This negative wave has also been reported by several groups studying auditory responses in children with language impairment or attention deficit disorders (Tonnquist-Uhlén, 1996; Korpilahti and Lang, 1994; Satterfield et al., 1994).

N1 wave in developmental disorders

Language disorders

The pathophysiology of language impairment in children with normal pure tone thresholds and without any obvious organic brain lesion is not fully understood. There is probably a close connection between impaired language development and central auditory processing disorders.

Electrophysiological methods have made it possible to show abnormalities in auditory processing in language impaired children. Courchesne and Courchesne (1988) studied children with receptive dysphasia, and reported unusually large amplitude responses for both brain stem components and the late cognitive response P300 (positive parietal wave elicited in detection tasks). No data on the N1 wave were reported but P2, the positive wave which immediately follows N1, was increased. The interesting result was that stimulus rate is a very important parameter for differentiation of dysphasic from normal and autistic children. These neurophysiological findings are consistent with Tallal's theory that dysphasia is linked to impairments in the processing of rapid acoustic information (Tallal and Piercy, 1973, 1978 Tallal et al., 1985).

Few data have been reported on the different components recorded in the N1 latency range. Mason and Mellor (1984) studied the peak to trough N1P2 and P2N2 amplitudes at T3 and T4. A contralateral hemisphere dominance after left or right ear stimulation was found in normal children, whereas amplitude asymmetry, with left hemisphere dominance, was observed in language impaired (LI) children. Dawson et al. (1988, 1989) studied right and left hemisphere speech-related AEPs looking at the latency of the N1 wave, in dysphasic children. Compared to control children, they displayed a reversed (right-dominant) pattern of hemisphere asymmetry unrelated to differences in language ability. This was interpreted as reflecting overactivation of the right hemisphere, which might interfere with normal left-hemisphere language processing, this dysfunction being inherent and stable in dysphasic children. The latency reported around 126 ms, the wide age range studied (6 to 15 years), and electrode locations (midway between C3-T5 and C4-T6) make it difficult to know which component was really studied (N1b or N1c). In a recent study of the topography of the N1 wave in LI children aged 9-15 years, Tonnquist-Uhlén (1996) focussed on responses obtained at temporal sites. The amplitude of Tb (corresponding to N1c) was higher over the hemisphere contralateral to the ear stimulated in both LI and control children but the latency of the peak was significantly longer in the LI group. The explanation proposed is a delay in maturation of the neuronal pathways and synaptic connections in these children. There were also more children without a T complex in the LI group; this was interpreted as indicating selective disturbance of the activity in the central auditory pathways of these children.

Autism

Autism is a behaviourally diagnosed disorder of early onset characterised by severe impairment of social relationships and a failure to develop verbal and nonverbal communicative skills. The inability to modulate sensory input adequately is also striking (Bergman and Escalona, 1949; Goldfarb, 1963; Ornitz and Ritvo, 1968) and has been shown to be a core symptom (Barthélémy et al., 1990, 1997). While all modalities are affected, these deficits are particularly evident in audition. One problem many parents have in the first stages of "knowing that something is wrong" is that some children are initially diagnosed as being deaf due to their lack of response to auditory stimuli, when they are later shown to be autistic. This hyporeactivity is apparent in disregard of both verbal commands and loud sounds. In contrast to this hyporeactivity are markedly exaggerated reactions to auditory stimuli both intense and mild in other children.

Specific neuropathological changes have not been demonstrated in the auditory system of autistic subjects. Brain stem and midlatency AEPs are normal (Courchesne, 1985; Grillon et al., 1989). There are several lines of evidence indicating that late AEPs recorded when subjects perform complex cognitive tasks display abnormalities (Courchesne, 1987). However, the components of the N1 wave which correspond to earlier steps in auditory processing, and whose characteristics are mainly influenced by physical parameters, are of interest. Previous studies have shown that the N1 peak recorded at midline sites displays lower amplitude and a significant shift in peak latency in autistic subjects as compared to controls (Small 1971; Lelord et al., 1973; Novick et al., 1980; Niwa et al., 1983; Courchesne et al., 1985; Martineau et al., 1987; Bruneau et al., 1987; Lincoln et al., 1995). These studies gave data from adults and children aged up to 10 years in whom frontocentral N1 is a reliable response. None reported data on temporal responses. Using the same AEP method as that used in dysphasic children, Dawson et al. (1988, 1989) studied hemisphere differences in the speech related AEP (latency of N1 wave) and found a similar pattern in dysphasic children and autistic children. However, in autistic children, the reversed pattern strongly correlated with poor language ability. It was suggested

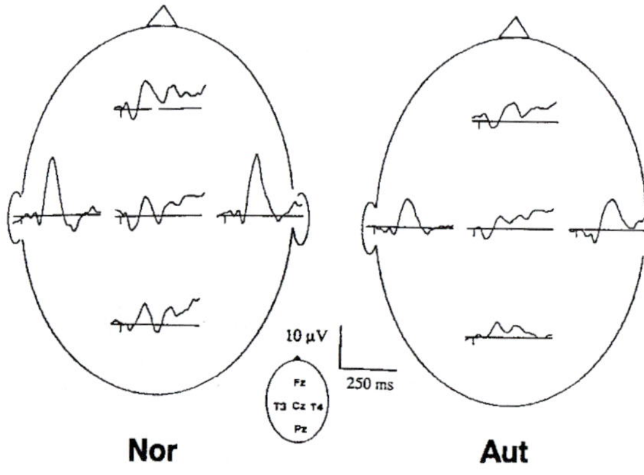

Fig. 3. Grand averaged AEPs across 20 normal (NOR) and 26 autistic (AUT) children for binaural stimuli (750 Hz, 200 ms, 70 dBSPL). All children were 4 - 8 years old.

that reversed asymmetries in autism may reflect transient abnormal function of the language areas of the left hemisphere which changes as the child develops greater language abilities. The left dysfunction is also supported by our data on the temporal N1 responses in 4- 8-year-old autistic children. At this age, normal children display prominent a N1c at temporal sites whereas central N1b is of very small amplitude. Using a similar paradigm to that used in normal children in Bruneau et al (1997) i.e. binaural tone stimuli (750 Hz; 250 ms, varying in intensity from 50 to 80 dB SPL), we showed a lack of significant difference in N1b recorded at midline sites in 4-8-year-old autistic children compared to controls, whereas significant differences were found on N1c recorded at temporal sites: the responses were of smaller amplitude and longer latency in autistic than in controls.

Moreover, the intensity effect found in controls (increasing amplitude and decreasing latency with increasing stimulus intensity) at both temporal sites was not found on the left side in autistic children (Bruneau et al., in preparation). Figure 3 illustrates these results and presents the responses obtained in 26 autistic children compared to 20 normal controls of the same age.

Conclusion

The different components of the AEP which occurred in the 80-200 ms period have been less extensively studied in children than in adults.

Nevertheless the data reported in this chapter indicate that these different auditory responses are useful not only to elucidate the different steps of cortical auditory processing but also to indexe cortical maturation in children. Indeed our findings demonstrate a clear evolution of the scalp potential distribution of the different components of the N1 wave with age. Further studies are necessary using more recent electrophysiological techniques (scalp current density mapping and dipole sources localization) to specify the subcomponents involved in the different components recorded in the N1 latency range and their evolution with age. This have to be studied on larger samples of children with narrow age grouping to obtain more informations on the development of brain organization and function throughout all childhood.

Such approaches will be essential for further studies of possible aberrant development associated with the wide variety of neurobehavioral and language disorders of childhood.

References

Alcaini M, Giard MH, Thévenet M, Pernier J (1994) Two separate frontal components in the N1 wave of the human auditory evoked response. Psychophysiology 31: 611-615

Allison T, Hume AL, Wood CC, Goff WR (1984) Developmental and aging changes in somatosensory, auditory and visual evoked potentials. Electroencephalogr Clin Neurophysiol 58: 14-24

Barthélémy C Adrien JL, Tanguay P, Garreau B, Fermanian J, Roux S, Sauvage D, Lelord G (1990) The Behavioral Summarized Evaluation: validity of reliability of a scale for the assessment of autistic behaviors. J Autism Dev Disord 20: 189-204

Barthélémy C, Roux S, Adrien JL, Hameury L, Guerin P, Garreau B, Lelord G (1997) Validation of the revised Behavior Summarized Evaluation scale (BSE-R). J Autism Dev Disord 27 2: 139-153

Bergman P, Escalona SK (1949) Unusual sensitivities in very young children. Psychoanal Study Child 3-4: 333-352

Borg E, Spens KE, Tonnquist I (1988) Audiology brain mapping, effects of age. Scandinav Audiol (Suppl) 30:161-164

Bruneau N, Dourneau MC, Garreau B, Pourcelot L, Lelord G (1992) Blood flow response to auditory stimulations in normal, mentally retarded, and autistic children: A preliminary transcranial Doppler ultrasonographic study of the middle cerebral arteries. Biol Psychiat 32: 691-699

Bruneau N, Garreau B, Roux S, Lelord G (1987) Modulation of auditory evoked potentials with increasing stimulus intensity in autistic children. In: Johnson R, Parasuraman R, Rohrbaugh JW (eds), Current trends in evoked potential research (EEG Suppl 40). New York: Elsevier, p 584-589

Bruneau N, Roux S, Garreau B, Lelord G (1985) Frontal auditory evoked potentials and augmenting-reducing. Electroencephalogr Clin Neurophysiol 62: 364-371

Bruneau N, Roux S, Guerin P, Barthelemy C (1997) Temporal prominence of auditory evoked potentials in 4-8 year old children. Psychophysiology 34: 32-38

Cacace AT, Dowman R, Wolpaw JR (1988) T complex hemispheric asymmetries: effects of stimulus intensity. Hearing Res 34: 225-232

Callaway E, Halliday RA (1973) Evoked potential variability: Effects of age, amplitude and methods of measurement. Electrencephalogr lin Neurophysiol 34: 125-133

Case R (1992) The role of the frontal lobe in the regulation of cognitive development. Brain Cognition 20: 51-73

Celesia GG (1976) Organization of auditory cortical areas in man. Brain 99: 403-414

Chelune GJ, Baer RA (1986) Developmental norms for the Wisconsin Card Scoring Test. J Clin Exp Neuropsychol 8: 219-228.

Connolly JF (1993) The influence of stimulus intensity, contralateral masking and handedness on the temporal N1 and the T complex components of the auditory N1 wave. Electroencephalogr clin Neurophysiol 86: 58-68

Courchesne E (1977) Event-related brain potentials: Comparison between children and adults. Science 197: 589-592

Courchesne E (1978) Neurophysiological correlates of cognitive: Changes in long-latency event-related potentials

from childhood to adulthood. Electroencephalogr Clin Neurophysiol 45: 468-482.
Courchesne E (1987) A neurophysiological view of autism. In: E Schopler and GB Mesibov (eds). Neurobiological issues in autism, Plenum Publishing Corp, New York, p 285-324
Courchesne E (1990) Chronology of postnatal human brain development: Event related potential, positron emission tomography, myelinogenesis and synaptogenesis studies. In: Rohrbaugh J, Parasuraman R, Johnson R (eds), Event-related brain potentials. Oxford University Press, New York
Courchesne E, Courchesne RY (1988) Event-related brain potentials. In: Rutter M, Tuma AH, Lann IS (eds), Assessment and Diagnosis in Child Psychopathology, Guilford Press, New York: p 265-299
Courchesne E, Courchesne RY, Hicks G, Lincoln AJ (1985) Functioning of the brain stem auditory pathway in non-retarded autistic individuals. Electroencephalogr Clin Neurophysiol 61: 491-501.
Dawson G (1988) Cerebral lateralization in autism: Clues to its role in language and affective development. In: Segalowitz S, Molfese D (eds). Developmental implications of brain lateralization, Guilford, New York
Dawson G, Finley C, Philips S, LEVY A (1989) A comparison of hemispheric asymmetries in speech-related brain potentials of autistic and dysphasic children. Brain Language 37: 26-41
De Crévoisier A, Peronnet F, Girod J, Challet E, Revol M (1975) Topographie des potentiels évoqués auditifs chez l'enfant éveillé. Rev EEG Neurophysiol Clin 45: 303-306
Dekaban A (1970) Developmental anatomy and physiology of the central nervous systems from birth to six years of age. In Williams and Wilkins (eds.), Neurology of early childhood. Baltimore: p 1-49
Giard M, Perrin F, Echallier JF, Thévenet M, Froment JC, Pernier J (1994) Dissociation of temporal and frontal components in the human auditory N1 wave: a scalp current density and dipole model analysis. Electroencephalogr Clin Neurophysiol 92: 238-252
Giedd JN, Snell JW, Lange N, Rajapakse JC, Casey BJ, Kozuch PL, Vaituzis AC, Vauss YC, Hamburger SD, Kaysen D, Rapoport JL (1996) Quantitative magnetic resonance imaging of human brain development: ages 4-18. Cerebral Cortex 6: 551-560
Goldfarb W (1963) Self-awareness in schizophrenic children. Arch gen Psychiat 8: 47-60
Goodin DS, Squires C, Henderson BH, Starr A (1978) Age-related variations in evoked potentials to auditory stimuli in normal human subjects. Electroencephalogr Clin Neurophysiol 44: 447-458
Griffin SA (1992) Young children's awareness of their inner world: a neo-structural analysis of the development of intrapersonal intelligence. In: Case R (ed.) The mind's staircase: exploring the conceptual underspinnings of children's thought and knowledge. Erlbaum. Hillsdale NJ p 189-206
Grillon C, Courchesne E, Akshoomoff (1989) Brainstem and middle latency auditory evoked potentials in autism and developmental language disorder. J Autism Dev Disord 19: 255-269
Hari R, Aittoniemi K, Järvinen ML, Katila T, Varpula T (1980) Auditory evoked transient and sustained magnetic fields of the human brain. Localization of neural generators. Exp Brain Res 40: 237-240
Hari R, Kaila K, Katila T, Tuomisti T, Varpula, T (1982) Interstimulus interval dependence of the auditory vertex response and its magnetic counterpart: implications for their neural generation. Electroencephalogr Clin Neurophysiol 54: 561-569.
Huttenlocher PR (1979) Synaptic density in human frontal cortex developmental changes and effects of aging. Brain Res 163: 195-205
Huttenlocher PR (1990) Morphometric study of human cerebral cortex development. Neuropsychologia 28: 517-527
Jernigan TL, Tallal P (1990) Late childhood changes in brain morphology observable with MRI. Dev Med Child Neurol 32: 379-385
Johnson, Ray, Jr. (1989). Developmental evidence for modality-dependent P300 generators: A normative study. Psychophysiology 26: 651-667
Knight R, Hillyard SA, Woods DL, Neville HJ (1980) The effects of frontal and temporal parietal lesions on the auditory evoked potential in man. Electroencephalogr Clin Neurophysiol 50: 112-124
Knight RT, Scabini D, Woods DL, Clayworth C (1988) The effects of lesions of superior temporal gyrus and inferior parietal lobe on temporal and vertex components of the human AEP. Electroencephalogr Clin Neurophysiol 70: 499-509
Korpilahti P, Lang HA (1994) Auditory ERP components and mismatch negativity in dysphasic children Electroencephalogr Clin Neurophysiol 91: 256-264
Kurtzberg D, Hilpert PL, Dreuzer JA, Vaughan HG Jr (1984) Differential maturation of cortical auditory evoked potentials to speech sounds in normal fullterm and very low-birthweight infants. Dev Med Child Neurol 26: 466-475
Lelord G, Laffont F, Jusseaume P, Stephant JL (1973) Comparative study of conditioning of averaged evoked responses by coupling sound and light in normal and autistic children. Psychophysiology 10: 415-427
Lincoln AJ, Courchesne E, Harms L, Allen M (1995): Sensory modulation of auditory stimuli in children with autism and receptive developmental language disorder: event-related brain potential evidence. J Autism Dev Disord 25: 521-529
Martin L, Barajas JJ, Fernandez R, Torres E (1988) Auditory event-related potentials in well-characterized groups of children. Electroencephalogr Clin Neurophysiol 71: 375-381
Martineau J, Garreau B, Roux S, Lelord G (1987) Auditory evoked responses and their modifications during conditioning paradigm in autistic children. J Autism Dev Disord 17: 525-539
Mason MS, Mellor DH (1984) Brainstem, middle latency and late cortical evoked potentials in children with speech and language disorders. Electroencephalogr Clin Neurophysiol 59: 297-309
McCallum WC, Curry, SH (1980) The form and distribution of auditory evoked potentials and CNVs when stimuli and responses are lateralized. In H.H. Kornhuber, L. Deecke (eds), Progress in brain research, volume 54. Motivation, motor and sensory processes of the brain: Electrical potentials, behaviour and clinical use. Elsevier, Amsterdam, p 767-775
Näätänen R, Picton T (1987) The N1 wave of the human electric and magnetic response to sound: a review and an analysis of the component structure. Psychophysiology 24: 375-429
Niwa S, Ohta M, Yamazaki K (1983) P300 and stimulus evaluation process in autistic subjects. J Autism Dev Disord 13: 33-42

Novick B, Vaughan HG, Kurtzberg D, Simon R (1980) An electrophysiologic indication of auditory processing defects in autism. Psychiat Res 3: 107-115

Ornitz EM, Ritvo ER (1968) Perceptual inconstancy in early infantile autism. Arch gen Psychiat 18: 76-98

Passler MA, Isaac W, Hynd, GW (1985) Neuropsychological development of behavior attributed to frontal lobe functioning in children. Dev Neuropsychol 1: 349-370

Peronnet F, Michel F, Echallier JF, Girod, J (1974) Coronal topography of human auditory evoked responses. Electroencephalogr Clin Neurophysiol 37: 225-230

Perrin F, Bertrand O, Pernier J (1987) Scalp current density mapping: value and estimation from potentials date. IEEE Trans. Biol. Eng 34: 283-288

Perrin F, Pernier J, Bertrand O, Echallier JF (1989) Spherical spines for scalp potential and current density mapping. Electroencephalogr Clin Neurophysiol 72: 184-187

Picton TW (1990) Auditory evoked potentials. In Daly DD, Pedley TA (eds) Current Practice of Clinical Electroencephalography, Second Edition. Raven Press, Ltd., New York

Picton TW, Hillyard SA (1988) Endogenous event-related potentials. In: Picton TW (ed.). Handbook of Electroencephalography and Clinical Neurophysiology, Vol 3, Human Event-Related Potentials. Elsevier, Amsterdam p 361-426

Picton TW, Woods DL, Baribeau-Braun J, Healey TMG (1977) Evoked potential audiometry. J Otolaryngol 6: 90-119

Picton W, Goodman WS, Bryce DP (1970) Amplitude of evoked responses to tones of high intensity. Acta Otolaryngol 70: 77-82

Polich J, Ladish C, Burns T (1990) Normal variation of P300 in children: age, memory span, and head size. Int J Psychophysiol 9: 237-248

Prescott J, Connolly JF, Gruzelier, JH. (1984) The augmenting-reducing phenomenon in the auditory evoked potential. Biol Psychol 19: 31-44

Regan D (1989) Human Brain Electrophysiology. Evoked potentials and evoked magnetic fields in science and medecine. Elsevier, Amsterdam p 250-271

Satterfield JH, Schell AM, Nicholas T (1994) Preferential neural processing of attended stimuli in attention-deficit hyperactivity disorder and normal boys. Psychophysiology 31: 1-10

Scherg M, Von Cramon D (1985) Two bilateral sources of the late AEP as identified by a spatio-temporal dipole model. Electroenceph Clin Neurophysiol 62: 32-44

Scherg M, Von Cramon D (1986) Evoked dipole source potentials of the human auditory cortex. Electroencephalogr Clin Neurophysiol 65: 344-360

Shepard DA (1968) A two dimensional interpolation function for irregular spaced data. Proc Acad Nat Conf: 517-524

Small JG (1971) Sensory evoked responses of autistic children. In: Churchill DW, Alpern GD, De Myer MK (eds), Infantile autism. Charles C Thomas, Springfield, Illinois, p 224-242

Steinmetz H, Rademacher J, Huang YX, Hefter H, Zilles K, Thron A, Freund HJ (1989) Cerebral asymmetry: MR planimetry of the human planum temporale. J. Comput Assist Tomogr 13: 996-1005

Steinschneider M, Kurtzberg D, Vaughan VG (1992) Event-related potentials in developmental neuropsychology. In: Rapin I, Segalowitz SJ (eds) Handbook of Neuropsychology. Vol 6, Elsevier, Amsterdam, p 239-299

Stuss DT.(1992). Biological and psychological development of executive functions. Brain Cognition 20: 8-23

Tallal P, Piercy M (1978) Defects of auditory perception in children with developmental dysphasia. In: Wyke M (ed.). Developmental dysphasia. Academic Press, Orlando, FL, p 63-84

Tallal P, Stark R, Mellitis F (1985) The relationship between auditory temporal analysis, and receptive language development: Evidence from studies of developmental language disorder. Neuropsychologia 23: 314-322

Tallal P, Piercy M (1973) Defects of non-verbal auditory perception in children with developmental aphasia. Nature 241: 468-469

Taylor MJ (1995) The role of event-related potentials in the study of normal and abnormal cognitive development. In: Handbook of Neuropsychology, vol 10, Elsevier, Amsterdam, p 581-605

Tonnquist-Uhlén (1996) Topography of auditory evoked long-latency potentials in children with severe language impairment: the T complex. Acta Otolaryngol (Stockh) 116 (in press)

Tonnquist-Uhlén I. Borg E. Spens KE (1995) Topography of auditory evoked long-latency potentials in normal children, with particular reference to the N1 component. Electroencephalogr Clin Neurophysiol 95: 34-41

Vaughan HG Jr. Ritter W (1970) The sources of auditory evoked responses recorded from the human scalp. Electrencephalogr Clin Neurophysiol 28: 360-367

Velasco M, Velasco F (1986) Subcortical correlates of the somatic, auditory and visual activities. II Referential EEG responses Electroencephalogr Clin Neurophysiol 63: 62-67

Weitzman ED, Graziani LJ (1968) Maturation and topography of the auditory evoked response of the prematurely born infant. Dev Psychobiol 1: 79-89

Wolpaw JR, Penry JK (1975) A temporal component of the auditory evoked response. Electroencephalogr Clin Neurophysiol 39: 609-620

Wolpaw JR, Cacace AT (1994) The influence of stimulus intensity, contralateral masking and handedness on the temporal N1 and the T complex components of the auditory N1 wave, by John F. Connolly. Electroencephalogr Clin Neurophysiol 91: 71-73

Wood CC Wolpaw JR (1982) Scalp distribution of human auditory evoked potentials. II. Evidence for overlapping sources and involvement of auditory cortex. Electroencephalogr Clin Neurophysiol 54: 25-38

Woods DL, Alho K, Algazi A (1992) Intermodal selective attention. I. Effects on event-related potentials to lateralized auditory and visual stimuli. Electroencephalogr Clin Neurophysiol 82: 341-355

Woods DL, Knight RT, Scabini D (1993) Anatomical substrates of auditory selective attention: behavioral and electrophysiological effects of posterior association cortex lesions. Cognitive Brain Res 1: 227-240

Woods DL. (1995) The component structure of the N1 wave of the human auditory evoked potential. Electroencephalogr Clin Neurophysiol (Supp) 44: 102-109

Yakovlev P, Lecours A (1967) The myelogenetic cycles of regional maturation of the brain. In: Minkowski A, (ed.), Regional Development of the Brain in Early Life. Blackwell, Oxford, p 3-70

Part two

Neurophysiological investigations and pathophysiology

1. Structural neuroimaging in Gilles de la Tourette's syndrome

M. ROBERTSON

Gilles de la Tourette's syndrome (GTS) is a genetically determined movement disorder characterised by multiple motor and one or more vocal tics (World Health Organisation, 1992; American Psychiatric Association, 1994; Robertson, 1994). Associated behaviour and psychopathology include coprolalia (inappropriate uttering of obscenities) in approximately 30% of clinic patients, echophenomena (copying behaviour) in roughly 40% (Robertson, 1989; 1994) and attention deficit hyperactivity disorder (ADHD) in 20%-90% of clinic patients (Robertson and Eapen, (1992). The most specific psychopathology, which is probably also genetically related, is obsessive compulsive disorder (OCD) (Robertson, 1995). Although GTS is genetically-determined, and the Most likely inheritance pattern is autosomal dominant transmission (Eapen et al., 1993), environmental influences are also important. Thus, prenatal events including maternal illness, eg., severe nausea and/or vomiting during the first trimester and maternal life stress during pregnancy, as well as the sex of the child, may lead to changes in the sensitivity of some dopaminergic receptors, and this could partially determine the eventual severity of expression of the syndrome (Leckman et al., 1990).

The precise brain pathology is, as yet, unknown, in part due the lack of adequate post-mortem (PM) studies. However, in general, PM studies have implicated the basal ganglia. The first PM undertaken on a patient with "Ilidiopathic" GTS was normal (Dewulf and van Bogaert (1941). Subsequent studies, however, have implicated the striatum (Balthasar, 1957; Singer et al., 1991) and the globus pallidus (Haber et al., 1986; Haber and Wolfer, 1992).

Structural neuroimaging allows us to examine anatomy in vivo and provides evidence complementary to these PM studies. Functional neuroimaging, examining regional blood flow, metabolism and receptor function, provides another avenue of exploring the neuropathological lesions of GTS. In this chapter, I confine myself to a description of structural neuroimaging studies, including computed tomography (CT) and magnetic resonance imaging (MRI).

In order to gain as comprehensive review of the literature as possible, MEDLINE and PSYCHLIT searches were performed using the titles "Tourettes", X RAY, CT scan and MRI scan. No articles involving GTS and X ray examinations were found. The literature on CT and MRI scans in patients with GTS will be reviewed. When considered relevant,, in some cases, more details will be given about individuel cases or the study, to illustrate the areas possibly involved in the pathogenesis of GTS.

Individual CT case reports

The first report of CT scan in GTS was by Yeragani et al (1983), who documented a 12-year-old girl with GTS, whose CT showed mild increase in the density of the caudate nuclei, thought to be due to calcification. There was no relevant family history. The patient had elevated levels of beta-phenylethylamine and the catecholamine metabolites normetanephrine, MHPG and 3-methoxytyramine, and a decrease in urinary 5-HT.

Soon afterwards, Shaenboen et al. (1984) reported the CT appearances in a 16 year old girl with GTS who had a brief acyanotic spell at 30 h of age, and delayed speech, but an otherwise unremarkable history. CT showed markedly enlarged occipital horns of both lateral ventricles. Lakke and Wilmink (1985) reported a 27 year old man with GTS whose CT showed a pineal tumour and calcification in the region of the third ventricle and periaqueductal grey matter. Kjaer et al. (1986) described the CT of a 28 year old woman with GTS, which showed a large porencephalic cyst in the right hemisphere, virtually replacing the temporal lobe and involving the basal ganglia, and contrast enhancement in the region of the left basal ganglia. The patient had been born 4 weeks premature, had a left sided clonic seizure at weeks old and a hyperactive stretch reflex on the left.

Vieregge (1987) documented monozygotic (MZ) twins concordant for GTS. Both had unremarkable gestations and births. In preschool age both were hyperactive and "destructive"; developmental milestones were normal. From the age of 6 years both showed compulsive behaviour. Motor tics began at the age of 12 (B) and 13 (A) years, followed soon after by vocal tics. The more severely affected twin (B) showed marked asymmetrical left involvement and soft neurological signs. There was a positive family history of GTS. Neurophysiological investigations (eg., visual evoked responses) were normal, as was the EEG, apart from muscle artefacts. CT revealed some ventricular asymmetry in both, without observable differences.

An interesting, acquired Tourette-like syndrome was reported by Northam and Singer (1991) in a 6 year old girl following presumed herpes encephalitis. She had no prior neuropsychiatric history and no family history of tics or OCD. After a 3 day prodrome of headaches, malaise, nausea and vomiting, she developed a fever (39.5.c) and presented, with focal motor seizures involving the left side of the face and left arm. CT without contrast medium was normal. She was treated with diazepam and phenytoin. Repeat CT on hospital day 3 showed an acute haemorrhagic lesion in the right mesial temporal region, and MRI on day 5 a small high-signal lesion in this region, involving both grey and white matter, and progressive oedema in the right temporal lobe, basal ganglia and thalamus.

After a presumptive diagnosis of herpes encephalitis, the patient was treated with acyclovir and maintained on phenytoin. At discharge 2 weeks later she had obvious neurological signs (eg., mild left facial and arm paresis), marked anxiety, personality change, emotional lability and hyperactivity. Two weeks later she developed both motor and vocal tics. CT two months after the onset showed encephaloclastic change in the right temporal lobe. Four months later she had no neurological abnormalities apart from the tics, which responded to small doses of pimozide.

Of course, individual case studies, while useful, are limited by difficulty in knowing the relevance the pathological findings in specific individuals with GTS, when most do not have any abnormalities. Thus, studies of series of patients with GTS allow us to determine whether any more systematic abnormalities are to be found.

CT studies in patients with GTS

Caparulo et al. (1981) reported CT abnormalities in (6) 38% of 16 patients with GTS, including mildly enlarged lateral ventricles (in 2 cases), substantially enlarged, symmetrical or asymmetrical ventricles (in 3) and an enlarged right Sylvian fissure. No systematic relationship was found between EEG and CT scan abnormalities. No mention was made of family history.

In a controlled study (Harcherik et al. 1985) CT was performed on 19 patients with GTS and compared with studies of patients with infantile autism, ADHD, and a language disorder, and a control group of medical patients (with headaches, post concussion or inner ear problems) . No significant difference was found between groups or controls with respect to total ventricular volume, right/left ventricular volume ratio, ventricular asymmetry, ventricle/brain ratios or brain density.

Chase et al. (1986) reported seven normal CT studies in a cohort of nine patients with GTS. The only abnormalities were mild ventricular dilatation in a 21 year old man, and mild, diffuse cortical atrophy in a 40 year old man.

Regeur et al. (1986) reported 47 normal CT examinations in a cohort of 53 patients with GTS. Abnormalities included a small occipital arachnoid cyst, a suprasellar epidermoid, a large defect in the right temporo parietal region, slight cortical atrophy, and asymmetry of the ventricles in two cases.

The largest CT study is that of Robertson et al. (1988) who found 71 of 73 patients to have normal CT examinations. The only abnormalities were a cavum of the septum pellucidum and two patients, both of whom had a history of head banging. The report of normal CT studies by Lees et al. (1984) included the same patients.

Thus, although some groups have found subtle abnormalities of ventricular size or symmetry, and there are occasional reports of cerebral anatomical abnormalities or structural pathology, the overall conclusion must be that there are no structural abnormalities are systematically revealed by CT in patients with GTS. The literature reviewed, reveals that 154/177 (87%) of the CT studies were normal. The mutation abnormalities described, may not distinguish GTS from other neuropsychiatric disorders presenting in childhood. It is of course possible that more subtle structural abnormalities are not detectable with CT.

MRI case reports in patients with GTS

To date, there have been five reports of normal MRI. Chase et al. (1986) reported two men aged 21 and 40 years, and a woman of 28 years who had normal MRI. Robertson and Trimble (1991) reported a 21 year old woman with typical symptoms with no associated behaviours, whose MRI was also normal, as were the neurological examination and EEG. Relevant family history was that a paternal aunt had facial tics. Hartman and Yuvarajan (1994) described an 82 year old woman who presented with motor and vocal tics, and coprolalia, which had developed in the months following an acute confusional state associated with posterior neck pain 10 years earlier, presumed to be encephalitis lethargica; the patient would therefore not fulfil criteria for "Ilidiopathic" GTS both because of her age and the organic insult. Nevertheless, despite her age and "Ilorganic" insult, MRI was normal.

Two case reports have documented MRI abnormalities. Sandyk (1988) reported a 7 year old boy who also had coprolalia, abnormal sexual behaviour and ADHD. At the age of 5 years he was prescribed methylphenidate (ritalin) for his ADHD. Neurological examination was normal. MRI being showed asymmetry of the cerebral peduncles, the left being larger than the right.

Robertson et al. (1990) documented a 19 year old man with severe GTS, obsessive compulsive (OCB) and self-injurious behaviours (SIB) and coprolalia, whose symptoms were so severe that he required psychosurgery, in the form limbic leukotomy. He was born at term by caesarian section following an antepartum haemorrhage due to placenta praevia; he was nursed in an incubator for the first four days of his life. His presurgical MRI revealed a single high signal focus in the right globus pallidus; CT and EEG were both normal.

MRI studies in GTS

There have been several MRI studies in GTS patients, although some have not been on patients with "pure" GTS and have included patients with, for example, GTS plus ADHD and Asperger's syndrome (AS). Nevertheless all studies will be reviewed and conclusions drawn where possible.

A preliminary MRI study of 10 children with GTS who also had ADHD found significantly larger ventricles (6.0% vs 3.2% of total brain volume; $p=0.007$), larger caudate nuclei (2.7% vs 2.5% of total brain volume; $p=0.05$) and trends toward a smaller globus pallidus compared with normal controls (Denkla et al., 1991).

Demeter (1992) compared 10 adult patients with 10 medical controls using MRI: no quantitative differences were found. However, two of the patients with GTS had focal abnormalities involving the basal ganglia, one of whom had a family history of tics.

Berthier et al. (1993) investigated nine males with GTS, and compared them to seven with concurrent GTS and AS using MRI. Eight of the patients with GTS had normal MRI; the only one patient with abnormal MRI had moderate enlargement of lateral ventricles. In contrast, five of the seven (71%) with both GTS and AS had abnormal imaging. Peterson et al. (1993) used MRI to examine 14 caucasien patients with GTS aged 18-49 years (11 men, 3 women) who had minimal lifetime neuroleptic exposure (10 had never received neuroleptics), and compared them with age- and sex- matched controls, who had no personal or family history of tic or obsessive compulsive symptoms. All patients were medication free for a month prior to imaging. Results showed a significant reduction in the volume of the left (but not the right) lentiform nucleus. Post hoc analyses revealed smaller mean volumes of the caudate and lentiform nuclei and globus pallidus then in controls on both the right and the left. Further analyses of basal ganglia asymmetry indices suggested that in GTS the basal ganglia do not have the volumetric asymmetry (left greater than right) observed in normal controls. In contrast, the patients had lateral ventricular asymmetry not seen in the normal subjects, which appeared to be due to a 33% increase in mean volume of the right lateral ventricle over control values, compared with a 12% increase the left lateral ventricle. Interestingly, vocal but not motor tic severity correlated positively with all basal ganglia volumes (globus pallidus excepted), on both right and left sides.

Singer et al. (1993) performed an MRI study on 37 outpatient children with GTS (29 boys, 8 girls; age range 7-16, mean 11.5 years) and compared them with 18 controls (14 boys, 4 girls; age range 6-15, mean 9.8 years). Of the patient 78% had a family history of either tics or OCD; of the controls none had a family history of tics or GTS. At the time of MRI 25 patients (68%) were receiving medication, most commonly desipramine (in 14); 6 were receiving neuroleptics. There were no statistically significant differences in the size of the right or left caudate nucleus, putamen, globus pallidus or lateral ventricles between the groups. In contrast, there were significant differences in symmetry in the putamen and lentiform nucleus. Virtually all the controls had a left-sided predominance of the putamen, whereas in 13/37 patients (35%), a right predominance exceeded that of any control. Statistical comparisons of 18 patients with and 19 without ADHD and the controls showed significant differences in volume of the left globus pallidus and lenticuform nucleus asymmetry. In the GTS+ADHD group, the left globus pallidus was significantly smaller than the right, and the lenticuform asymmetry was due to a greater right-sided predominance in the GTS+ADHD group.

Peterson et al. (1994) measured the midline cross-sectional area and other morphological features of the corpus callosum (CC) on MRI of 14 medication free patients with GTS (11 men; 3 women) and 14 normal controls (matched for age, sex, socio economic status and handedness; all were right handed); the ages ranged between 18 and 49 years. Exclusion criteria in the patient group included history of head trauma causing loss of consciousness, past or current depressive or psychotic illness, neurologic illness, pregnancy and a history of alcohol or drug abuse. No control subject gave any reported no personal or family history of tics or obsessive-compulsive symptoms. The cross-sectional area of the CC correlated positively with brain size and basal ganglia volumes. Overall, CC area was 17.7% less in the patients than in the controls ($p < 0.006$); there was also a 10% reduction in the circumference of the CC. The reduction in area was similar in degree throughout the CC. Analyses of covariance with total midsagittal area of the head revealed the reductions in the overall CC area of the CT and all its subsections to be statistically significant. The width of the CC tended to be insignificantly less throughout (5%-11%); its overall length from rostrum to splenium was significantly reduced (by 5.3%). The bending angle and mean curvature of the CC were both increased in GTS, suggesting that the CC was less rounded than that of normal controls. Worst-ever motor tic symptoms showed the strongest significant correlation with the length of the CC in the patients. These findings suggested that structural interhemispheric connectivity may be aberrant in the central nervous system in GTS, and the authors suggested that they provide indirect supportive evidence for the presence of altered cerebral lateralisation in GTS.

A careful monozygotic (MZ) twin study was undertaken by Hyde et al. (1995) who performed morphometric analyses of MRIs of 10 MZ twin pairs concordant for tic disorders, but discordant for tic severity. Twins were considered to be MZ only if their blood samples matched on all 19 blood antigens tested. The mean age of the group was 16.3 years (range 9-31). No focal neurologie abnormalities were found other than tics, and no patient had abused drugs. The right caudate nucleus volume was slightly (6%) but significantly reduced in the relatively more severely affected twins compared with the less affected ($t=3.34$; $p < 0.009$). Most of the difference was attributable to reduced volume of the anterior right caudate nucleus ($t=2.26$; $p < 0.02$), which was smaller in the more severely affected twin in nine out of ten sets. There was also a trend for the left anterior caudate nucleus to be smaller in the more severely affected twin sets. In addition, the mean volume of the left lateral ventricle was 16% less in the more severely affected than in the less severely affected twins ($t=2.86$; $p < 0.01$). In eight of ten sets, the more severely affected twin had a smaller left lateral ventricle. The normal left greater than right asymmetry of the lateral ventricles was not present in the more severely affected twins ($t=-3.39$; $p < 0.008$). In addition, the difference within a pair in the degree of loss of the normal ventricular asymmetry correlated with the difference within a pair in the severity of the tic disorder. In contrast to the maintenance of the normal ventricular asymmetry in the less severely affected twins, both less and more severely affected twins had a predominance of the caudate nuclei and striatum as a whole. The authors suggested that because MZ twins are genetically identical, the structural abnormalities must reflect adverse environmental events.

The nost recent study is from our group (Moriarty et al. submitted for publication). In brief, MRI was used to assess 17 patients with GTS and eight normal controls. There were no differences in volume between patients and controls in the amygdala or caudate nuclei and no difference in whole brain index. There was, however, loss of the normal caudate asymmetry in the patients. The area of the corpus callosum was significantly greater in patients than in controls and there was a loss of the normal correlation between it and whole brain index.

In summary, and not unexpectedly, the MRI studies reveal substantially more abnormalities than the CT investigations. These include primarily those in the basal ganglia and lateral ventricles: abnormalities of caudate nucleus size (mostly decrease) and loss of normal caudate nucleus asymmetry: in the asymmetry of other basal ganglia (eg., putamen and lentiform nucleus); and in the size of the lateral ventricles, with loss of normal ventricular asymnetry. Finally, two studies have found abnormalities of the corpus callosum, likely to reflect abnormalities in the development of cerebral lateralisation (Witelson 1993). However, one group found an increased cross-sectional area of the corpus callosum in GTS patients, while the other found it lobe reduced, reinforcing the fact that structural neuroimaging studies have methodological limitations, and further systematic investigation will be needed to clarify these findings.

Conclusions

While PM and earlier CT studies did not show convincing or consistent abnormalities in patients with GTS, recent studies with the more sophisticated techniques of MRI show a reasonable consistency in abnormalities of cerebral lateralisation, affecting particularly the basal ganglia. Whether or not these structural abnormalities are genetically determined, or, as suggested by Hyde et al. (1995), are the result of environmental factors is as yet unknown. More controlled studies and more twin studies are called for. The next phase of neuroimaging investigations in GTS be functional MRI studies, which might bridge the gap between the traditional functional studies such as single-photon emission tomography and positron emission tomography (PET) and traditional MRI, and allow further insights into the pathophysiology of GTS.

Acknowledgements

I wish to thank Dr John Moriarty for his helpful comments.

References

American Psychiatric Association (1994) Diagnostic and Statistical Manual of Mental Disorders (4th Edition) (DSM IV), Washington DC

Balthasar K (1957) Uber das anatomische Substrat der generalisierten Tic-Krankheit (maladie des tics, Gilles de la Tourette): Entwicklungshemmung des Corpus striatum. Arch Psychiat Nervenk 195: 531-549

Berthier ML, Bayes A, Tolosa ES (1993) Magnetic resonance imaging in patients with concurrent Tourette's Disorder and Asperger's syndrome. J Am Acad Child Psychiat 32 3: 633-639

Caprulo BK, Cohen DJ, Rothman SL (1981) Computed tomographic brain scanning in children with developmental neuropsychiatric disorders. J Am Acad Child Psychiat 20: 338-357

Chase GN, Geoffrey V, Gillespie M, Burrows GH (1986) Structural and functional studies of Gilles de la Tourette's syndrome. Rev Neurol 142: 851-855

Demeter S (1992) Structural imaging in Tourette's syndrome. Advan Neurol 58: 201-206

Denckla MB, Harris EL, Aylward EH, Singer HS, Reiss AL, Reader MJ, Bryan RN, Chase GA (1991) Executive function and volume of the basal ganglia in children with Tourette's syndrome and attention deficit hyperactivity disorder. Ann Neurol 30: 476

Dewulf A, van Bogaert L (1941) Etudes anatomo-cliniques de syndromes hypercinetiques complexes - Partie 3. Une observation anatomo-clinique de maladie des tics (Gilles de la Tourette). Monat Psychiat Neurol 104: 5361

Eapen V, Pauls DL, Robertson MM (1993) Evidence for autosomal dominant transmission in Gilles de la Tourette's syndrome - United Kingdom cohort study. British J Psychiat, 162: 593-596

Haber SN, Kowall NW, Vonsattel JP, Bird ED, Richardson EP (1986) Gilles de la Tourette's syndrome: a postmortem neuropathological and immunohistochemical study. J Neurol Sci 75: 225-241

Haber SN, Wolfer D (1 992) Basal ganglia peptidergic staining in Tourette's syndrome. Advan Neurol 58 145-150

Harcherik DF, Cohen DJ, Ort S (1985) Computed tomographic brain scanning in four neuropsychiatric disorders of childhood. AmJ Psychiat 142: 731-743

Hartman JA, Yuvarajan R (1994) Tourette's syndrome in the elderly. Int J Geriat Psychiat 9 2: 157-159

Hyde TM, Stacey ME, Coppola R, Handel SF, Rickler KC, Weinberger DR (1995) Cerebral morphometric abnormalities in Tourette's syndrome. Neurology 45: 11761182

Kjaer M, Boris P, Gadegaard Hansen L (1986) Abnormal CT scan in a patient with Gilles de la Tourette's syndrome. Neuroradiology 28 362-363

Lakke JP, Wilrrunk JT (1985) A case of Gilles de la Tourette's syndrome with midbrain involvement. J Neurol Neurosurg Psychiat 48: 1293-1296

Leckman JF, Dolansky ES, Hardin MT, Clubb M, Walkup JT, Stevenson J, Pauls D (1990) Perinatal factors in the expression of Tourette's syndrome: an exploratory study. J Am Acad Child Psychiat 29 2: 220-226

Lees AJ, Robertson MM, Trimble MR, Murray NNM (1984). A clinical study of Gilles de la Tourette's syndrome in the United Kingdorn J Neurol Neurosurg Psychiat 47: 1-8.

Moriarty J, Varma AR, Stephens J, Fish M, Trimble MR, Robertson MM (1996) Subcortical abnormality in Gilles de la Tourette's syndrome: an MRI study. Submitted for publication

Northam RS, Singer HS (1991) Postencephalitic acquired Tourette-like syndrome in a child. Neurology 41: 592-593

Peterson B, Riddle MA, Cohen DJ, Katz LD, Smith JC, Hardin MT, Leckman JF (1993) Reduced basal ganglia volumes in Tourette's syndrome using three-dimensional reconstruction techniques from magnetic resonance images. Neurology 43: 941-949

Peterson BS, Leckman JF, Duncan JS, Wetzles R, Riddle MA, Hardin MT, Cohen DJ (1994) Corpus callosum morphology from magnetic resonance images in Tourette's syndrome, Psychiat Res Neuroimag 55: 85-99

Regeur L, Pakkenberg B, Fog R (1986) Clinical features and long-term treatment with pimozide in 65 patients with Gilles de la Tourette's syndrome. J Neurol Neurosurg Psychiat 49: 791-795

Robertson MM (1989) The Gilles de la Tourette's syndrome: the current status. British J Psychiat 154: 147-169

Robertson MM (1994) Annotation: Gilles de la Tourette's syndrome - an update. J Child Psychol Psychiat 35 4: 597-611

Robertson MM (1995) The Relationship between Gilles de la Tourette's syndrome and obsessive compulsive disorder. J Serotonin Res, Suppl 1: 49-62

Robertson MM and Eapen V (1992) The pharmacologic controversy of CNS stimulants in Gilles de la Tourette's syndrome. Clin Neuropharmacol 15 5: 408-425

Robertson MM, Doran M, Trimble MR, Lees AJ (1990) The treatment of Gilles de la Tourette's syndrome by limbic leucotomy. J Neurol Neurosurg Psychiat 53: 691-694

Robertson MM, Trirnble MR, Lees AJ (1988). The psychopathology of the Gilles de la Tourette's syndrome: a phenomenological analysis. British J Psychiat 152: 383-390

Robertson MM, Trimble MR (1991) Gilles de la Tourette's syndrome in the Middle East. British J Psychiat 158: 416-419

Sandyk R (1988) A case of Tourette's syndrome with midbrain involvement. Int J Neurosci 43: 171-175

Shaenboen MJ, Nigro MA, Martocci RJ (1984) Colpocephali and Gilles de la Tourette's syndrome. Arch Neurol 41: 1023

Singer HS, Hahn I-H, Moran TH (1991) Abnormal dopamine uptake sites in postmortem striatum from patients with Tourette's syndrome. Ann Neurol 30: 558-562

Singer HS, Reiss AL, Brown JE, Aylward EH, Shih B, Chee E, Harris EL, Reader MJ, Chase GA, Bryan RN, Denckla MB (1993) Volumetric MRI changes in basal ganglia of children with Tourette's syndrome. Neurology 43: 950-956

Vieregge P (1987) Gilles de la Tourette's syndrome in monozygotic twins. J Neurol Neurosurg Psychiat 50: 1554-1556

Witelson SF (1 993) Clinical neurology as data for basic neurosciences Tourette's syndrome and the human motor system. Neurology, 43: 859-861

World Health Organisation (1992) International classification of diseases and health related problems (tenth revision). Geneva

Yeragani VK, Blackman M, Baker GB (1983) Biological and psychological aspects of a case of Gilles de la Tourette's syndrome. J Clin Psychiat 44: 27-29

2. SPECT studies in Tourette's syndrome

J.K. BUITELAAR, W.I. DE BRUIN, P.P. VAN RIJK

Tourette's syndrome (TS) is a chronic neuropsychiatric disorder that is primarily characterised by multiple motor and vocal tics and has its onset in childhood. Although tics can affect virtually any muscle group, they most commonly start in the orofacial region. When the disorder progresses the tics usually move along a cephalocaudal and proximal-distal gradient. Family genetic and twin studies support a genetic aetiology, with a probable sex influenced autosomal dominant mode of inheritance and variable expressivity as TS, chronic motor tic disorder or obsessive-compulsive disorder (Cohen and Leckman, 1994; Robertson, 1994). In addition to the wide range of tics, subjects with TS often present with other disorders such as attention deficit hyperactivity disorder (ADI-ID) in children and adolescents and obsessive-compulsive disorder (OCD) in adults.

A substantial body of data implicates the basal ganglia and related cortical and thalamic structures in the pathophysiology of TS (Leckman et al., 1992). Circumstantial evidence implicating dysfunction within the basal ganglia includes its established role in other movement disorders, such as Huntington's chorea and Parkinson's disease. There is a paucity of postmortem studies of classical TS; the reports available have not established specific abnormalities, except for one case with smaller neurons in the putamen and caudate nuclei (Richardson, 1982). This suggests hypoplasia of parts of the basal ganglia, which may be putamen and caudate nuclei (Richardson, 1982). This can be due to some developmental arrest. The intensity and frequency of tics can be modified by stimulating or lesioning the afferent and efferent pathways of the basal ganglia. For example, lesions made in the thalamus, cingulum and prefrontal cortex attenuate tic and related complex motor phenomena in humans. Finally, in vivo neuroradiological studies provide support for the involvement of the basal ganglia in the pathophysiology of TS. Structural neuroimaging by means of three-dimensional reconstructed MRI has pointed to smaller volumes of the caudate nuclei and lentiform and globus pallidus in patients with TS than in controls and to an absence of the normal volumetric asymmetry (left greater than right) (Peterson et al., 1993; Singer et al., 1993).

The focus of this chapter is the contribution of single photon emission computed tomography (SPECT) studies to the elucidation of the pathophysiology of TS. A number of SPECT studies have examined blood flow in the basal ganglia and related structures in TS using technetium 99m-hexamethylpropylene amine oxide (HMPAO), a lipophilic compound which rapidly crosses the blood-brain barrier. The ligand enters the brain within 2-3 minutes of injection and remains stable for hours, the redistribution effect is negligible. The radioactivity measured then reflects regional cerebral blood flow, which under most conditions corresponds to brain metabolism. Further SPECT studies have investigated the status of the dopaminergic neurotransmitter system by using either a radiotracer (^{123}I-IBZM) which binds to the dopamine D2-receptor, or a ligand (^{123}I-βCIT) with high affinity for the dopamine transporter. We will first review the literature on SPECT in TS and then report pilot data from study of children and adolescents with TS in Utrecht University Hospital.

Review of SPECT studies in TS

The first HMPAO-SPECT study compared nine drug-free, right-handed adults with TS (age mean - SD 29.6 - 6.9 years) and nine person-to-person age- and sex-matched controls (Riddle et al.1992). Scanning time was about 45 min, following injection of 20 mCi HMPAO. Regions of interest (ROI) were drawn manually on the basis of the anatomical information of the SPECT images and an anatomical atlas. The dependent variables were the weighted averages of the number of counts per pixel, based on relative area, for each ROI. The ROI data were related to the activity measured in the whole brain, and expressed as ROI-to-whole-brain minus cerebellum ratios. Cerebral perfusion as reflected by HMPAO uptake was significantly reduced in the left putamen and globus pallidus of the patients with TS. Furthermore, the severity of motor tics appeared to be positively correlated with HMPAO uptake in the left thalamus.

A second study included 20 unmedicated patients with TS 23.8 - 12.0 years old and 8 control subjects aged 34.7 - 12.5 years (George et al., 1992). The two groups were not matched for age and for sex; 10 of the individuals with TS had concurrent obsessive-compulsive disorder. Regional cerebral blood flow was examined by means of HMPAO during a scanning time of 15 minutes which started about 10-30 minutes after injection. The ROI analysis was performed on 4 × 4 non overlapping pixel regions, outlined using an anatomic atlas. The uptake of HMPAO in different ROI was calculated and cxpressed as a ratio to visual cortex values, and as a ratio to whole brain uptake. The patients with TS showed greater right frontal activity than control subjects, both when the ratio to visual cortex and when the ratio to whole brain was taken as dependent variable. This finding should be interpreted with caution, however, since the analysis did not include a correction for multiple comparisons and the frontal perfusion in controls was unusually low. The presence of concurrent obsessive-compulsive symptoms did not affect this result. No differences between the two groups were found in radioactivity measured over the basal ganglia.

A third study is only available in abstract form (Dimitsopulos et al., 1993). Six drug-free adults with TS (aged 26 to 54 years) and 9 normal controls were included in an HMPAO-SPECT study. Radioactivity was expressed as counts per pixel, and symmetry indices (right/left ratios) of activity the two groups were compared. The right/left ratio of the basal ganglia for the patients with TS was significantly lower than in controls, indicating that they had relatively decreased perfusion of the non dominant basal ganglia. No differences across the frontal regions were reported. Recently, a fourth HMPAO study (Moriarty et al., 1995), with a relatively large sample size, including 50 individuals with TS (mean age 24 years, range 7-65 years) and 20 controls. The controls had a mean age of 23 years, and although the report fails to present details, presumably were all young adults. Of the patients 34 were drug-free, the others were on neuroleptics. All were injected with 550 MBq HMPAO and scanned for a maximum of 30 minutes. ROI were determined by means of visual inspection and expressed a ratio relative to visual cortex. The Bonferroni correction for multiple comparisons was applied. In two regions, the left caudate nucleus and anterior cingulate area, the HMPAO uptake relative to visual cortex was significantly lower in the patients than in the controls, using the Bonferroni correction. There was a trend towards reduced perfusion in the left dorsolateral frontal area in the TS group. Additional findings were that a greater degree of severity of tics appeared to be associated with somewhat lower perfusion in the left caudate nucleus and cingulum, and in the left dorsolateral prefrontal and left anterior temporal regions.

The HMPAO studies mentioned predominantly included adults; unfortunately, Moriarty et al., (1955) failed to indicate how many patients below 18 years of age they studied. There are a number of methodological problems with all the studies, such as the absence of MR images for coregistration and the lack of a sufficiently large, matched control group. Furthermore, methods applied to define ROI and to calculate activity within them relative to a reference region and the instruments used to measure tic severity differ widely across the studies. Hence, it is not surprising that some of the findings show discrepancies. Both Riddle et al., (1992) and Moriarty et al., (1995) found low perfusion in the left basal ganglia areas of caudate nucleus, putamen and globus pallidus, whereas Dimitsopulos et al., (1993) reported perfusion to be lower in the right basal ganglia. These discrepant findings are not necessarily in contradictors, however, since Dimitsopulos et al. (1993) did not relate HMPAO uptake in the basal ganlgia area to an ipsilateral reference region. In any case, these findings support the hypothesis that the basal ganglia are involved in the pathogenesis of TS.

Another point of discrepancy is the relationship between regional perfusion and tic severity in TS. Increased tic severity is reported to bec associated with increased perfusion of the left thalamus (Riddle et al., 1992) and decreased perfusion of the left caudate nucleus and cingulate area and the prefrontal and anterior temporal cortex (Moriarty et al., 1995). It is possible to reconcile these discrepancies by reference to the cortico-striatothalamo-cortical circuits which connect all these structures (Alexander and Crutcher, 1990). The thalamus is part of the direct pathway between the prefrontal and motor cortex and the motor output structures in the striatum, and has an overall facilitating influence on ongoing

Table 1
Description of subjects

variable	ADHD (n = 19)	TS (14)	TS + ADHD (n = 8)	statistic
age (yrs)	9.3 ± 1.5	11.2 ± 2.3	11.0 ± 2.6	F (2,40) = 4.33, p < .05
FSIQ (WISC-R)	96 ± 9	98 ± 16	87 ± 13	
TSGS				
sum	– –	44 ± 7	58 ± 17	
tic		18 ± 7	18 ± 6	
CBCL (T-scores)				
inattentiveness	71 ± 7	65 ± 11	74 ± 9	F (2,40) = 6.38, p < .05
sum	71 ± 7	64 ± 7	70 ± 13	
TRF (T-scores)				
inattentiveness	64 ± 5	57 ± 5	56 ± 9	F (2,40) = 7.52, p < .05
sum	68 ± 11	57 ± 8	56 ± 7	
boys:girls	18:1	10:4	8:0	
handedness R:L	16:3	12:2	6:2	

note : TSGS Tourette's syndrome Global Scale; CBCL Child Behavior Checklist; TRF Teacher Report Form

motor activity. This fits with the finding that coagulation of parts of the thalamus abolishes tics, whereas stimulation of thalamic nuclei leads to an exacerbation of tic severity (Leckman et al., 1993). On the other hand, the prefrontal cortex and the cingulate area have an inhibiting influence on the limbic striatum; when metabolic activity in these inhibiting structures decreases may the overall effect be an increase in involuntary movements. A final point is that intragroup variability in regional HMPAO uptake, is considerable both in patients and normal controls, is considerable and may casily mask specific relationships between behavioural parameters and perfusion measures.

Although the neurobiochemical basis of TS is unknown, the dopaminergic neurotransmitter system has been pinpointed as the possible biochemical locus of disease. Arguments in support of this hypothesis are, among others, that dopamine-blocking agents, including neuroleptics such as haloperidol, reduce the frequency and intensity of tics, whereas psychostimulants which increase dopaminergic turnover aggravate or even induce tics and other symptoms of TS (Singer and Walkup, 1991). One possibility is supersensitivity of postsynaptic dopamine receptors, due to increased number or increased affinity of the receptor. To examine this possibility, George et al., (1994) administered the radioactive dopamine-D2 ligand ^{123}I-IBZM intravenously to 15 patients with TS (mean age 23 years, range 10-47 years) and 6 normal controls (mean age 24 years). Seven patients were on medication, mostly neuroleptics, and some were also taking clomipramine for OCD. Scanning started immediately following injection and continued for at most 55 minutes. ROI were drawn manually and regional uptake in the basal ganglia was expressed as both basal ganglia to visual cortex and basal ganglia to frontal cortex ratios. The ^{123}I-IBZM binding curves of the right and left basal ganglia relative to visual cortex proved not to differ between unmedicated patients and controls. The patients on medication, however, had significantly lower ^{123}I-IBZM binding than control subjects in both right and left basal ganglia. This latter finding was anticipated since neuroleptics block D2 receptors, decreasing binding of ^{123}I-IBZM. The hypothesis of supersensitive postsynaptic D2 receptors was not supported by this study.

Another approach was followed by Malison et al., (1995) who administered ^{123}I-βCIT, a radioactive probe of the striatal dopamine transporter, to five adults with TS and five normal controls. All patients were drug-free. Image acquisition started 4 hours after injection and lasted 36 minutes. Striatal ^{123}I-βCIT binding was higher in all patients than in the individually age- and sex-matched controls. This finding is accordance with post-mortem data on increased numbers of the dopamine transporter in TS (Singer et al., 1991), and indicates that abnormalities in dopaminergic function in TS may be ascribed to presynaptic compolients.

HMPAO-SPECT study of children and adolescents with TS in Utrecht

About 40% of children and adolescents with TS also have an attention deficit hyperactivity disorder (ADHD). Abnormalities in the fronto striatal regions have also been implicated in the pathophysiology of ADHD. For example, MRI studies have shown that children with ADHD have a smaller corpus callosum and decreased volumes of the caudate nuclei (Castellailos et al., 1994; Giedd et al., 1994). Furthermore, SPECT studies showed decreased perfusion in the tronto striatal areas (Lou et al., 1984). For these reasons, we were interested in whether regional cerebral perfusion was different in TS and in ADHD. Another question we attempted to address was whether the pattern of cerebral perfusion of children with the combination of TS and ADHD was different from that in the uncomplicated disorders, i.e. TS and ADHD.

We have so far studied 41 children and adolescents with ages ranging from 8 to 15 years. Ethical concems on radiation exposure precluded the use of a normal control group. All children and their parents gave informed consent to participate in this study, which was approved by the ethical committee of the Utrecht University Hospital. The participants were children referred to the outpatient child psychiatric unit, where they underwent extensive diagnostic procedures, including standardised psychiatric examinations, developmental history and neuropsychological testing. On the basis of DSM-IV criteria the subjects were categorised into three groups: TS without ADHD (14), TS and ADHD (8) and ADHD without TS (19). The subjects were further characterised by their scores on the Childhood Behavior Checklist and the Teacher Report Fonn (Achenbach and Edelbrock, 1983; 1986), completed by their parents and teachers respectively. Severity of tics was measured on the Tourette's syndrome global scale, rated by the clinician (Harcherik et al. 1984). Details of the sample are summarised in Table 1. The mean age of the children with pure ADHD was two years less than that of the children with a tic disorder ($p <.05$). All subjects were on medication. ADHD subjects were treated with methylphenidate (14) or clonidine (5). The patients with TS were taking either clonidine (7) or low doses of neuroleptics (7).

To measure cerebral perfusion, we gave an intravenous injection of 600-800 MBq Tc 99m-HMPAO (the dose depending on age and weight) under resting conditions in a quiet room. Image acquisition started 20 minutes after injection, using a 3-head high-resolution Prism 3000 camera. and with a scanning time of 30 minutes. The data were analysed in MedView on a Apple working station. The raw data were reconstructed along the canthomeatal line and ROI were aligned on oblique axial slices 3.91 cm thick. Six regions of interest were drawn manually, bilaterally, on the basis of visual interpretation: frontal, parietal and temporal cortex (each in 2 slices), and the thalamus (6 slices), putamen (3 slices) and globus pallidus (5 slices). The cerebellum was drawn as region of reference. The interrater re-

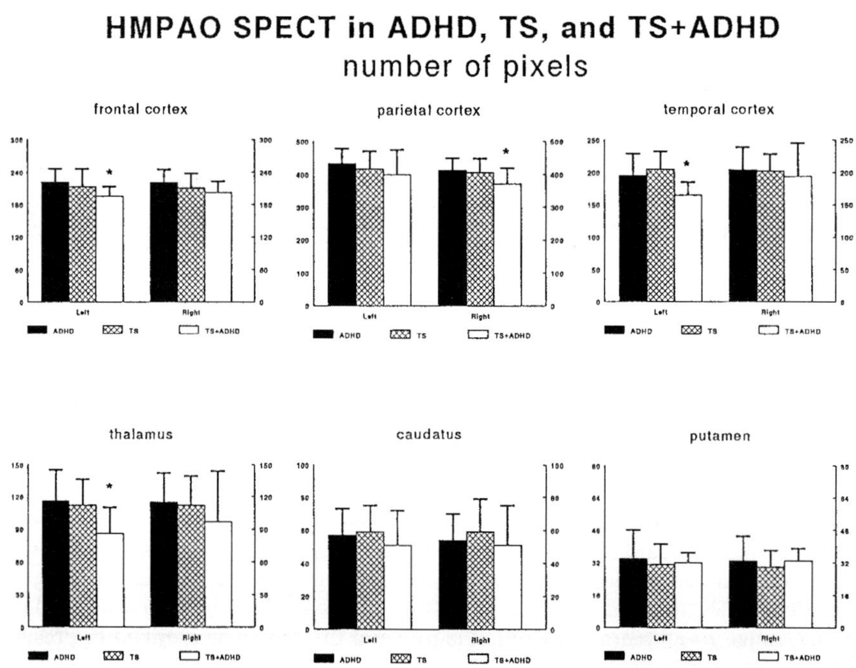

Fig. 1
Group data (mean - SD) of number of pixels in various ROIs for childrcn with ADHD, TS and a combination of TS and ADHD. Significant differences arc indicated by an asterisk ($p < .05$). For details of statistical analysis, see text.

liability across two raters in establising the regions was good (ICC -.80). The activity measured was expressed as counts per pixel averaged over the slices of a specific ROI. Dependent variables were the number of pixels and regional perfusion ratios relative to whole brain. To analyse the interdependence of regional perfusion in various ROI of the same subjects, Spearman-rank-correlation coefficients were computed between the ratios of the various regions and compared between the three groups of children.

As a first step it was established that neither the number of pixels nor the perfusion ratios relative to whole brain were dependent on age or type or dosage of medication used. Then an omnibus MANOVA was run with within-subjects factors region (6 levels), and side (2 levels) and between subject factor diagnostic group (3 levels). We found a main diagnostic group effect on the number of pixels [$F(2,40) = 3.76$, $p < .05$], of course a main ROI effect [$F(5,145) = 1106.8$, $p < .001$] and interaction effects "region × side" [$F(5,145) = 7.82$, $p < .001$) and "group × region × side" [$F(10,145) = 1.99$, $p < 051$. Follow-up tests revealed that the children with both TS and ADHD differed from the other two groups of children in showing a significantly reduced number of pixels in the left frontal and temporal cortex, left thalamus and right parietal cortex (Figs 1, 2). There were no significant effects in the overall OVA on the ratios of regional perfusion.

When the pattern of correlations of regional activity across the diagnostic groups was compared, the subjects with the combination of TS and ADHD were left out of the analysis because of the small size of this sub-sample. Clear differences emerged in the pattern of correlations between children with pure TS and those with pure ADHD. For example, the correlations between the crosslateral regions were: frontal cortex R-L in TS .93 ($p < 01$), in ADHD .08 (ns); thalamus R-L in TS .17 (ns) and in ADHD .76 ($p < .01$); caudate nucleus R-L in TS .35 (iis) and in ADHD -.73 ($p < .01$). The simplest way to take account of differences in the complex pattern of inter-region correlations between the two groups is simply to calculate the number of significant correlations of each region (out of a total number of 12 correlations) (Fig 3). It appears then that in TS radioactivity in the right thalamus failed to correlate with activity in any other region in both hemispheres, whereas in ADHD the perfusion in the left frontal region was independent of the perfusion in other regions. Finally, severity of tics, indexed by the total tic score on the TSGS proved to be correlate significantly with the perfusion ratio in the left caudate nucleus (Spearman $r = -.34$, $p < .05$) and left frontal cortex (Spearman $r = -.32$, $p < .05$). The absence of a normal group limits the conclusions to be drawn from this study. Nonetheless, our data indicate that patients with the combination of TS and ADHD clearly stand out from both pure disorders in having less radionuclide uptake at three regions on the left of the brain (thalamus, frontal and temporal cortex) and one on the right (parietal cortex). Since the number of pixels was used as the dependent variable, this indicates that the area in which radioactivity was measured was much smaller in the combined group. The more severe combination of psychopathological symptoms proves to be associated with more severe disturbances in cerebral perfusion, particularly on the left side of the brain, in the fronto-striato-thalamo-cortical circuits. Differences between pure TS and ADHD are more subtle, and were not found in the areas of radioactivité measured nor in the intensity of radioactivity (ratios of counts per pixel relative to whole brain). However, when we recognise that functional output of the brain seems to be dependent on the interdependence of and coordination between activity within various areas, it is important to examine correlations in brain perfusion between various areas. A head-to-head comparison of patients with pure TS and pure ADHD enables us to pinpoint neurobiology abnormalities that probably are more specific to each of these disorders. Our data suggest that TS is linked to dysfunction in the thalamus and ADHD to a problem in the left frontal cortex, i.e. at different nodes in the cortico-striato-thalamo-cortical circuit. This is in accordance with data on executive function in individuals with TS and ADHD, which point to frontal lobe deficits in ADHD but not in TS (Pennington and Ozonoff, 1996).

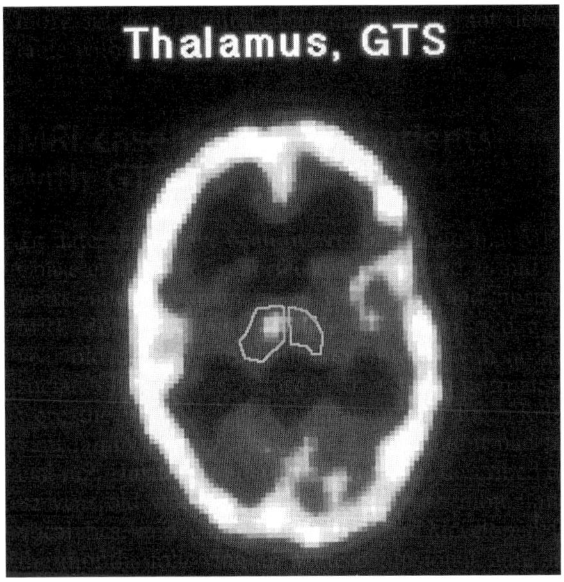

Fig. 2. SPECT of 13-year old boy with TS and ADHD and decreased number of pixels in left thalamus.
See colour illustrations appendix

We are currently enlarging our samples and analysing coregistered MRI data. The latter will be matched with SPECT images, and individually aligned ROI will be used as a template for SPECT analysis.

Advances in functional MRI with superior temporal and spatial resolution and absence of radiation exposure will probably result in decreased use of HMPAO-SPECT in future studies of cerebral metabolism and perfusion. In contraste for in vivo study of neurobiochemistry, i.e., of the density of receptors and transporters, SPECT may be the most cost-effective and rewarding method, particularly in children and adolescents in view of the radiation exposure inherent in PET.

Note

All zero-order correlations between age and the dependent measures were nonsignificant. When age was dichotomised (below or above 12 years) and included in an overall MANOVA as a between-subjects factor, the age by region interaction approached significance with the number of pixels as dependent variable ($p = .07$). There were no significant interactions between age and diagnostic group. Follow-up tests showed that the number of pixels in both the right and left putamen was significantly lower in the younger age group.

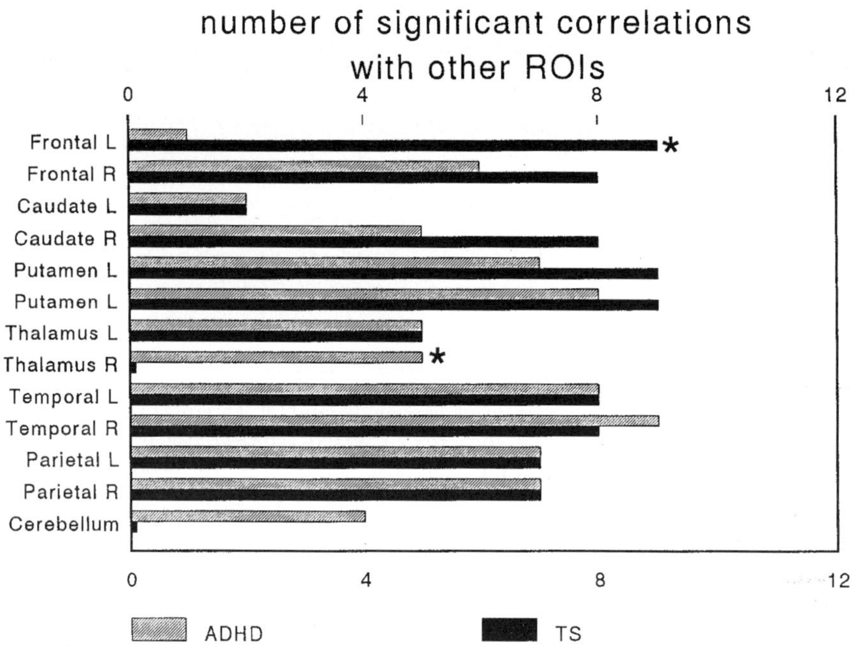

Fig. 3
Number of significant correlations in perfusion which each ROI has with all other ROI. Significant differences are found for the right thalamus in TS and the left frontal cortex in ADHD.

References

Achenbach TM, Edelbrock CS (1983) Manual for the child behavior checklist and revised profile. University of Vermont, Department of Psychology, Burlington

Achenbach TM, Edelbrock CS (1986) Manual for the teacher's report form and the teacher version of the child behavior profile. University of 'Vermont, Department of Psychology, Burlington

Alexander GE, Crutcher MD (1990) Functional architecture of basal ganglia circuits: neural substrates of parallel processing. Trends Neurosci 13: 266271

Castellanos FX, Giedd JN, Eckburg P, Marsh WL, Vaituzis AC, Kaysen D, Hamburger SD, Rapoport JL (1994) Quantitative morphology of the caudate nucleus in Attention deficit hyperactivity disorder. Am J Psychiat 151 1791-1796

Cohen DJ, Leckman JF (1994) Developmental psychopathology and neurobiology of Tourette's syndrome. J Am Acad Child Adolesc Psychiat 33 2-15

Dimitsopulos T, Klieger P, Kurlan R (1993) Asymmetry of basal ganglia perfusion in Tourette's syndrome shown by single photon emission tomography (abstract). Movement Dis 8: 415-416

George MS, Trimble MR, Costa DC, Robertson MM, Ring HA, Ell PJ (1992) Elevated frontal cerebral blood flow in Gilles de la Tourette's syndrome: a 99 Tecn HMPAO SPECT study. Psychiat Res Neuroimag 45: 143-151

George MS, Robertson MM, Costa DC, Ell PJ, Trimble MR, Pilowsky L,Verhoeff NPLG (1994) Dopamine receptor availability in Tourette's syndrome. Psychiat Res 55: 193-203

Giedd JN, Castellanos FX, Casey BJ, Kozuch P, King AC, Hamburger SD, Rapoport JL (1994) Quantitative morphology of the corpus callosum in attention deficit hyperactivity disorder. Am J Psychiat 151: 665-669

Harcherik DF, Leckman JF, Detlor J, Cohen DJ (1984) A new instrument for clinical studies on Tourette's syndrome. J Am Acad Child Psychiat 23: 153160

Leckman JF, Pauls DL, Peterson BS, Riddle NM, Anderson GM, Cohen DJ (1992) Pathogenesis of Tourette's syndrome: clues from the clinical phenotype and natural history. Advan Neurol 58 -.15-23

Leckman JF, De Lotbinière AJ, Marek K, Gracco C, Scahill L, Cohen DJ (1993) Severe disturbances in speech, swallowing, and gait following stercotactic infrathalamic lesions in Gilles de la Tourette's syndrome. Neurology 43: 890-894

Lou HC, Hendriksen L, Bruhn P (1984) Focal cerebral hypofusion in children with dysphasia and/or attention deficit disorder. Arch Neurol 41 825-829

Malison RT, McDougle CJ, Van Dyck CH, Scahill L, Baldwin RM, Seibyl JP, Price LH, Leckman JF, Innis RB (1995) [123I]-CIT SPECT imaging of striatal dopamine transporter binding in Tourette's disorder. Ani J Psychiat 152: 1359-1361

Moriarty J, Campos D, Costa C, Schmitz B, Trimble MR, Ell PJ, Robertson MM (1995) Brain perfusion abnormalities in Gilles de la Tourette's syndrome. British J Psychiat 167: 49-254

Pennington BF, Ozonoff S (1996) Executive functions and developmental psychopathology. J Child Psychol Psychiat 37: 51-87

Peterson B, Riddle MA, Cohen DJ, Katz LD, Smith JC, Hardin MT, Leckman JF (1993) Reduced basal ganglia volumes in Tourette's syndrome using 3-dimensional reconstruction techniques from magnetic resonance images. Neurology 43: 941-949

Richardson EP (1982) Neuropathological studies of Tourette's syndrome. Advan Neurol 35: 83-87

Riddle MA, Rasmusson AM, Woods SW, Hoffer PB (1992) SPECT imaging of cerebral blood flow in Tourette's syndrome. Adv Neurol 58: 207-212

Robertson MM (1994) Annotation: Gilles de la Tourette's syndrome - un update. J Child Psychol Psychiat 35: 597-611

Singer HS, Hahn IH, Moran TH (1991) Abnormal dopamine uptake sites in postmortem striatum from patients with Tourette's syndrome. Advan Neurol 30 558-562

Singer HS, Reiss AL, Brown JE, Aylward EH, Shih B, Chee E, Harris EL, Reader MJ, Chase GA, Bryan RN, Denckla MB (1993) Volumetric MRI changes in basal ganglia of children with Tourette's syndrome. Neurology 43: 950-956

Singer HS, Walkup JT (1991) Tourette's syndrome and other tic disorders. Diagnosis, pathophysiology, and treatment. Medicine Baltimore 70: 15-32

3. Electrical brain activity and motor control in Tourette's syndrome and attention deficit hyperactivity disorder

A. ROTHENBERGER

Disordered control of movement patterns is a key feature of both Tourette's syndrome (TS) and attention deficit hyperactivity disorder (ADHD). While in TS motor and vocal tics are the main problem, in ADHD general motor restlessness and often clumsiness can be recognised. Cognitive, emotional and social aspects cannot be ignored within the clinical and research framework of both disorders. Nevertheless, we will focus on the motor aspects of TS and ADHD: firstly, because TS is defined by its motor features and, secondly, because hyperactivity (HA) as part of ADHD seems to be insufficiently considered in most recent clinical and research work (Steinhausen 1995, Sandberg 1996, Rothenberger 1995, 1996). It may be thus worth taking a closer look at the neurodynamics of motor control in TS and ADHD. Recording electrical brain activity (here, event-related potentials; ERP) with surface electrodes on the scalp seems appropriate, since brain mapping not only reflects topographical changes over time but, in contrast to MRI and SPECT or PET, also offers high temporal resolution and, in addition, allows recording in parallel of time-locked task performance (Brandeis 1995, Brandeis et al., in press).

Motor circuits

Movement-related neurodynamics involve the interaction of several parts of the brain. Together they are called "motor circuit" or,"motor loops". The cortico-striato-pallido-thalamo-cortical circuit can be affected at different locations, which may lead to several distinct dyskinetic syndromes (e.g., dystonia, parkinsonism, Huntington's diseased Sydenham's chorea).

Within this motor circuit, both voluntary and involuntary movement patterns can be processed. A cognitively-based intention for a voluntary motor action is usually developed through co-operation of fronto lateral and parietal association cortex ("what to do") and forwarded to fronto medial cortex with its supplementary motor area (SMA), where the necessary programming and timing of the sequential movement pattern is arranged ("how to do") and the right moment for starting it ("when to do") is determined (Rothenberger 1990a, Dinners and Lüders, 1995, Garcia, 1993).

The somatotopic organisation of the motor circuit (composed of many mini circuits) continues from

SMA to the motor parts of the basal ganglia (putamen, modulated by the substantia nigra; globus pallidus, modulated by the nucleus subthalamicus), to the motor nuclei of the thalamus and after that to motor cortical areas. It is forwarded to the primary motor cortex as the last relay station before the movement volley initiates peripheral action at the muscles; there is feedback, closing the motor circuit to prefrontal and premotor cortex and SMA for online adaptive motor regulation of slow voluntary movements. In addition, influences on the motor circuit by intracortical circuits connected with association areas, the somatosensory circuit and the motor loop activity via the cerebellum may modify the primarily planned or unplanned movement. The latter includes tics in TS and general motor restlessness in ADHD. However, the will of the patients to suppress or downregulate these motor disturbances (mainly based on frontal lobe sensitive executive functions) shows that interference between involuntary motor action and voluntary motor control i.e., between motion and cognition may play an important role concerning visible symptomatology and coping behaviour in these groups of patients.

We will first describe anatomically which parts of the motor circuit may be disturbed in TS and ADHD, there present the neurodynamics, i.e., the interplay between functional motor deficits and possibilities for their cognitive compensation of both disorders.

Movement-related electrical brain activity

Active movement-related information-processing in the primary motor cortex and SMA can be easily recorded.

Recording *Bereitschaftspotential* (BP; also known as readiness potential) appears to be a suitable method for describing changes in brain electrical activity occurring prior to a voluntary action. The BP is a slow, continously rising negative potential which starts about 500 to 1500 ms prior to the first muscle activity. This "premotor" negative potential developing prior to the movement is interpreted in terms of an increase in neuronal activity and facilitation of the movement related neuronal networks. It is associated with preparatory processes such as preprogramming and initiation of an intended motor action. The BP can be recorded on both sides of the scalp. In adults, a negative amplitude is seen most clearly over central recording sites, whereas a smaller negative, sometimes even positive, amplitude is normally observed over frontocortical areas. In general, the BP starts by developing with an almost symmetrical amplitude over the primary motor cortex and then displays a larger amplitude over the central brain area contralateral to the movement prior to the onset of EMG activity.

A more passive form of information processing in the primary motor cortex can be evoked by the novel technique of *transcranial magnetic stimulation* (TMS), which tells us about cortical excitability, i.e., the inhibitory and facilitatory properties of the motor cortex. Introduced by Barker et al. (1985), TMS is now readily established as a non invasive, painless tool for studying the human motor system in health and disease. In addition to the conventional measurement of motor threshold, motor-evoked potential (MEP) amplitudes and central motor conduction time, it allows determination of other parameters thought to be specifically related to motor cortex inhibitory mechanisms: the cortical silent period (CSP), and the intracortical (cortico cortical) inhibition obtained in a paired-stimulus conditioning test paradigm (Ziemann et al., in press).

Interaction between the primary motor cortex, SMA, dorsolateral frontal cortex and posterior association cortex becomes evident when several other measures of electrical brain activity, i.e., the *slow cortical negative potentials* (SNP) are investigated: the contingent negative variation (CNV) and post imperative negative variation (PINV) are thought to be reliable correlates of cognitive functions which underly behavioural control (e.g., early CNV or CNV1: orientating; late CNV or CNV2: expectancy and motor preparation; PINV: contingency evaluation and stimulus control) (Dumais-Huber and Rothenberger, 1992; Dumais-Huber, 1993).

The CNV is a slow negative cortical potential change elicited during a paired-stimulus reaction time task (S1-S2-R-paradigm) and developing after the warning stimulus (S1) but prior to the imperative stimulus (S2). The PINV appears after S2 and appears sensitive to the emotional content of the imperative stimulus (S2) and the evaluation of contingencies between the imperative stimulus S2 and the associated motor response i.e., control versus non-control of terminating S2 by the motor response. When motor control of S2 becomes unpredictable, performance declines because the contingent relationship between S2 and the motor response cannot be established. In such experimental conditions, healthy individuals exhibit a particularly high PINV amplitude over frontal recording sites. In contrast, patient with frontal brain damage fail to show a similar increase in negativity. Observations of this sort led to the suggestion that PINV activity reflects the dynamics of frontocortical neuronal pools.

In order to reconcile the findings from different methodological approaches and provide a frame of reference for the elaboration of a unified model of motor control integrating information from various slow cortical negative potentials (SNP) it is important to compare and contrast the properties of all wave forms under given experimental conditions. When this is done many experiments have demonstrated a *parallelism between the BP and the late CNV* (CNV2) and an analogous topography over the midline recording sites, both having a maximal amplitude over the vertex in normal subjects. However, despite their similarity, the two phenomena should at present be considered as reflecting distinct preparatory processes differentially sensitive to motor and non specific psychological factors; a sharp awareness of the limitations of an oversimplified model of the neurophysiological mechanisms is necessary when bridging the gap between BP and late CNV results.

With these considerations in mind, *we assessed the function of the motor cortex and frontocortical system in TS and ADHD*. Non cortical parts of the motor circuit (e.g. the basal ganglia) can be investigated only indirectly by SNP. For example, changes in SNP topography caused by D2 receptor blocking agents acting at the level of the basal ganglia can help us to draw conclusions about the neurodynamics of cortical-subcortical interaction (Rothenberger 1990b).

Furthermore, SNP are measures of neural activation with millisecond resolution and allow tracking of covert information processing. One advantage of ERP studies is that they can reveal both specific neurophysiological correlates of poor performance, and specific differences in covert neural processing in the absence of performance differences. Neuroelectric mapping of these ERP provides detailed spatio-temporal measurement of covert processes. It combines the high temporal resolution of ERP with the spatial resolution needed to detect brief (50-500 ms) segments of the ERP characterised by distinct map distributions. These *microstates* are determined by adaptive segmentation procedures. Such procedures divide the map series into topographically stable time-segments of variable duration. Microstates reflect distinct patterns of neuronal activity and have been related to different information processing activities. Separate measures of map topography, such as locations of map extrema or centroids and of map strength, e.g., global field power (GFP) have been developed to clarify whether differences in task conditions or clinical groups reflect qualitative (strength or timing) aspects of information processing (Leeuwen van et al., in press, Brandeis, 1995).

Tourette's syndrome

A substantial body of evidence implicates the basal ganglia and related cortical and thalamic structures of the motor circuit in the pathobiology of motor and vocal tics. These data include the beneficial effects on tic behaviour observed after lesions of thalamic nuclei which receive afferents from the "motor" portion of the internal segment of the globus pallidus and the pars reticulata of the substantia nigria. Beneficial effects on tics have also been reported after procedures isolating regions of the prefrontal cortex. In addition, recent PET studies have demonstrated altered regional metabolic activity in the caudate nuclei and a variety of cortical areas (orbital, prefrontal, cingulate and sensorimotor). These results need to be regarded with caution since very often the psychopathological selection criteria of the groups investigated were not applied thoroughly enough and, therefore, a mixture of tics, motor restlessness, attentional deficits, obsessive-compulsive behaviour and anxious-depressive symptoms were present.

Nevertheless, it can be hypothesised that the motor aspect of TS is associated with a failure to inhibit at least subsets of the cortical-striatal-thalamic-cortical motor mini circuit. On the basis of this hypothesis, it can be anticipated that the frequently encountered facial tics are associated with a failure of inhibition of certain mini circuits including probably the ventromedian areas of the nucleus (probably) and mainly the putamen, which receive topographic projections from the orofacial regions of the primary motor and premotor cortex (Leckman et al., 1991).

In our past studies on *motor control* in tic disorders (Rothenberger 1984, 1990a and b, 1991) we showed four main features, by recording BP: 1 its latency did not differ between children with tics and normals; 2 the asymmetry of its amplitude between left and right primary motor cortex tended to be smaller in children with tics than in normals; 3 children with tics showed higher amplitude over the SMA than normals; and 4 this difference was clearly reduced (towards normality) when children with tics were successfully treated with D2 receptor blocking agents acting at the level of the basal ganglia.

It follows that children with tics may need the same time as normals to prepare a voluntary movement, but that this movement may lack precision because the motor *cortex* neuronal activity in children with tics seems to be less focussed than in normals probably, because of insufficient inhibitory properties in the motor cortex. To compensate for this functional "premotor" deficit, online adaptive regulation by the *SMA and prefrontal cortex* has to be enhanced. For the latter process an additional, and even stronger, factor may play a role. There is a lack of motor inhibition at the level of the *basal ganglia* which leads to strong interference between involuntary tic-related and voluntary goal-directed movement. This interference may be reduced by drug treatment. Hence, cortical-subcortical neurodynamics of motor control in TS could be shown indirectly by neuroelectric mapping.

To further test the hypothesis of decreased inhibition in the primary motor cortex we recently used TMS (Ziemann et al., submitted). In 20 adult patients with TS and 21 age-matched healthy control subjects. Local TMS was applied to the left motor cortex and a surface electromyogram was recorded from the right abductor digiti minimi (ADM) muscle. Motor threshold, cortical silent period and intracortical inhibition and facilitation were studied as parameters of motor cortex excitability. The peripheral silent period and the maximum M-wave after supramaximal electrical stimulation of the ulnar nerve at the wrist were also determined.

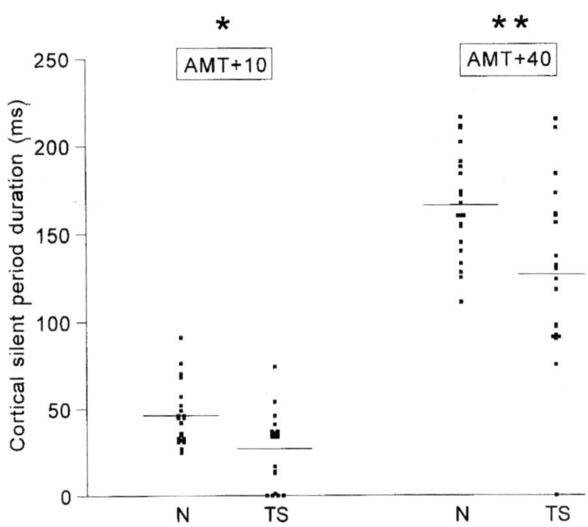

Fig. 1. Comparison of the duration of the cortical silent period in patients with Tourette's syndrome and age-matched controls Each dot shows the cortical silent period duration (in ms) of an individual subject at magnetic stimulation intensities of 10 or 40% of maximum stimulator output above the individual active motor threshold (AMT). Horizontal bars indicate mean values for the respective groups and stimulus intensities. N = normal subjects; TS = patients with Tourette's syndrome. Asterisks indicate significant differences between N and TS at the respective stimulus intensities (* $p < .05$; ** $p < .01$). Note that in one Tourette patient no cortical silent period was elicitable, not even at the high stimulus intensity.

We showed that patients with TS had normal motor thresholds and normal peripheral motor excitability, but their cortical silent period was shortened (Fig. 1) and the intracortical inhibition was less than in the control group. A subgroup analysis of patients revealed that these abnormalities were mainly seen when tics involved the ADM. Other features of the patients, such as age, sex, attention deficit hyperactivity disorder, obsessive-compulsive disorder, sensory urges or use of neuroleptics, had no significant effect on motor excitability. These findings indicate that tics in TS are associated with defective motor impulse control in the primary motor cortex. Whether this is due to a primary subcortical disorder affecting the motor cortex through disinhibited afferent signals and/or impaired inhibition in the primary motor cortex itself remains an unresolved question.

To underline the close relationship between primary motor cortex and SMA in tic disorder (TD) we can refer to the introspective descriptions of Bliss (1980), who emphasised, like many other patients with TS, that tics may be a "voluntary capitulation" to the sensory experiences which precede them. Other writers have also linked sensory urges and the voluntary nature of tic production (Rothenberger, in press). Subthreshold stimulation of the SMA in humans may produce an urge to make a movement (Lim et al., 1994, Dinners and Lüders, 1995). This is of particular interest, since the SMA is thought to play a key function in the planning and self-paced initiation of voluntary movements. If it is true that sensory urges and the voluntary aspect of tic production are intimately connected, the finding that sensory urges had no significant effect on motor hyperexcitability in TS could be taken as evidence that volition had no important contribution to the shortened cortical silent period and the reduced intracortical inhibition. Nevertheless, in addition to detective inhibitory mechanisms in the motor cortex, the shortened cortical silent period may indicate an enhanced voluntary "motor drive" or facilitated accessibility of a motor command to the motor cortex in TS, since the duration of the cortical silent period also depends on the accessibility of these neurons to the motor command when increasing the level of tonic muscle contraction (Wilson et al., 1993).

To give more weight to the *cognitive parts* of motor control we investigated another group of 13 children with tics and 15 healthy children (Dumais-Huber and Rothenberger 1992). We chose SNP, namely the CNV and PINV, as electrophysiological indicators of cognitive functions associated with behavioural control. An auditory paired-stimuli reaction time task (S1-S2-R) was run under two conditions: control and non control. In the latter, the 28 boys carrying out the task were kept from effectively stopping the imperative stimulus S2 (white noise) despite adequate motor reaction. Under the non control condition, the maximum amplitude of PINV showed a similar relative topographical shift towards frontal areas in both groups of children (i.e., the children with tics — like the healthy controls — were able to focus their electrical brain activity over frontal leads). A focussing over frontal leads was also found for the orientating response (early CNV). On the other hand, there was no differential topographic distribution over midline frontocentral areas in either group with respect to anticipation (late CNV).

We suggest that the proficiency of children at compensating for their deficits in motor control and coping with environmental changes depends on their ability to activate circumscribed frontocortical neuronal assemblies. This regulatory capacity seems to be preserved in children with tics.

Attention deficit hyperactivity disorder

In attention deficit hyperactivity disorder (ADHD) disturbances in the basal ganglia are recognised (Rothenberger 1990a). In our studies on motor control at the cortical level in ADHD (Rothenberger et al. 1986, Voss 1986, Rothenberger 1990a), children were instructed to press a lever of a toy speed controller every 15 whenever they wished, while the movement-related electrical brain acitivity was recorded. In both hyperkinetic children and healthy controls we found a BP waveform which corresponded to that of adults, with a maximum negative peak at the start of the movement, and a maximum BP amplitude over the vertex.

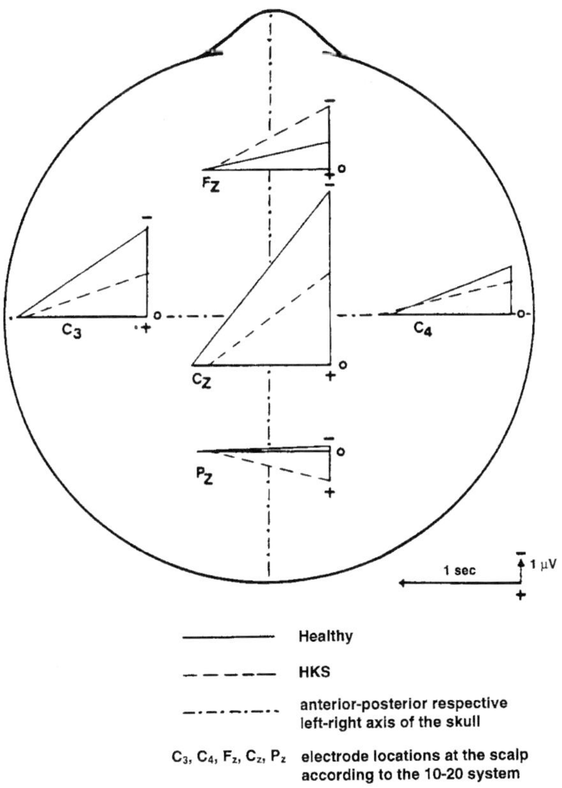

Fig. 2. Bereitschaftspotential in healthy children (n = 12) and children with hyperkinetic syndrome, HKS (n = 12): topographical distribution of latency (in ms) and amplitude (× in µV over 250 ms before EMG onset).
Note: Reduced anterior-posterior (Cz-Fz) as well as left-right (C3-C4) difference of BP-amplitude, but similar BP-latency.

With respect to topography (Fig. 2), two main findings describe the abnormalities occurring along the left-right axis (electrode difference: C3-C4) and in the midline anterior-posterior direction (electrode difference: Cz-Fz).

A reduced topographical differentiation was identified along the left-right axis, as shown by the differences in BP amplitude. Amplitudes at C3 and C4 (*primary motor cortex*) tended to be smaller in hyperkinetic than in healthy children. In the latter, the BP was clearly larger over C3, i.e. over the primary motor cortex contralateral to the dominant hand used for motor responses. However, the BP recorded over C4 in hyperkinetic children was not much smaller than that of healthy controls. Hyperkinetic children and healthy controls did not differ in BP latency. Thus, we found similar preparatory activity before the movement over the primary motor cortex in tic hyperkinetic children and those with tics. Our assumption that the reduced left-right differentiation might correlate with a lack of precision in voluntary movements may be supported by the clinical observation that many hyperkinetic children show difficulties in motor co-ordination (Gillberg and Gillberg 1990) and many of those with tics show-low level signs of ADHD (Rothenberger 1996).

The anterior-posterior difference (Cz-Fz) of BP amplitude was also significantly smaller in hyperkinetic children than in healthy controls. In the former, the BP amplitude measured over *frontal cortex* (Fz) reached, on average, almost the amplitude obtained over Cz; in contrast, healthy controls exhibited larger BP amplitudes over Cz than over Fz.

The poor topographical differentiation of the BP identified along the anterior-posterior axis in hyperkinetic children seems to reflect a reduced ability to focus neuronal activity. At the same time, it suggests an increased cortical activation or facilitation children over the frontal leads. This may indicate that hyperkinetic children need to activate their available frontal regulatory functions (e.g., inhibition of motor impulses and irrelevant sensory stimuli when preparing for voluntary action) to a greater extent than healthy children confronted with a similar task. On the other hand, they seem to be unable to focus their movement-related neuronal activity at frontal sites, as observed in children with tic disorders.

Thus, hyperkinetic children seem to have a *deficit of motor control in the primary motor cortex as well as at the level of the frontal lobe.* They do not regulate the neuronal networks responsible for voluntary motion with selective activation and sufficient precision. This possibly applies even more to "spontaneous" movements, which are badly under voluntary control. Hence, their tendency for associative mirror movements could be better clarified by using specific experimental tasks such as lateralised BP, aimed at assessing premotor processes (De Jong et al., 1990). Such studies could help to determine whether the disturbance in motor control processes is attributable to a lack of selective neuronal ability to choose adequate motor programs or to energety deficits in the early information processing steps which translate these programs into the intended movement, or to a combination of these. It should be noted here that methylphenidate not only improves the writing skills of hyperkinetic children but also leads to an increase in BP amplitude, thus exerting an influence on preparatory motor processes. Clearly, the motor control of movement patterns is tightly bound to regulatory cognitive processes (Rothenberger 1995).

A similar result was obtained in another study, in which an S1-S2-R task was used to record early and late CNV and PINV in normal and hyperkinetic children (Dumais-Huber 1993). Hyperactive children had difficulties in focussing their *frontal brain activity*. This difference in brain dynamics applied to orientating (CNV1) and contingency evaluation after response to the imperative stimulus S2 (PINV). These two processes are not based on the evaluation of a given temporal frame. The hypothesis of a frontal lobe deficit in hyperkinetic children is thus supported. Furthermore, since a constant timeframe is used for CNV2, i.e., the interstimulus interval between S1 and S2 remains constant, the lack of group differences for this late CNV component may be taken as a sign that external cues are particularly helpful for hyperkinetic children, a finding which parallels clinical observations of the effectiveness of behavioural instructions for these children.

The data accumulated by our research group on orienting (CNV1) and anticipation (CNV2) are largely compatible with earlier experiments carried out in healthy children and children with attentional deficits (Grünewald-Zuberbier and Grünewald 1982). The latter manifested their deficit only with increasing complexity of the task. Such observations in hyperkinetic children are known not only in everyday situations but also from studies involving specific psychological tests.

In a recent co-operative study (van Leeuwen et al. in press), two separate samples of 11 ADD and 16 ADHD children were compared with 9 and 16 healthy controls respectively in a CPT-AX-task (warning stimulus: letter A; imperative stimulus: letter X). Mapping the event-related EEG activity in such a task reveals a characteristic sequence of brief (50-500 ms) segments with stable map distribution called neuroelectric microstates. Topographical change marks the transition between successive microstates and indicates that information processing triggers a sequence of distinct patterns of neuronal activity.

As expected, children with ADD or ADHD showed less accurate and more variable performance than the control children, and their already lower perceptual sensitivity declined rapidly with time and task. Sensitivity is thought to be a reflection of neuronal efficiency, a process not under voluntary control; i.e., this and their poor motor response inhibition parallel their decreased ability to focus electrical brain activity.

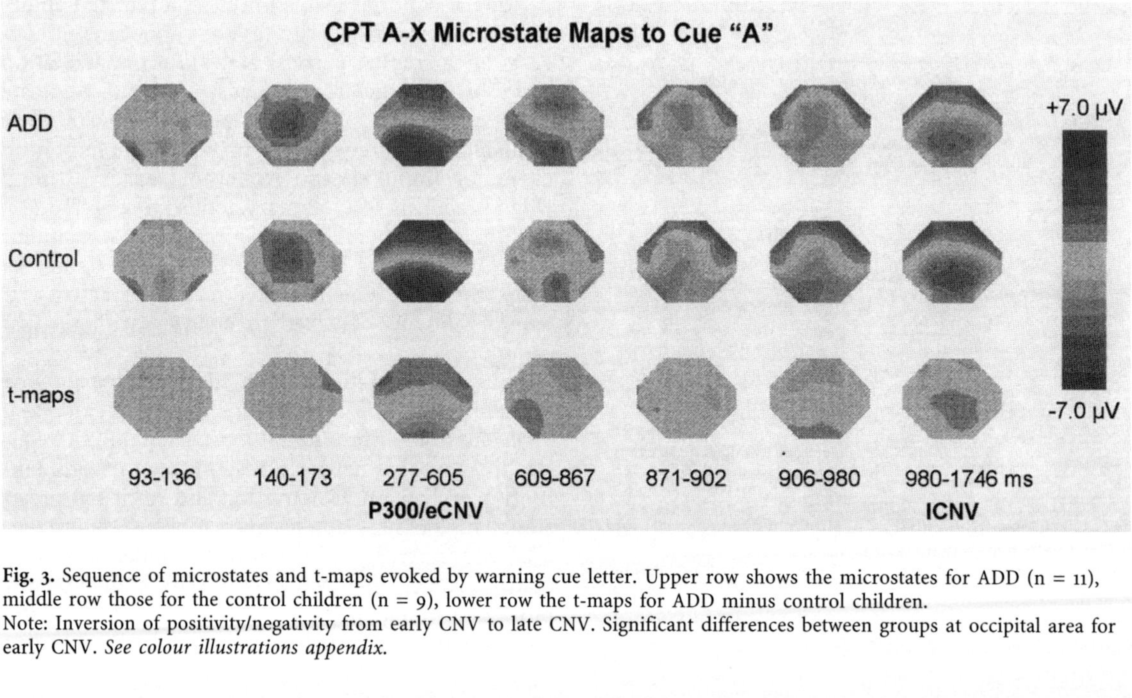

Fig. 3. Sequence of microstates and t-maps evoked by warning cue letter. Upper row shows the microstates for ADD (n = 11), middle row those for the control children (n = 9), lower row the t-maps for ADD minus control children.
Note: Inversion of positivity/negativity from early CNV to late CNV. Significant differences between groups at occipital area for early CNV. *See colour illustrations appendix.*

Inspection of the microstate maps of SNP amplitude confirmed the reversal in the topographical distribution of positivity and negativity between the early and late CNV amplitude microstates (Fig. 3). Negativity was frontally distributed in the early, but more posterior in the late CNV microstate. Positivity was posteriorly distributed for the early CNV, but more frontal in the late segment. There are no significant differences between the groups in the topographical distribution in the early and late CNV microstates, which argues against qualitative differences between groups.

A significant interaction with groups, the two CNV microstate, and stimulus letters was found for differences in global field power, which means there are highly specific group differences in map strength. The latter was significantly attenuated in the children with ADD or ADHD in only the early CNV microstate evoked by the warning letter A. This suggests that there are group differences in strength of preparatory (orientating, rather than executive) task-processing because the effect was obtained for the warning stimulus A, rather than the target X.

A comparable specific effect was obtained by Brandeis et al. (in press) in a stop-and-go task with the same ADD and control children. This task requires that subjects stop responses to a primary task if a second signal follows. However, it is not clear whether problems with is performance reflect impairment of the stopping process per se, whether they are related to reduced frontal lobe activation, or are confined to severe and pervasive forms of ADHD. In 11 healthy and 9 control children, neuroelectric microstates were mapped in a stop- and delayed go-task. In both tasks, reliable group differences in neuroelectric processing were found despite matched performance. Children with ADD showed specific early processing deficits on trials in which they failed to stop. The timing of this microstate is too early to reflect deficits in actual stop-signal processing and instead suggests deficient initial orientating of attention. Imaging with low resolution tomography (LORETA) (Pascual-Marqui et al., 1993) during this microstate to stop failures indicated mainly posterior activation for both groups, and increased rather than reduced frontal activation in children with ADD. For a later (around 550 ms) microstate LORETA indicated strong frontal activation after successful stopping, but no group differences. These results suggest that information processing of children with ADD in relation to motor control deviates during activation of posterior mechanisms which may be related to the orienting towards the motor task, and which precede and partly determine inhibitory control problems in ADD. This supports the notion that there are not only functional deficits in the motor cortex and/or frontal lobes in hyperkinetic children, but also posterior contributions which can be seen in both electrical brain activity and SPECT data (Sieg et al., 1995). Since the *posterior deficits* reported in hyperkinetic children were seen in a visual task and have no sufficient statistical backing (Brandeis et al. in press) they should be replicated and controlled for dyslexia (Rothenberger and Moll, 1994) before a possible relationship to the posterior attention system and posterior norepinephrine projection of locus coeruleus can be suggested

Association of TS and ADHD

One important issue in daily child psychiatric practice is the association of tic disorder (TD), including TS and chronic motor or vocal tics and hyperactivity (HA), the latter being a major part of ADHD. Although no genetic relationship seems to exist between these two hypermotility conditions, the frequency of their co-existence is very high, i.e., about 50 %. Yet, it remains an open question whether coexistent TD and HA represent two independent pathologies, a separate united nosological entity, or a subgroup of one of the two contributing diseases manifested by both tics and hyperactivity (Rothenberger 1991, 1995, Rothenberger et al., 1994).

To elucidate this, it seemed necessary to clarify whether the additive effects of TD and ADHD as manifest by the combination of tics and hyperactivity (TD + HA) observed clinically in children would also be present in a similar additive way in electrophysiological investigations. In pursuing this goal, the following main questions were addressed: 1. do TD and ADHD in children relate differently to primary motor cortex and/or frontal lobe function as reflected by SNP?; 2. is there an independent (additive) effect of TD and ADHD on SNP amplitude in cases of combined TD + HA disturbance?; 3. or does a qualitatively specific (non additive) pattern of frontal lobe activity characterize the TD + HA association?

Thus, a further objective of our work was to study the effects of TD and HA on SNP of children with combined TD + HA. As it is related to neuronal processes of the primary motor cortex, we recorded the BP at left and right central sites. Different processes of frontal lobe control over preparatory cortical activity were examined by measuring BP, early and late CNV and PINV at fronto central leads. BP and SNP amplitudes were analysed as reflecting the adequacy of preparatory cortical activation; scalp distribution of SNP its and relationship to reaction times were studied as revealing the efficiency of task-related region specific activation. The aspect of motor control evaluation by frontal lobe resources was analysed by choosing the PINV as an indicator of frontal lobe function which is closely related to the self regulation behaviour.

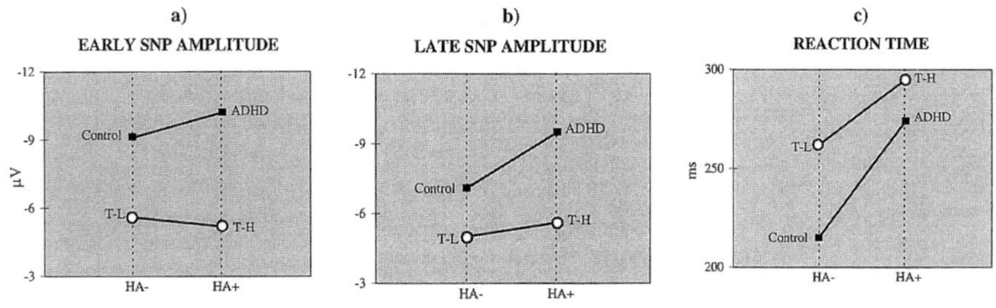

Fig. 4
Main effects of tic disorder (TD) and hyperactivity disorder (HA) on (a) early SNP amplitude, (b) late SNP amplitude, and (c) reaction time.

In each of two different studies (Rothenberger 1984, 1991, Yordanova et al. 1996, in press), four groups of children were investigated: healthy controls, pure TD, pure attention deficit hyperactivity disorder (ADHD), and combined tic and hyperactivity (TD + HA). SNP were recorded in a BP task in one study and an auditory-warned reaction time task (S1-S2-R) in the other, to measure early and late SNP (similar to CNV) and PINV.

There was no difference in BP latency. The reduced left-right asymmetry at the *motor cortex* seen in TD and HA was almost absent in the group with TD + HA (healthy: -2.6 µV; TD: -1.0 µV; HA: -0.8 µV; TD + HA: ± 0.0 µV). This may be interpreted as an additive effect in parallel to the psychopathological symptoms (Rothenberger 1984). But, this view has to be modified when looking at the anterior-posterior (*frontocentral*) distribution of the SNP. Coexistence of tics and hyperactivity in children did not show an additive effect at the psychophysiological level (Rothenberger 1984, Yordanova et al. 1996, in press). As in TD, the increased midfrontal BP amplitude could also be seen in TD + HA (healthy: +0.2 µV, TD: -5.5 µV; HA: -2.9 µV; TD + HA: -5.5 µV). Furthermore, the frontally-focussed BP amplitude (Cz-Fz-difference of BP amplitude) was observed in TD and even more significantly in TD + HA, but not in HA (healthy: -5.8 µV; TD: + 2.3 µV; HA: -1.6 µV; TD + HA: + 3.8 µV).

In the study of Yordanova et al. (1996, in press), cortical excitability was assessed with respect to its adequacy as reflected by the magnitude of early and late SNP and PINV, efficiency as reflected by the task-specific scalp distribution of preparatory activation, and by the association of SNP with behavioural responses.

The studies clearly demonstrated that children with TD had significantly lower early SNP amplitudes than children without TD. A similar trend for lower amplitudes in children with tics was found for the late SNP (Fig. 4 and 5). These findings are in accordance with the prediction of attenuated slow cortical potentials in tic disorder. The lower SNP amplitude in children with TD may reflect some additional processing in the period between the warning and imperative stimulus. As it is suggested that compensatory involvement of the *frontal areas* is employed by these children to suppress tics intervening during task conditions, a virtual frontocortical performance during the warned reaction task may coincide with development of the SNP, thus reducing its amplitude in this group.

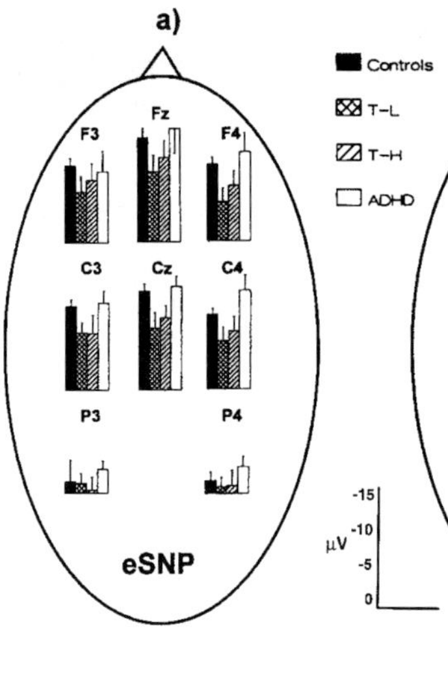

Fig. 5. Group means (± 1 SE) of (a) early SNP, and (b) late SNP amplitudes at 8 electrode locations in 4 groups of children: controls; T-L, tic disorder with low level of hyperactivity; T-H, tic disorder with high level of hyperactivity; ADHD, attention deficit hyperactivity disorder. SNP, slow negative potentials.
Note: lower amplitude in tic-disorders. Early SNP is more frontally distributed.

On the other hand, reduced SNPs could also result from inadequate cortical activity due to a disregulation in the fronto cortical-thalamo-basal ganglia system. Hence, the lower SNP amplitude of children with TD may also indicate some pathophysiological disregulation in the axis including the basal ganglia, thalamus and frontal cortex. It may be argued that disregulation of cortical excitability would affect both the adequacy of activation as expressed in magnitude of the SNP, and efficiency as associated with specific topographical patterns and level of performance. The finding that children with TD had topographical patterns of SNPs similar to those of control subjects points to a preserved potential of these chil-

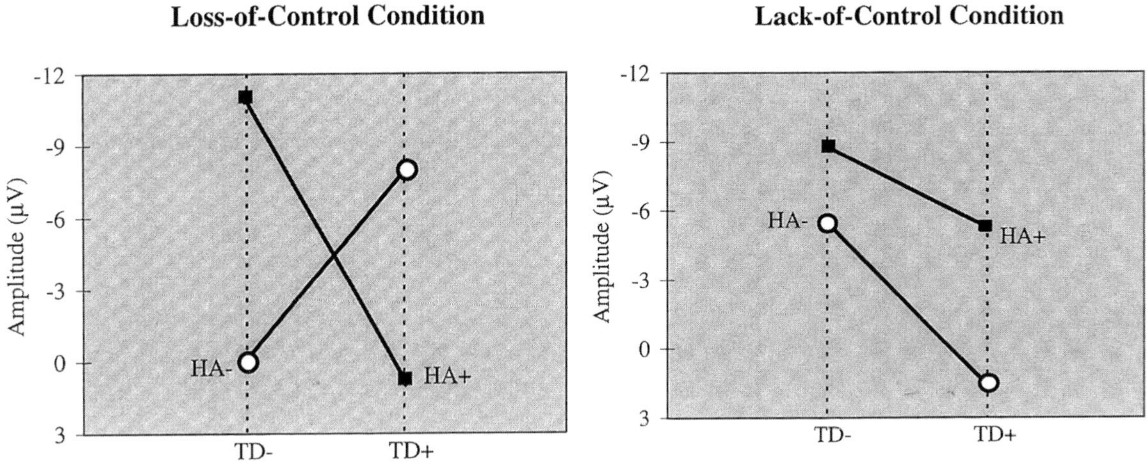

Fig. 6. Effects of tic disorder (TD) and hyperactivity disorder (HA) on postimperative negative variation (PINV) amplitude (in μV) in the loss-of-control condition (left) and lack-of-control condition (right). TD-, without tics; TD+, with tics; HA-, without hyperactivity, HA+, with hyperactivity; ordinate: average of Fz and Cz amplitudes in μV.

dren to distribute the preparatory activity across the scalp. Therefore, additional interfering internal processing related to tic suppression seems to be responsible for the lower SNP amplitudes in TD. In contrast, over motor responses of both groups of children with TD were not related to the SNP. These results suggest that the brain electrical processes investigated seem to be similar in pure TD and TD + HA. Furthermore, in view of the findings on amplitude, topography and correlation criteria, it appears that pathological processes underlying ADHD are different from those in patients with combined TD and HA (Yordanova et al., 1996).

Whether tic and attention deficit hyperactivity disorders are differentially related to *frontal brain function* was tested by PINV measurements at the same locations, as a general indicator of frontal lobe function. There were prominent effects of both tic and hyperactivity disorder on its amplitude and responsiveness. Thus, the hypothesis emphasising the role of the frontal lobes in these childhood psychiatric disorders is supported, although no group behavioural differences were found as indicated by reaction times.

Effects of TD and ADHD on the frontal lobe processes associated with the PINV were found to depend strongly on the condition-specific processing demands. Under conditions of controllability and consistent contingency between the motor response and its outcome, no significant influence of TD or ADHD on PINV was detected; however, processing of steady non controllability (lack of control) was differentially affected by TD and HA. Since TD was associated with reduced, and HA with enhanced PINV amplitudes, this may be interpreted as an independent contribution similar to the one observed at the psychopathological level. Between group comparisons under this condition favour the neurodynamic hypothesis that children with TD, require less fronto neuronal activity than those with HA to control for a steady stimulus interference (Fig. 6).

When, on the other hand, a sudden demand of contingency change processing (loss of control) was imposed, it became evident that qualitatively different modes of frontal lobe activity occur, depending on the presence of pure TD, pure ADHD or combined TD + HA. By applying this condition of high requirements of frontal lobe processing, it was possible to demonstrate that, in contrast to the clinical examination, the psychophysiological effects of TD and ADHD were interdependent but not additive (Fig. 6). Thus, when TD and ADHD coexist in children they seem to show a differentiated and complex interplay, depending on the task demands the child has to meet. When compared to pure children with ADHD, those with TD + HA children (although showing two disorders) nevertheless seem to be at least as efficient with respect to reaction times and performance in other neuropsychological tasks (Rothenberger et al., 1994), and may be more able to activate frontal lobe resources to regulate their behaviour.

Conclusions

Psychophysiological experiments with recording and topographical mapping of SNP (such as BP, CNV, and PINV) seem very useful not only for clarifying where the specific functional deficits within the brain may be found. Beyond this, they contribute to an understanding of the neurodynamic processes of motor control which take place before, during and after a movement pattern in children with movement disorders such as TS and ADHD. In particular, their inhibitory deficits within the motor circuit at the cortical level (primary motor cortex, frontal lobe, parietal areas), the subcortical level (e.g., striatum, pallidum, thalamus), and their possible cortico-cortical and cortico-subcortical interaction, can be elucidated.

Finally, the SNP data (in combination with neuropsychological assessment of the children in question) can lead to a better insight and more differentiated understanding of comorbidity, when TS and ADHD in the same individual. This may enable us to tune our available diagnostic and therapeutic knowledge and to develop new approaches to help the afflicted children and their families.

References

Barker AT, Jalinous R, Freeston IL (1985) Non-invasive magnetic stimulation of the human motor cortex. Lancet; i: 1106-1107

Bliss J (1980) Sensory experiences of Gilles de la Tourette's syndrome. Arch Gen Psychiat 37: 1343-1347

Brandeis D (1995) Psychophysiologie der hyperkinetischen Störung. In: Steinhausen HC (ed.), Hyperkinetische Störungen im Kindes- und Jugendalter (S. 71-89). Stuttgart: Kohlhammer

Brandeis D, van Leeuwen TH, Rubia K, Vitacco D, Steger J, Pascual-Marqui RD, Steinhausen HC (in press). Neuroelectric mapping reveals precursors of failures to stop in children with attention deficits. Brain Behav Res

Dinners DS, Lüders HO (1995) Electrical stimulation and movement-related potential studies. In: Jasper HH (eds.), Epilepsy and the functional anatomy of the frontal lobe. Raven Press, New York p 261-271

Dumais-Huber C, Rothenberger A (1992) Psychophysiological correlates of orienting, anticipation, and contingency changes in children with psychiatric disorders. J Psychophysiol 6: 225-239

Dumais-Huber C (1993) Electrical brain activity and stimulus control. A study on the regulatory processes of the frontal cortex in psychiatric disordered children. Doctoral Thesis, University of Heidelberg, Germany

Garcia C (1993) Supplementär-motorisches Areal (SMA). Fortsch Neurol Psychiat 61: 383-389

Gillberg C, Gillberg I (1990) What becomes of clumsy children with attention deficits? Some data and reflections from a population-based study in Sweden. In: Rothenberger A (ed.), Brain and behavior in child psychiatry. Springer, New York p 283-301

Grünewald-Zuberbier E, Grünewald G (1982) Event-related EEG changes in children with different abilities to concentrate. In: Rothenberger A (ed.), Event-related potentials in children: Elsevier, Amsterdam p 295-316

Jong de R, Coles MGH, Logan GD, Gratton G (1990) In search of the point of no return: the control of response processes. J Exp Psychol 16: 164-182

Leckman JF, Knorr AM, Rasmusson AM, Cohen DJ (1991) Basal ganglia research and Tourette's syndrome. Trends Neurosci 14: 94 (letter)

Leeuwen van TH, Brandeis D, Overtoom CCE, Pascual-Marqui RD, van't Klooster B, Rothenberger A, Sergeant JA, Steinhausen CH (in press) The Continuous Performance Test revisited with neuroelectric mapping: impaired orienting in children with attention deficits. Brain Behav Res

Lim SH, Dinners DS, Lüders H, Pillay PK, Morris HH, Klem G, Wylie E, Awad IA (1994) Functional anatomy of human supplementary sensorimotor area: result of extraoperative electrical stimulation. Electroencephalogr Clin Neurophysiol 91: 179-193

Pascual-Marqui RD, Michel CM, Lehmann D (1993) Low resolution electromagnetic tomography: a new method for localizing electrical activity in the brain. Int J Psychophysiol 18: 49-65

Rothenberger A (1984) Bewegungsbezogene Veränderungen der elektrischen Hirnaktivität bei Kindern mit multiplen Tics und Gilles de la Tourette's syndrom. Postdoctoral Thesis, University of Heidelberg, Germany

Rothenberger A (1990a) The role of the frontal lobes in child psychiatric disorders. In: Rothenberger A (ed.), Brain and behavior in child psychiatry: Springer, Heidelberg p 34-58

Rothenberger A (1990b) Dopamine receptor blockers and Bereitschaftspotential (BP) in tic children. In: Brunia CHM, Gaillard AWK, Kok A (eds.), Psychophysiological brain research, vol. 2: Tilburg University Press, Tilburg p 116-119

Rothenberger A (1991) Wenn Kinder Tics entwickeln — Beginn einer komplexen kinderpsychiatrischen Störung. Stuttgart, New York: Fischer

Rothenberger A (1995) Electrical brain activity in children with hyperkinetic syndrome: evidence of frontal cortical dysfunction. In: Sergeant J (ed.), European approaches to hyperkinetic disorder: Trümpi, Zurich p 255-270

Rothenberger A (1996) Tourette's syndrom und assoziierte neuropsychiatrische Auffälligkeiten. Z Klin Psychol 25: 259-279

Rothenberger A (in press). Sensory aspects in tic disorders. Bibliotheca Psychiatrica 167

Rothenberger A, Kemmerling S, Schenk GK, Zerbin D, Voss M (1986) Movement-related potentials (MRPs) in children with hypermotoric behavior. In: McCallum WC, Zappoli R, Denoth R (eds.), Cerebral Psychophysiology: Studies in Event-Related Potentials. Electroencephalogr Clin Neurophysiol, Suppl., 38: 496-498

Rothenberger A, Woerner W, Dumais-Huber C, Moll G, Röhrkohl N, Yordanova J (1994) Welche Bedeutung haben Merkmale des hyperkinetischen Syndroms bei Kindern mit Tic-Störungen? In: Todt H, Heinicke D (eds.). Aktuelle Neuropädiatrie 1993 (S. 52-71). Wehr: Ciba-Geigy

Rothenberger A, Moll G (1994) Standard-EEG and dyslexia in children — new evidence for specific correlates? Acta Paedopsychiat 56: 209-218

Sandberg S (1996) Hyperkinetic or Attention Deficit Disorder. British J Psychiat 169: 10-17

Sieg KG, Gaffney GR, Preston DF, Hellings JA (1995) SPECT brain imaging abnormalities in attention deficit hyperactivity disorder. Clin Nucl Med 20: 55-60

Steinhausen HC (1995) Hyperkinetische Störungen im Kindes- und Jugendalter. Kohlhammer, Stuttgart
Voss MK (1986) Das Bereitschaftspotential bei Kindern mit Hyperkinetischem Syndrom. Doctoral Thesis, University of Essen, Germany
Wilson SA, Lockwood RJ, Thickbroom GW, Mastaglia FL (1993) The muscle silent period following transcranial magnetic cortical stimulation. J Neurol Sci 114: 216-222
Yordanova J, Dumais-Huber C, Rothenberger A (1996) Coexistence of tics and hyperactivity in children: no additive effect at the psychophysiological level. International J Psychophysiol 21: 121-133
Yordanova J, Dumais-Huber C, Rothenberger A, Woerner W (in press) Frontocortical activity in children with comorbidity of tic disorder and attention deficit hyperactivity disorder. Biol Psychiat
Ziemann U, Rothwell JC, Ridding MC (in press) Interaction between intracortical inhibition and facilitation in human motor cortex. J Physiol
Ziemann U, Paulus W, Rothenberger A (submitted) Neurobiological basis of deficient motor impulse control in Tourette syndrome: decreased inhibition at the level of the motor cortex

4. SPECT in attention deficit hyperactivity disorder (ADHD). Implications for the understanding of awareness

H.C. LOU, T.W. KJAER

The neurophysiological basis of consciousness is hotly debated in the neurobiological literature at present. The subject is often confused by imprecise terminology. One of the core issues is the definition of consciousness. According to one standard English dictionary (Webster, 1989), consciousness has three aspects, or meanings: awareness of one's own existence, sensations, thoughts and surroundings in the past, present and future (for which we might use the term qualitative concsciousness); fully active mental faculties (quantitative consciousness), and voluntary activity. The present discussion, like most others, although often implicity, will be limited to the examination of consciousness as awareness.

The history of medicine and physiology offers many examples of how insights into basic mechanisms may be gained through the study of pathological examples of malfunction and its consequences. One such example, we believe, may be attention deficit hyperactivity disorder (ADHD) which can be seen as a syndrome of deficient awareness. ADHD is a common syndrome of disturbed behaviour in childhood, particularly among boys (Gillberg, 1995). The aetiology if often genetic, but in many instances lesional factors play a role. One such factor is prematurity and deficient oxygenation of the immature brain (Lou, 1997). The affected child is impulsive, distractible and hyperactive. The available neuropsychological data suggest that impulsiveness is the core disturbance, constituting the basis of attention deficit and of hyperactivity. Impulsiveness, or disinhibition, is characterised by acting without awareness or contextual attention, whether in time or space. Particularly informative is the performance on the so-called go-no go test, which requires the subject to execute a simple motor response to one stimulus (the "go") while inhibiting this response in the presence of another (the "no go" stimulus). On this test the patient with ADHD is apt to fail (Trommer et al., 1991). During the last decade or so we have been examining the neurophysiological basis of that disorder by means of single-photon emission tomography (SPECT) and ^{133}Xe inhalation (Lou 1984, 1989, 1990).

The patients were selected from the Department of child psychiatry, national university hospital, Copenhagen, and from a special school for children with neurological and neuropsychological handicaps. The following criteria of the American Psychiatric Association (DSM-IIIr) were used: attention deficit, impulsiveness, hyperactivity and temper, as substantiated by reports from teachers and parents. The diagnosis was confirmed by examination by a neuropsychologist, a paediatric neurologist and a child psychiatrist. Seven boys and two girls had relatively monosymptomatic (i.e., "pure") ADHD whereas eight boys had ADHD with phonological-syntactical dysphasia (ADHD+). The control group consisted of 15 children aged 7-15 years, mainly siblings of the children in the study groups. All patients in the study had normal, without evidence of ventricular enlargement. All children were studied at rest with open eyes. Three dimensional regional CBF (rCBF) and flow distribution were determined. Four children from the ADHD group and nine from the ADHD+ group received methylphenidate. They were examined before and 30-60 min after oral ingestion of their daily dose of 10-30 mg methylphenidate hydrochloride. The average flow distribution before and after medication was compared, and changes in regional perfusion were calculated.

Regional CBF in the ADHD group differed from the control group in the following respects: the striatal regions appeared hypoperfused, whereas the primary sensory and the sensorimotor regions appeared relatively hyperperfused. This impression was substantiated by the followig deviations from normal: right striatum ($p<0.002$), occipital lobe ($p<0.005$), and left sensorimotor and primary auditory region ($p<0.05$) while other areas failed to reach significance. In the more heterogeneous ADHD+ group, the deviation from normal flow distribution was essentially similar, but the central low-flow region appeared more extensive, and the increase in occipital lobe and sensorimotor regions less conspicuous. Statistical analysis showed a highly significant decrease in both striatal regions. The decrease in the left posterior periventricular region was close to statistical significance ($0.05<p<0.1$). A significant increase was seen in the occipital lobe. No other deviations attained statistical significance.

Administration of methylphenidate appeared to increase flow in the central regions, with a less conspicuous decrease in cortical areas. This increase paralleled definite clinical improvement. Calculation showed an increase in both striatal (left, 7%, right, 2%) and posterior periventricular regions (both 7%). The increase in the right striatal region failed to achieve significance. Thus, the common denominator for children with pure ADHD or with ADHD+ was hypoperfusion and, most likely, low neural activity in the striatal regions. The appearance of a more extended low-flow region centrally in ADHD+ is probably an indication of more extended neural dysfunction, characterized by more extensive neuropsychological and neurological signs. These deviations from normal were partly reversible with methylphenidate (Lou et al., 1989). A subsequent larger study confirmed the hypoactivity of the striatum and, less conspicuously, the thalamic region (Lou et al., 1990). Recently, morphological abnormalities in the striatum have been demonstrated by volumetric MRI (Hynd et al., 1993; Castellanos et al., 1994).

Requirements for a theory of awereness

To assess the striatum as a possible candidate for a crucial role in the physiological basis of qualitative consciousness we must whether the theory could fulfil a tentative list of conditions with which any such theory should comply (Churchland, 1996):

- Involvement with short term memory
- Variable or steerable attention
- Alternative interpretation of ambiguous data
- Independence of sensory input
- Disappearance in sleep
- Reappearance in dreaming
- Unity across modalities
- Fictive reasoning and exploration of the environment.

If such criteria were accepted as a framework, a recurrent neural network would be well suited for the purpose. One major argument in favour of a recurrent network is the time factor: experimental research by Libet et al. (1975) indicates that time is critical for neural processes to become conscious and several of the characteristics listed above (for instance, variability and flexibility) require time. To ensure stable but flexible neural activity a recurrent network would be ideal. One might then ask what kind of recurrent network would include the striatum.

The striatum is functionnally tightly coupled to the frontal cortex. This is seen not only on single cell recordings, but also from the fact that experimental lesions in the frontal lobe and striatum, in particular the caudate nucleus, may give rise to almost identical symptoms (Iversen, 1977). This concept has been carried further recently, in particular by Alexander et al. (1986), who described segregated circuits linking (frontal) cortex, striatum, thalamus, and cortex in cortico-subcortical loops. Cummings (1993) describes at least five separate frontal-subcortical loops, each with a distinct neurobehavioural function and associated deficiency syndromes.

It is of interest that disinhibition and poor performance on the go-no go test may be seen in experimental and clinical lesions in several structures which could constitute a loop of awareness: the medial frontal lobe, with the anterior cingulate gyrus (Drewe, 1975; Leimkuhler, 1985), ventral striatum (Inversen, 1977), and the medial thalamic region (Eslinger, 1991). Heilman et al. (1991) have hypothetically attributed the clinical phenomenology of

ADHD to disturbance of fronto-subcortical circuits, an interpretation fully compatible with our earlier demonstration of deficient striatal function in ADHD.

We tested that hypothesis in a group of 6 normal boys (age range 6-11, median age 8 years) and 12 hyperactive boys (age 5-12, median age 9,5 years) with ADHD, fulfilling the DSM-IIIr criteria. The children were of normal intelligence (IQ (WISC) < 85) and had normal physical and neurological examination. Each was examined three times with single-photon emission computed tomography (SPECT). They were awake but motionless, with eyes open in a quiet room with subdued lights. The ears were covered by soft-padded earphones through which auditory stimuli were presented from a tape recorder. The following auditory/linguistic stimuli, calibrated to the same intensity level, were presented in random order: "white noise", containing a spectrum of frequences between 500 and 10 000 Hz and "animal series", a series of names of animal to which the subjects were instructed to attend carefully. In a separate section an additional requirement was that the subject press a button with a movement of the right index finger each time the name of a dangerous animal was presented. Regional CBF was measured with the ^{133} xenon inhalation technique in a fast-rotating, brain-dedicated SPECT tomograph. Radiation was recorded simultaneously from two parallel transverse slices of the brain 50 and 90 mm above the orbitomeatal plane. The spatial resolution in the transverse plane was 12 mm. The technique, with pCO_2 corrections, is described in detail elsewhere. The estimated absorbed radiation dose per study was 0.37 mSV.

A set of regions of interest (ROI) was defined, as previously described. Factor analysis of the rCBF data was performed to identify brain regions co activated by stimuli, to define functionnally interconnected regions. To eliminate the effect of influences such as genetics, age, etc., a grand mean for each subject was calculated as a reference. It consisted of the mean of all of the subject's rCBF values (28 ROI x 3 tasks). In an analysis of the effect of stimulation by verbal awareness on striatal flow, this "mean rCBF" was subtracted from the regional flow values for each subject and task. Differences between striatal flow and "mean rCBF" were positive for both subject groups and tasks, indicating a high rCBF in the striatal regions. The most conspicuous finding, however, was that in both groupss there was a trend for bilateral higher striatal flow with increased demands on verbal awareness (F analysis $p = 0.015$). This effect is largely explained by the difference between the two language activation conditions and white noise ($p = 0.030$). Striatal flow was generally lower in ADHD than in normals (F analysis, $p = 0.03$, pooled across ROI and tasks). Factor analysis identified one major with correlation coefficients < 0.50, explaining 21 per cent of the variance. It was symmetrical and included the anterior cingulate and dorsal prefrontal cortical regions, the striatal regions and the inferior frontal gyri. The activity of the factor, like the striatum itself, was dependent on the demands on verbal awareness by the task. The striatum contributed significantly less to the factor in ADHD than in normals. The investigation therefore seemed to confirm the idea of a frontal subcortical symmetrical network subserving verbal awareness, which is dysfunctional in ADHD.

Thus, the clinical phenomenology of ADHD is that of a disorder of consciousness, not in the sense of wakefulness as seen in certain lesions of the ascending reticular system, but in the sense of awareness. The core behavioural feature is impulsiveness, with actions uninfluenced by contextual attention. We have presented evidence that ADHD is characterised by striatal dysfunction, and that the striatum has a key role in a network activated by verbal awareness. Thus, both indirect and direct evidence points to the existence of a frontal-subcortical circuit subserving awareness in normals as well as in ADHD, but partially impaired in the latter through striatal dysfunction.

References

Alexander GE, Deong MR, Strick PL (1986) Parallel organization of functionally segregated ciruits linking basal ganglia and cortex. Ann Rev Neurosci 9: 257-281

Castellanos FX, Gjedd JN, Eckburg BS, Marsh WL, Vaituzis AG (1994) Quantitative morphology of caudate nucleus in attention deficit hyperactivity disorder. Am J Psychiat 151: 1791-1796

Churchland PM (1996) Eighteenth Annual Conference of the Cognitive science society, San Diego, (oral presentation)

Drewe EA (1975) Go-no go learning after frontal lobe lesions in humans. Cortex 11: 8-16

Eslinger PJ, Warner GC, Grattan LM et al (1991) "Frontal lobe" utilization behavior associated with paramedian thalamic infarction. Neurology 41: 450-452

Gilberg C (1995) Clinical child neuropsychiatry. Cambridge University Press, Cambridge

Heilman KM, Voeller KK, Nadean SE (1991) A possible pathophysiologic substrate of attention deficit hyperactivity disorder. J Child Neurol 6 (Suppl.): 576-581

Hynd GW, Hern KL, Novey ES, Eliopulos D, Marshall R, Gonzales JJ, Voeller KK (1993) Attention deficit-hyperactivity disorder in asymmetry of the caudate nucleus. J Child Neurol 8: 339-347

Iversen SD (1977) Behavior after neostriatal lesions in animals. In Divac I, Oberg TGE (eds) The neostriatum. Pergamon Press Elmsford, p 1995-2210

Leimkuhler ME, Mesulam MM (1985) Reversible go-no go deficits in a case of frontal lobe tumor. Ann Neurol 18: 617-619

Libet B, Kobayashi H, Tanaka T (1982) Synaptic coupling into the production and storage of a neuronal memory trace. Nature 258: 155-157

Lou HC, Henriksen L, Bruhn P (1984) Focal cerebral hypoperfusion in children with dysphasia and/or attention deficit disorder. Arch Neurol 41: 825-829

Lou HC, Henriksen L, Bruhn P (1990) Focal cerebral dysfunction in developmental learning disabilities. Lancet 335: 8-11

Lou HC (1997) Etiology and pathogenesis of ADHD - significance of prematurity and perinatal hypodtic hemodynamic encephalopathy. Acta Paediatrica (in press)

Tromner BL, Hoepner JAB, Zecker SG (1991) The go-no go test in attention deficit disorder is sensitive to methylphenidate. J Child Neurol, 6 (Suppl.): 128-131

Webster's encyclopedy unabridged dictionary of the English Language (1989) Gramercy Books, New York

5. Neuroanatomical and neurophysiological clues to the nature of autism

M. BELMONTE, R. CARPER

Of all the developmental brain disorders, autism is perhaps the most fascinating, the most mysterious, and the most telling fascinating, because of its impact on absolutely every aspect of a child's perception of and interaction with the surrounding world; mysterious, because of the complexity of the many interacting brain systems it perturbs; telling, because it strikes at the social, cognitive, and linguistic abilities that seem, at least on the surface, so essential to one's very humanity. During the past few decades, the riddle of autism has begun to yield to advances in the study of autistic behaviour and the biological foundations which affect it. The examination of brain anatomy, physiology, histology and function in people with autism continues to supply new information on the nature and ætiology of this complex syndrome. This chapter will focus primarily on the neuroanatomical and neurophysiological abnormalities found in autistic subjects, particularly those seen in magnetic resonance imaging (MRI) and event-related potential (ERP) studies.

A plethora of proposals

Many regions of the cerebrum have been posited as loci of autism. In fact, autism impacts upon so many abilities and behaviours that it is difficult to find any brain region which has not been put forth as a possible site of dysfunction. Sites proposed have included the limbic system, brain stem, basal ganglia, vestibular system and cerebellum. Damasio and Maurer (1978), focussing on autistic deficits in executive function, pointed to the medial frontal lobes and the basal ganglia as sites of dysfunction. In their discussion of the medial frontal lobes they placed particular emphasis on the role of the cingulate gyrus, an important part of the limbic system. This hypothesis was based on similarities between the behaviour observed in people with autism and in adults with acquired medial frontal or basal ganglia lesions. A hypothesis put forth by Ornitz (1983) suggested that autistic difficulties with sensory modulation and sensorimotor response could best be explained by a malfunction of brain stem and diencephalic networks which gate sensory input. Deficits in higher-order capacities such as language, he proposed, are consequences of the abnormal input supplied to the cerebrum by these malfunctioning gating systems. (As we shall see, this notion of a cascade of dysfunction, in which one malfunctioning brain system perturbs its functional consequents, is a recurring theme in theories of autistic neuropathology). Another possible explanation for the stimulus-overselectivity manifest in autism is a developmental spatial neglect syndrome et akin to the acute spatial neglect which follows parietal lobe injury. Bryson et al. (1990) reviewed a number of autonomic, electrophysiological and behavioural studies indicating the existence of attentional anomalies in people with autism and described similarities between the behaviour of people with autism and of patients with left-sided neglect. Hetzler and Griffin (1981) and DeLong (1992), recognising the similarities between autistic behaviour and the Klüver Bucy syndrome, characterised autism as the effect of developmental dysfunction in structures of the medial temporal lobe, especially the hippocampus and amygdala. This theory incorporates an observation that is sure to figure in any explanation of autism: the effect of a lesion in a developing brain is often more severe than or distinct from the effect of a similar lesion in a mature brain, because brain systems downstream from the lesion may depend on correct input for their proper maturation. This is supported by finding of Bachevalier's (1994) that lesions of medial temporal lobe structures induced in neonatal monkeys result in behaviours more typical of autism than similar lesions induced in adult monkeys.

As well as these anatomical systems, a number of chemical systems have been thought to underlie autism. The finding of hyperserotonaemia in some people with autism has been widely replicated (Cook, 1990). Levels of other monoamines also have been found to be higher than normal in people with autism (Martineau et al., 1992). Panksepp (1979), on the basis of autistic insensitivity to pain, suggested dysfunction of opiatergic systems, and others have confirmed elevated levels of opiate activity in cerebrospinal fluid (Gillberg et al., 1985) and urine (Gillberg et al., 1982; Gillberg, 1988; Reichelt et al., 1991, Reichelt et al., 1994; Williams et al., 1991; Shattock and Lowdon, 1991) of people with autism.

Cerebellar anatomy in autism

Each of these theories seems to contain at least a grain of truth, but how can they all be unified? Is there a single brain structure or system which could produce secondary malfunctions in all these other structures and systems? What region is consistently abnormal in autistic brains? So far, the most consistent neuropathological abnormalities have been found in an area which no one would have considered until recently: the cerebellum.

While the most noticeable and diagnostic characteristics of autism are cognitive (e.g., impaired social interaction and communication, restricted range of interests (American Psychiatric Association, 1992), a number of motor abnormalities have also been noted, although they receive relatively little attention clinically and scientifically. For instance, autistic children are universally dyspraxic (Jones and Prior, 1985), and manifest disturbances of gait (Vilensky et al., 1981) which persist, to some extent, into adulthood (Hallett et al. 1993). Motor anomalies are clear enough that Adrien et al. (1992) found that blinded raters were able to differentiate autistic children from normal children on the basis of motility and other factors appearing in home movies taken before autism was suspected. In a more recent study using a battery of tests taken from a standard neurological examination, Haas et al. (1996) found that autistic patients showed abnormalities indicative of cerebellar and parietal lobe dysfunction, but no significant abnormalities on tests of pyramidal motor and cranial nerve abilities. Furthermore, classical eyeblink conditioning, a hallmark of cerebellar functioning, is abnormal in autism, in both the amplitude and latency of conditioned responses and the rate of extinction (Sears et al., 1994).

The first indication of the neuropathological bases of these functional abnormalities came a decade and a half ago, when Williams et al. (1980) detected a low count of Purkinje cells in the cerebellum of one of four autistic brains at autopsy. Ritvo et al. (1986) confirmed this finding, reporting a 41 % loss of Purkinje cells in the vermis and a 35 % loss in the hemispheres in four autistic brains compared to normal brains. In a more comprehensive autopsy study, Bauman (1991) reported depletion of Purkinje cells and granule cells in autistic brains, with no evidence of the gliosis which ensues when neurons degenerate after infancy. In the cerebellar deep nuclei, the destinations of Purkinje cell axons, abnormally enlarged cells were found at autopsy in children and a depletion of cells in adults. In the inferior olive, the source of climbing-fibre input to Purkinje cells, small cell bodies were found in the lateral portion, but no apparent loss of cells. This absence of retrograde cell death in the inferior olive, like the absence of gliosis in the cerebellar cortex, points to a time of onset early in fetal life. Bauman and Kemper (1993) later speculated that the olivary and deep nuclear abnormalities might be a consequence of the retention of a fetal pattern of cerebellar circuitry in which climbing fibres synapse directly on cells of the deep nuclei, without sending the major branches of their axons into the cerebellar cortex. Such a short-circuited pattern of connections would sabotage the regular topography of the cerebellar cortical map. The climbing fibres which do extend to the cerebellar cortex may innervate multiple Purkinje cells inappropriately, because of the depletion of granule cells which somehow mediate the formation of the correct, one-to-one or one-to-few mapping of climbing fibres to Purkinje cells (Crepel, 1982).

By the late 1980s, MRI studies began to reinforce the autopsy findings. The depletion of cells at the microscopic level was manifest as a deficit in size at the macroscopic level, specifically, as a reduction in the cross-sectional area of the cerebellar vermis. Courchesne et al. (1987) reported this finding in a single case, and Gaffney et al. (1987) extended the finding to a group of eight subjects. In a larger study of 18 autistic subjects, Courchesne et al. (1988) localised this hypoplasia to vermian lobules VI and VII. Subsequent work in the same laboratory demonstrated that hypoplasia could be found not only in the vermis of the autistic cerebellum, but also in the cerebellar hemispheres (Murakami et al. 1989). In the largest MRI study of the autistic cerebellum to date, Hashimoto et al. (1995) found hypoplasia of lobules VI and VII when a group of 102 people with autism were compared to 112 control subjects. This difference was found even in children less than 2 years old who were later diagnosed as having autism. In contrast, studies from several other laboratories (e.g., Holttum et al., 1992; Hashimoto et al., 1993; Kleiman et al., 1992), using similar anatomical methods, failed to replicate these findings. There are a number of possible explanations for this discrepancy, including small sample size (none of the studies which obtained negative results used more than 18 autistic subjects), and the use of patient controls (Hashimoto et al., 1992; 1993, Kleiman et al., 1992) unstead of healthy volunteer (Courchesne et al., 1988; Piven et al., 1992; Holttum et al., 1992; Garber et al., 1992).

It is also possible that non specific IQ effects play a role in these findings. While some of the aforementioned studies chose control groups with IQs comparable to those in their autistic groups (e.g., Piven et al., 1992; Holttum et al., 1992) most, including the studies which found significant differences in vermian area (Courchesne et al., 1988; Hashimoto et al., 1995), did not. It has therefore been suggested (Piven and Arndt, 1995; Filipek, 1995) that these differences were due to confounding differences in IQ rather than to a specific effect of autism. In fact, Schaefer et al. (1996) have presented evidence that a number of disorders can result in vermian hypoplasia, including disorders which do not show autistic-like behaviours. Needless to say,this is an important result and emphasises the necessity of including IQ-matched control groups in future studies. However, we must not forget that a single macroscopic difference (i.e., vermian hypoplasia) could result from a wide variety of distinct microscopic differences (e.g., loss of Purkinje cells in autism, loss of granule cells in Down's syndrome). Additional research is necessary to assess the specificity of both macroscopic and microscopic differences. We must also keep in mind that even a non specific finding may give us an insight into the nature of the causal abnormalities of the autistic syndrome.

Another possible explanation for the discrepancies between studies as to the presence of significant differences was suggested when Courchesne et al. (1994) described the possibility of a hyperplastic subgroup in addition to the hypoplastic group described previously. Their analysis of 50 autistic subjects showed a bimodal distribution in the areas of lobules VI and VII with 5 individuals being more than 2 standard deviations above the mean in normal controls (Fig. 1). If this result is verified in additional studies with large samples, this mix of subgroups would, as demonstrated by Courchesne et al. (1994a,b), explain the inability of smaller studies to

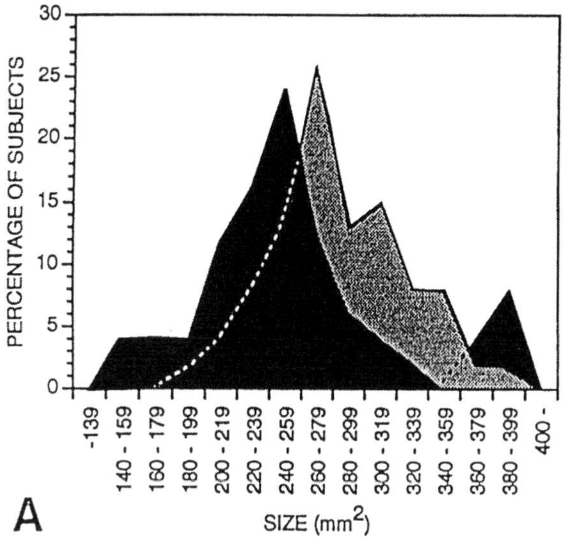

Fig. 1. Midsagittal area of vermian lobules VI-VII shows a normal, Gaussian distribution for the control group (n=53, stippled area), but a bimodal distribution for the autistic group (n=50, black area). A few individuals in the latter group have enlargement of lobules VI-VII, but in most they are smaller than in the control group (From Courchesne et al., 1994).

find significant differences between people with autism and control subjects.

While there has been a great deal of discussion (Courchesne et al., 1994; Piven et Arndt, 1995; Filipek, 1995; Schaefer et al., 1996) as to whether MRI studies demonstrate hypoplasia of the vermis in the autistic cerebellum and whether this effect is specific to the disorder, an appraisal of all the available data indicates that cerebellar abnormalities are an important aspect of autism. This includes both the neuropathological studies, all of which have found cerebellar abnormalities especially of the Purkinje cells, and the neuroimaging studies, in which those with the largest sample sizes (and therefore the greatest statistical power) have found cerebellar hypoplasia.

It is important to note that the cerebellar abnormality is not limited to the vermis. In reviews of this topic, the earlier work on the vermis often is cited without mention of the hemisphere findings (i.e., Murakami et al., 1989), this is an unfortunate omission since may suggest that the hemispheres are unaffected. In fact, the hemispheres are affected almost as much as the vermis. The only reason the vermis has been the focus the majority of research is that it is technically easier to measure: its anatomy provides a ready plane for the alignement of MRI sections such that any alignement error is immediately discernible from alteration of midsagittal cerebellar landmarks, and its borders are sufficiently obvious to make outlining its area straightforward. However, evidence of decreased size of the hemispheres does exist and future research and reviews should emphasise the full anatomical extent of cerebellar pathology in autism to give a more accurate perspective.

The cerebellum and cognition

It is easier to understand how cerebellar damage might produce autistic cognition and behaviour if we first understand the role of the normal cerebellum in cognition. Leiner, Leiner, and Dow (1986, 1991) were the first to argue forcefully for involvement of the cerebellum in non motor operations. They based their conjecture on the concomitant evolution of the prefrontal cortex and the neocerebellum, and on the idea that a single computational architecture could implement both motor and non motor representations. These influences could be achieved through the neuronal connections which exist between the cerebellum and multiple regions of the cerebrum. In monkeys, the cerebellum projects via the thalamus to the prefrontal cortex (Middleton and Strick, 1994). In cats, the cerebellum projects to the hippocampus via the thalamus, and appropriately timed stimulation of the cerebellar vermis potentiates hippocampal response to somatosensory input (Newman and Reza 1979). In rats, stimulation of the vermis modulates responses of the brain stem, tectum, and cerebral cortex to visual, auditory and somatosensory stimuli (Crispino and Bullock, 1984). In humans, cerebellar strokes can result in decreased metabolism in prefrontal cortex and temporal cortex (Attig et al., 1991). In short, the cerebellum is ideally placed to influence all the cognitive systems and anatomical regions which have been implicated in the various theories of autism.

Several functional imaging studies have carried this relationship a step further, by going beyond the static relationships of anatomy and examining the functional relationship between the cerebellum and the rest of the brain. Petersen et al. (1989) showed that the right lateral cerebellum is active during a semantic language task, but not during a language repetition task. Specifically, the cerebellum was active when subjects had to produce spoken verbs whose meanings were related to nouns they read, but not when the subjects had merely to speak the nouns. With practice, however, this cerebellar activation, along with prefrontal activation in the cerebral cortex, diminishes (Raichle et al., 1994). Especially in light of the anatomical projection of the cerebellum to prefrontal cortex, this suggests that a cerebello-thalamic-prefrontal control system is involved in the creation of novel cognitive strategies, but not for rote execution of such strategies. Similarly, in subjects attempting to solve a pegboard puzzle, activation of the dentate nuclei was three to four times as large as that occurring during simple, visually-guided movements of the pegs (Kim et al., 1994). In tasks requiring tactile discrimination, the dentate nucleus was again much more active than in cases of similar but passive palpation (Gao et al., 1996). In a visual 'oddball' task, which required simple visual discrimination without a motor response, the posterosuperior cerebellar cortex was strongly activated, but this area was only very weakly activated by a simple motor task. Similarly, when the discrimination task was combined with a contingent motor response, activation was no greater than in the non motor discrimination task (Allen et al., submitted). On the basis of these first few studies, the role of the cerebellum in cognition might be characterised in general as adaptive selection of cognitive strategies. Functional imaging of the cerebellum has not yet been attempted in people with autism, probably because they often have difficulty lying still in the scanner and because even the normal cerebellar contribution to cognition is only just beginning to be characterised. We can, however, look forward, to a growing understanding of cerebellar function, and the beginning of an inquiry into the specifics of its abnormal function in autism. Functional imaging techniques will be critical to the development of this understanding.

An important point about the role of the cerebellum in autism is the distinction between early developmental cerebellar malformation and other types of cerebellar abnormality. It might be argued that the cerebellum can not be responsible for autism, since people whose cerebellum becomes damaged or is congenitally absent do not behave like people with autism. This argument overlooks the developmental nature of the deficit. Time and time again in the study of neural systems, we find that appropriately structured input is required for correct development. The Purkinje cells of the cerebellar cortex are the sole inhibitory input to the deep cerebellar nuclei. Loss of appropriately patterned inhibition could produce constitutive activation of these deep nuclei, and, consequently, constitutive, nonspecific activation downstream in the cerebral cortex. Such a situation may very well be worse for development than having no cerebellum at all! Even aside from these biological considerations which may explain congenital or early developmental defects more damaging than acquired defects, there may be psychological considerations. How might congenital impairment of the attentional and other cognitive functions of the cerebellum differ from acquired impairment in the nature and scope of its effect?

The development of joint social attention is a major milestone in the maturation of a normal child. It marks the beginning of a baby's ability to learn the nature of its world under the guidance of its parents and other adults. The learning process is thus greatly accelerated. A properly-functioning attentional system is essential for the timely development of joint social attention, and on the later depends the explosion of learning which characterises every normal toddler. Imagine the following scene. A baby rests on his father's lap. Outside a window, a flash of sunlight glints from a fender, a car horn sounds, there is a crunch of gravel, and the throb of an engine grows and then abruptly ceases. The father strokes the baby, smiles at him, and announces that the baby's mother has arrived. The father has made an inference about the world, and a normal baby would learn eventually to make the same inference when presented with the same conjunction of stimuli. Implicit in this process is a tremendous degree of integration of sensory stimuli: the father's gentle touch, his tone of voice, the particular words he speaks, his smile, all figure in the representation of mother; the glint of light, the sounds of the engine, of the horn and of the gravel beneath the tire all point to the fact that a car is entering the driveway. Combine this with the stored knowledge that mother has been out in a car, and the inference is made. But if the baby has difficulty with attentional shifting or distribution, then only one or a few of these many stimuli may reach awareness. They come in rapid sequence, via various sensory modalities, and from diverse locations in space. Without a properly functioning mechanism for rapidly and automatically shifting and distributing attention, the task of integrating all of them into a coherent percept is rendered very difficult, to say the least. In a developing infant, who has no prior knowledge of the world, learning may become almost impossible. Thus amage to olivoponto-cerebello-thalamocortical control loops which optimise attentional dynamics although a rather innocuous deficit in itself, may begin a cascade of detrimental effects in profound alteration of cognitive and social development.

If this is the case, then it should be possible to observe the primary attention difficulty in brain-injured adults, without the profound, secondary, developmental effects that result from the congenital form of such damage. Akshoomoff and Courchesne (1992) have observed just such a dissociation. Their experiment consists of two 'oddball' paradigms running simultaneously. In the standard oddball paradigm, there are two types of stimulus, a relatively rare, target stimulus, and a common, background stimulus. The subject must produce a motor or mental response to each instance of the target, but not to the background stimuli. In a visual oddball experiment, for example, the target stimulus might be a red flash which occurs with 20% probability, and the background stimulus might be a green flash occurring with 80% probability. In an auditory oddball experiment, high and low tones might be used for the same purposes. In the attention-shifting experiment, visual and auditory oddball stimuli are presented concurrently, and subjects must attend to one modality, either vision or audition, while ignoring the other. A target stimulus in the attended modality cues not only an overt motor response but also a covert shift of attention to the previously unattended modality. The next target in this newly attended modality cues a shift back to the other modality, and so on. Akshoomoff's original experiment was a behavioural measure of the execution time of attention shifts between visual and auditory modalities. She found that patients with cerebellar damage were impaired specifically in detecting targets that occurred in a newly attended modality within the first few seconds following the cue to shift from the previously attended modality. Later, this result was replicated

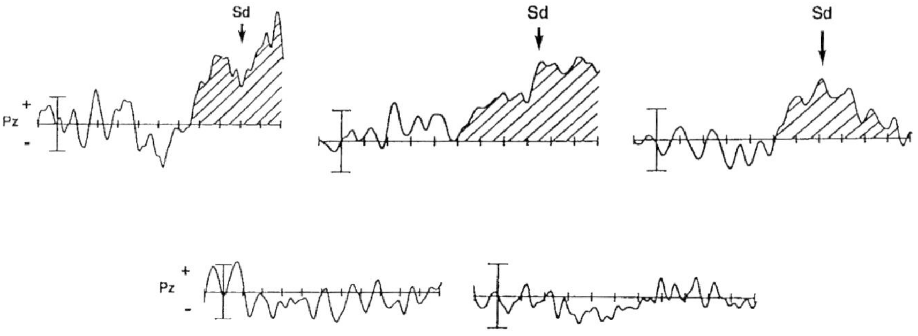

Fig. 2
In normal children, adults and three children with cortical lesions, there is a large Sd, the shifting attention related difference ERP response, at Pz (parietal scalp site) evoked by visual stimuli; the Sd may reflect neural activity elicited by the requirement to execute a shift of attention. In autistic adults and in children with cerebellar lesions, the Sd was greatly reduced in response to these visual cues. The horizontal scale is time, divided into 100 ms intervals; stimulus delivery at large vertical bar, which also represents amplitude ± 5mV (From Courchesne et al., 1994).

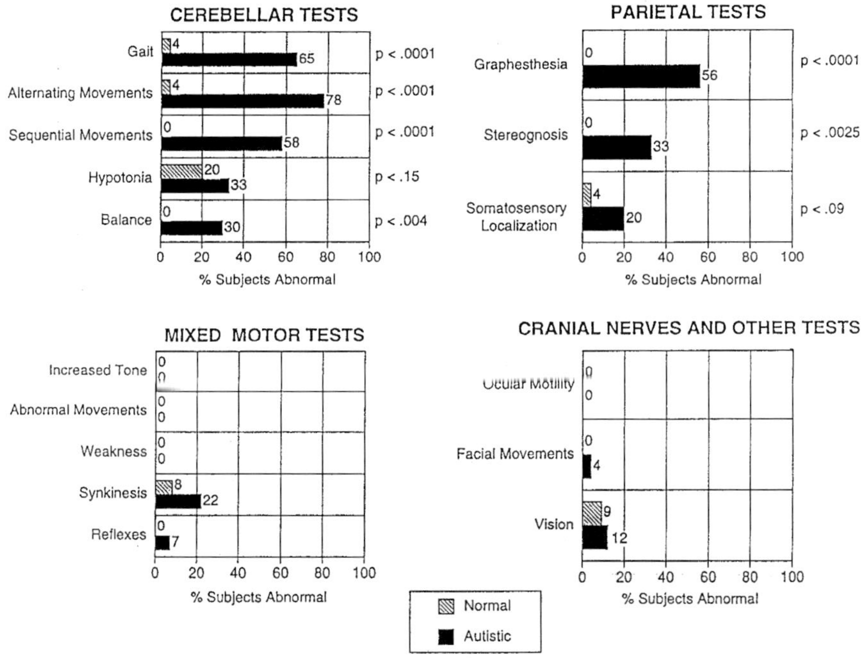

Fig. 3
Percentage of autistic (black bars) and normal control subjects (shaded bars) who performed in the clinically abnormal range on individual tests. Probabilities are shown for c2 neurological which tests were significant or near significant. Significantly more autistic subjects were judged to show abnormal function (From Haas et al., 1996).

in people with autism (Courchesne et al., 1994), and in tasks requiring division of attention between auditory and visual modalities and between several attributes of visual stimuli (Casey et al., 1993). (This latter study, however,used a heterogeneous group of subjects with either autism or some other pervasive developmental disorder, who had unusual calendar-calculating ability.) A second version of the shift experiment (Akshoomoff and Courchesne, 1994) tested intramodality shifts of attention, in which the attended features were the colour and form of visual stimuli presented at a single spatial location. A similar behavioural result was found.

Reinforcing this behavioural result was an absence, in patients with cerebellar deficits and people with autism, of the positive shift-difference (Sd) potential which in normal brains appears with a long latency (~700ms) after a cue to shift attention (Fig. 2). This difference potential may be akin to the late directing attention positivity (LDAP) reported by Harter (Harter et al., 1989; Harter and Anllo-Vento, 1991) in another attention-shifting experiment. Rather than using a continuous back-and-forth shifting paradigm, this experiment examined ERPs in response to an attention-directing cue in the centre of the visual field. A cue to shift attention was followed, in the hemisphere contralateral to the cued side, by an occipitoparietal negative potential at about 200ms, and then by the LDAP from about 400ms to 700ms. These effects arose in difference waves comparing responses at each electrode to left and to right cues.

In an experiment based on the spatial attentional cueing paradigm of Posner (1980), Townsend found in patients with cerebellar deficits and autistics the same behavioural deficit for short cue-to-target intervals as in the previous inte- and intramodality studies (Fig. 3)

That is, autistics and patients with cerebellar lesions patients are abnormally slow to shift attention in space or between or within sensory modalities. The behavioural and electrophysiological effects shown by the patients and people with autism in these experiments, which address selectively the capacity for rapid shifting of attention, support the hypothesis that cerebellar damage in autism produces a deficit in such shifting, which may further impair cognitive and social development.

The temporal lobe

The cerebellum seems the most consistently abnormal structure in the autistic brain, and it would simplify matters if the cerebellum were the only one, but the picture is not so straightforward. In the same studies in which they noted depletion of cerebellar granule cells and Purkinje cells, Bauman and Kemper (1985) also reported pathological changes in cell morphology in limbic structures. In the hippocampus, amygdala, anterior cingulate gyrus, entorhinal cortex and mamillary bodies they noted small, closely-packed cells. A Golgi analysis of two subjects also showed a decrease in dendritic branching of

CA1 and CA4 hippocampal neurons (Raymond, Bauman and Kemper, 1989). It was speculated that these changes, like those in the cerebellum, may reflect incomplete development (Bauman and Kemper 1993).

Additional evidence supporting temporal lobe dysfunction in autism comes from epilepsy research. Epilepsy is believed to be relatively common, affecting up to a quarter of people with autism (American Psychiatric Association, 1994), and some forms of temporal lobe epilepsy with onset in early childhood can mirror at least some of the symptoms of autism. The Landau-Kleffner syndrome (Landau and Kleffner 1957; Deonna, 1991), for example, involves a malformation of the temporal lobe which results in a loss of language as well as seizures. Since a seizure focus in the temporal lobe can mimic autistic symptoms, it seems logical to hypothesise that autism, in at least some of its forms, involves abnormal function of the temporal lobe. Reinforcing this hypothesis are several case reports of acquired autistic behaviours in older children (DeLong et al., 1981; C. Gillberg 1986), and even in one adult (Gillberg 1981) following acute encephalitis. In each of these cases an autism-like syndrome developed rapidly (in 1-3 months) in previously normal people and was presumed to be due to temporal lobe dysfunction, as evidenced by an abnormal temporal lobe EEG and, in two cases, CT or MRI. Two of these patients recovered fully from the autistic syndrome (DeLong et al., 1981). Another report (Hoon and Reiss, 1992) described a rather classic case of autism, with first signs at 1-2 years, associated with a unilateral temporal lobe tumour and seizures.

Another condition that seems to have some features in common with autism is the Klüver-Bucy syndrome. This has been described primarily in monkeys with temporal lobe lesions. It occurs rarely in humans, following bilateral lesions of the temporal lobe due to encephalitis, or, previously, psychosurgery. The features are severe visual agnosia, also known as 'psychic blindness', nonresponsiveness in social contexts, flatness of affect, and a tendency to oral and somatosensory exploration with relative disuse of vision and hearing. Bachevalier (1994) described a related but distinct disorder in monkeys in which temporal lobe lesions were produced neonatally rather than in adulthood. At two months of age, these monkeys showed greater passivity and less tendency to initiate social contact then normal monkeys. By six months of age the same monkeys showed an even greater degree of abnormality, actively avoiding social contact and demonstrating stereotyped locomotor activity. They monkeys did not demonstrate hypersexuality, a feature of the Klüver-Bucy syndrome not seen in autism, nor did they demonstrate the loss of fear characteristic of Klüver-Bucy syndrome.

While these diverse cases offer insight into the possible bases of autistic symptoms, imaging studies are in a unique position to demonstrate the location of the physiological abnormalities in classic autism. A detailed imaging study (Saitoh et al., 1995) showed no macroscopic decrease in cross-sectional area of the posterior hippocampus in people with autism compared to normals. The temporal lobe as a whole, is in fact, larger in people with autism (Osamu Saitoh, unpublished observations). These somewhat paradoxical findings illustrate the difficulty of mapping macroscopic imaging data onto microscopic, histoanatomical observations. Nevertheless, on the basis of the neuropathological data, it does seem that some process of abnormal development is occurring in the medial temporal lobe of the autistic brain. The neuronal connections between the cerebellum and the temporal lobe raise the possibility that temporal and limbic maldevelopment may, at least in some cases, be a consequence of cerebellar maldevelopment. Thus there is no shortage of possible mechanisms for the unification of the limbic theory of autism with the cerebellar theory.

Much more imaging work on the temporal lobe in autism is required. The posterior hippocampus is the only medial temporal lobe structure investigated quantitatively using MRI. More anterior regions,such as the amygdala, remain unexamined. Functional imaging may also contribute to our knowledge of the temporal lobe in autism. SPECT studies (George et al., 1992; Mountz et al., 1995) have demonstrated decreased perfusion of the temporal lobe, but in small samples. Furthermore, the progression of this abnormality over the course of development remains unclear.

The parietal lobe

The list of features of the Klüver-Bucy syndrome seems described above, at least superficially, to describe autism. Of the course, agnosia can to a large extent be mimicked by attentional neglect. Furthermore, the social and emotional abnormalities of autism may be developmental epiphenomena of a lack of attentional control. Thus, autism might be explained by either, or both, or neither of the temporal (gnostic) and the parietal (attention) theories. Hetzler and Griffin (1981) characterised autism as a deficit in the formation of cross-modal associations. Here again, though, the question is one of primacy: is there some defect in the associative processing that binds multimodal sensations into percepts, or is the apparent association deficit a product of a more fundamental lack of ability to distribute or to shift attention among several sensory modalities simultaneously?

Bryson et al., (1990), as mentioned at the beginning of this chapter, hypothesised that autism is a

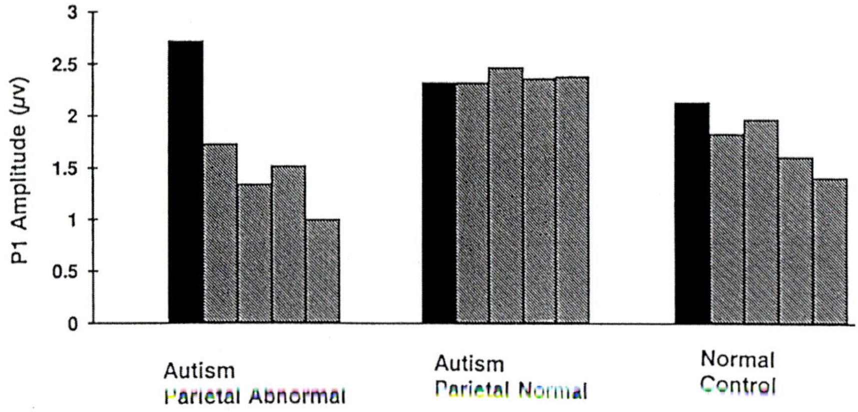

Fig. 4
Bar graphs for three groups, collapsed across the five locations, showing P1 peak amplitude at O1 to an attended spatial location (dark bar), compared to when attention was focussed one, two, three, and four locations away (light bars) (From Townsend, 1992).

developmental neglect syndrome, related to the hemisphere neglect in patients with parietal lesions. There is imaging evidence to support this theory, at least in some cases. Of the people with autism studied by Courchesne et al. (1993) 43 % had parietal sulcal widening, as determined in a blinded assessment by a neuroradiologist. If autism is a developmental version of parietal lobe lesions, then it is much more pervasive than the acquired version, as in the case of developmental cerebellar pathology. This could be due to downstream consequences of the deficit on the development of other brain regions and because of the absence of fully mature, alternative cognitive faculties which might be used to compensate for a deficit in one particular aspect of cognition. It is generally believed that the parietal cortex, especially the right hemisphere, is important in spatial attention (Heilman et al., 1985). While the parietal anatomical deficit in autism has been assessed qualitatively, it awaits quantitative study, which may reveal decreased parietal lobe volume in a larger proportion of autistic subjects.

Reinforcing the finding of a deficit in parietal lobe volume is the finding of narrowing of the posterior part of the corpus callosum (Egaas et al., 1995), the region which contains fibres crossing between the parietal lobes (Pandya et al., 1971). An MRI study of myelination of the corpus callosum in autism (Belmonte et al., 1995) detected no difference between people with autism and normals, even though its methods were sensitive enough to detect an age-related progression in myelination. This suggests that the axons present are myelinated to a normal extent, and that the deficiency in cross-sectional area must result from a deficiency in their number. It thus seems as if the normal complement of layer V pyramidal cells may be absent from the parietal lobes in at least some cases of autism. This hypothesis awaits histoanatomical study.

The parietal deficit shown by MRI is corroborated by behavioural and electrophysiological studies. In the neurological examination by Haas et al. (1996) mentioned previously, the only category of test other than cerebellar shown to be abnormal in people with autism was the group of parietal tests assessing graphaesthesia, stereognosis, and somatosensory localisation (Fig. 4). In the attention-shifting paradigm of Posner (1980), people with autism demonstrate a heightened validity effect at long cue-to-target intervals (Casey et al., 1993; Wainwright-Sharp and Bryson, 1993). That is, they take longer than normal to respond to a target at an unpredicted location when their attention has already been engaged at an erroneously predicted location. Townsend et al. (1996) showed that this effect is due specifically to the subgroup which parietal sulcal widening, and that the degree of the behavioural effect correlates with parietal volume loss.

In the normal brain, attention to the spatial location of a stimulus operates by a mechanism of 'early selection', that is, all stimuli at an attended location, whether their particular features are relevant or not, enhance neural response, even at relatively short latencies (Heinze et al., 1990). The competing theory, of late selection, would predict a dependence of brain response to stimuli at an attended location on whether or not the stimuli possessed attended features. So, for example, if an subject were instructed to respond to a square in the upper left corner of the screen, the brain electrical response would be stronger to that target stimulus than to a circle appearing in the same location. In fact, during the first few hundred milliseconds following the stimulus, this is not what is observed: the amplitude of the occipito-temporal P1 evoked potential is increased in response to any stimulus in the upper left corner, not just to the square. These data suggest that spatial attention operates independently, and in advance of attention to features. Such computational architecture makes sense, because the extraction of features is a much more complex procedure than the simple identification of the appearance of a new stimulus at a particular location.

Attention enhancement, instead of being organised in a 'spotlight' with distinct spatial boundaries, operates as a spatial gradient centered on the attended locus. For example, P1 amplitude is greatest for stimuli at the attended location, but is nearly as great in response to stimuli occurring close to it. Rather than a definite cutoff, there is a gradual decline in amplitude with increasing eccentricity from the focus of attention (Mangun and Hillyard, 1987, 1988). The close functional association of the P1 with attention processing is further supported by the fact that behavioural measures of accuracy, such as detectability and reaction time, covary with P1 amplitude (Mangun and Hillyard 1990). In people with autism, the story differs: they distribute visual spatial attention abnormally, even in conditions of static attention, without any requirement to shift from one location to another. In an experiment by Townsend and Courchesne (1994), autistic subjects were presented with brief flashes, at one of five separate locations. Subjects were asked to respond by pressing a button to flashes in one of the locations, but to ignore flashes in the others. Normal subjects responded with a spatial gradient of P1 amplitude enhancement. A subgroup of autistic subjects with parietal sulcal widening on MRI operated more in keeping with the spotlight metaphor; their P1 in response to stimuli at the attended location was actually larger than normal, but their P1 in response to stimuli even slightly eccentric to the attended location was much smaller than normal. This suggests an abnormally focussed allocation of attentional resources to one particular point in space, with a relative neglect for the surrounding space. In contrast, autistic patients without obvious volume reduction in the parietal lobe evidenced little enhancement of P1 to stimuli presented at an attended location as compared to surrounding locations (Fig. 5). This reult, however, needs to be verified with a larger group of autistic subjects with normal parietal lobes; work on this is in progress. It is typical of the pervasive nature of autism that a defect in one brain area, the parietal lobe, is best observed electrophysiologically by examining responses generated in another area, the occipital lobe. By observing the perturbed function of the visual system, it is possible to trace the dysfunction back to the attentional system.

The P1 experiment tells us a lot about dysfunction in statically-allocated attention, but it can not address the neurophysiology of shifts in attention. Shifts in attention are difficult to assay using conventional event-related potentials, because the latencies and durations of sensory evoked responses are in general comparable to or even greater than the time courses of attention shifts. Investigating rapid attention processes using such relatively slow signals would be like trying to repair a watch with a sledgehammer. To investigate attention dynamics using evoked responses, we have adopted the paradigm of the steady-state visual-evoked potential (SSVEP), an electrical resonance in the visual system which arises in response to stimuli flashed at regular intervals. Stimulus frequencies in the a band (about 8-12 Hz), the natural resonance frequency of the brain, produce particularly powerful SSVEP. In normal brains, allocation of spatial attention to a particular location modulates the brain responses in the occipito temporal region of the hemisphere contralateral to the newly attended stimulus. In particular, the amplitude of the SSVEP is augmented, while the amplitude of background activity which is not phase-locked to the flashing stimulus is diminished (Belmonte, 1997a). These differentials can be detected using specialised algorithms (Belmonte, 1997b), and changes can be observed as the subject shifts attention from one flashing stimulus to another at a different location.

The autistic brain, in contrast, manifests no such modulation. Rather, both the SSVEP and the background responses in both hemispheres are greater to stimuli in the left visual ofield than in the right (Belmonte, 1997c). This tendency does manifest in the normal brain, in that attentional augmentation of right-hemisphere responses to left-field stimuli is in general greater than that of left-hemisphere responses to right-field stimuli. It seems that what is missing in the autistic brain is the hemisphere specificity. It is quite possible and, we think, probable that this lack of hemisphere specificity is just the most obvious manifestation of a general lack of spatiotopy in attentional modulation of brain responses. This would agree with the lack of spatially specific P1 enhancement described by Townsend and Courchesne (1994).

The frontal lobe

The frontal lobe has yet to be addressed quantitatively by anatomical imaging studies, but results of functional imaging and event-related potential studies do suggest its involvement. Much has been made of the so-called 'theory of mind' deficit in autism (Baron-Cohen, 1989), and frontal dysfunction may underly a specific deficit in making abstract inferences about the social world which are often described as the essence of a theory of mind. In normal subjects, the orbitofrontal cortex seems selectively activated during a task involving theory of mind (Baron-Cohen et al., 1994), but it remains unclear whether this specifically reflects the second-order social inference characteristic of theory of mind tasks, or a more general difference in task complexity.

Ozonoff et al. (1991) hypothesised that the apparent deficits in theory of mind may be secondary to a general deficit in executive function. Such deficits are more universal than deficits in theory of mind among people with autism. Perhaps people with autism are more impaired at applying a theory of mind than at constructing one: they may be able to understand the theory-of-mind task, yet be unable to avoid responding in terms of what they themselves know rather than in terms of the knowledge they attribute to others. There does seem to be evidence for a more general deficit in executive dysfunction in autism. In a task similar to the Wisconsin card sorting test but whose changes of sorting criterion involved either a change in which feature was relevant or a reversal of the value of the relevant feature, people with autism were selectively impaired in responding appropriately to the changes between features (Hughes et al., 1994). This deficit in executive function is reminiscent of findings of stimulus overselectivity in autism (Lovaas et al., 1971), and stimulus overselectivity on the input side may contribute to perseverative classification on the output side.

The normal frontal negative potentials associated with auditory attention and visual attention are absent in autism (Courchesne et al., 1985; Ciesielski et al., 1990). People with autism also manifest a reduced auditory P3 component (Novick et al., 1979, 1980; Courchesne et al., 1984, 1985, 1989), and some of this reduction results from an increase in variability of the response: in single trials it is sometimes present, sometimes not. Interestingly, the behavioural performance of people with autism in vigilance tasks not involving shifts of attention is normal, despite the lack of these potentials. Either the P3 and the Nc do not reflect processes essential to behaviour, or people with autism develop some compensatory strategy which yields the same appropriate behaviour but uses alternative brain mechanisms.

A functional imaging study has added to the evoked potential evidence of frontal dysfunction in autism. A longitudinal study using SPECT (Zilbovicius et al., 1995) revealed an apparent developmental retardation of the frontal cortex. Three year old autistic children showed low levels of frontal cerebral blood flow, more resembling the levels of normal one year olds. By six years of age, however, frontal blood flow in the autistic children was normal. Normal frontal function in the intervening years may be critical for normal social development, that this transient dysfunction could do permanent damage.

Other anatomical findings

In addition to the diverse neuroanatomical findings already described, more general observations have been made with regard to the autistic brain. Piven et al. (1995) reported that total brain volume measured using MRI in people with autism was significantly larger than in normal control subjects. This agreed with a previous study finding from the same laboratory (Piven et al., 1992) of a larger midsagittal brain area in people with autism than in controls and with an abstract from Filipek et al. (1992) which reported an increased volume. It is to be hoped that additional research will be done to determine if these differences are due to localised differences in brain size, e.g., specific to a particular lobe or structure or represent a diffuse difference throughout the brain.

Another study from the same laboratory (Piven et al., 1990) examined MRI of autistic and control brains for evidence of gyral malformation. The images were assessed for abnormalities such as polymicrogyria, pachygyria, heterotopia and schizencephaly, i.e., defects in neuronal migration. One or more such malformations was found in 7 of 13 autistic subjects but in none of 13 controls. The malformations were not specific to any particular lobe or side of the brain nor did they all fall into a single category of malformation. This suggests that defects in cortical neuronal migration may play a role in some cases of autism and that such defects may have multiple ætiologies. Again, further research with additional subjects should shed light on the frequency of the various defects and possibly on the root causes of the abnormalities.

Biochemical bases of imaging results

So much is wrong in autism that it is difficult to single out a primary dysfunction. One candidate, cerebellar maldevelopment, may well be the explanation for many cases. But it would be naïve to suggest that the cerebellum might be the be-all and end-all of autistic disorder. Undoubtedly multiple ætiologies are at work, and these will be difficult to disentangle. Furthermore, the cerebellar theory itself demands its own explanation: if the cerebellum is developing abnormally, if Purkinje cells are dying, or failing to differentiate or to migrate, what cellular and molecular mechanisms are responsible?

As mentioned in the introduction, the cerebrospinal fluid and urine of many people with autism have high levels of opiate binding. Reichelt et al. (1991, 1994), and Shattock and his colleagues (Williams et al., 1991; Shattock and Lowdon, 1991), suggested that these opioids may result from incomplete digestion of gluten or casein and consequent passage of opioid peptides from the gut into the circulation, and thence across the blood-brain barrier. Whatever their source, these opioids are definitely present in the central nervous system in many people with autism. Since opioids act during development to inhibit neuronal growth, their presence to excess in the developing brain could produce the cellular effects noted in the autopsy studies discussed above. Morphine in low concentrations reduces dendritic arborisation in murine Purkinje cells in vitro, and in higher concentrations kills them (Hauser et al., 1994). In normally developing cerebellar cortex in the rat, messenger RNA for proenkephalin is expressed in Purkinje cells, in spatiotemporal gradients which match regional rates of maturation (Osborne et al., 1991, 1993). The enkephalins themselves are concentrated in the external germinal layer, where neural stem cells proliferate and differentiate (Zagon et al., 1985, 1987). This suggests a process of opioid-mediated signalling in proliferation or differentiation. The human z opioid receptor subtype is expressed in the cerebellum only in infants (Zagon et al., 1990), so it may be the most important in this process. Large, daily doses of the opioid antagonist naltrexone, sufficient to block opioid receptors continuously throughout postnatal development, result in cerebellar hyperplasia. Low doses of naltrexone which block opioid receptors only briefly and so produce an overall up-regulation of opiatergic transmission, result in cerebellar hypoplasia (Zagon and McLaughlin, 1986a, 1986b). This paradoxical effect suggests a tantalising link to the bimodal distribution of cerebellar size in autistic brains. The same, bidirectional effect occurs when Leu-enkephalin is added to cultured rat raphé cells (Davila-Garcia and Azmitia 1989). In addition to their cerebellar effects, opioids distort the development of the cerebrum. The same low dose which produces cerebellar hypoplasia also produces increased density of cell packing in the cerebrum, particularly the hippocampus. Such increased packing is exactly what Bauman and Kemper (1985) reported at autopsy in some autistic brains.

In addition, genetic factors are certain to play a modifying or contributing part in many cases of autism. This is demonstrated by the great difference in concordance for autism between monozygotic and dizygotic twin pairs (36 % of 11 vs. 0 % of 10 pairs respectively), (Folstein and Rutter, 1977), and by the clustering of affective disorders in relatives of people with autism (DeLong and Nohria 1994). The hyperserotonaemia common in autism occurs also in relatives of people with autism (Cook 1990), and correlates with levels of depressive and obsessive-compulsive symptoms (Cook et al., 1994). In a significant step towards a possible molecular genetic basis for this tendency, Comings et al. (1991) reported that the prevalence of the A1 allele of the dopamine D2 receptor gene in the autistic population is double that in controls. A peculiarity of the D2 receptor gene may be associated in particular with the regressive subtype of autism, in which children begin to develop normally but then lose language and social abilities (Lincoln, unpublished observations). Reiss et al. (1986) noted that the site of CGG repeats in Fragile X Syndrome, in which probands have some autistic features, is close to the location of several genes involved in cerebellar development. Daniels et al. (1995) reported an association of autism with C4B null allele of the major histocompatibility complex, suggesting a genetic basis for the immune abnormalities observed in autism.

None of these candidate modifying factors is mutually exclusive. Genetic liability may magnify the effects of damage due to opioids or malfunction of the immune system. The opiatergic neurotransmitter systems and aminergic neurotransmitter systems interact strongly with one another and can influence the immune system (Marchetti et al., 1990).

Futures directions

Over the last two decades a number of theories, anatomical and chemical, have been presented to explain the biological bases of autism. All of the arguments come with some supporting and some conflicting evidence, but none is conclusive. Of the data accumulated, the most extensive and consistent relate to the cerebellum and the limbic system. Theories regarding these structures have support from neuropathological, anatomical, physiological and behavioural studies. Discussion continues, however, and more studies must be done before we can draw any concrete conclusions.

A complete understanding of autism may lead not only to prophylaxis for future generations but also to more effective treatments and coping strategies for people who currently have autism. This understanding can arise only from a synthesis of developmental neuroanatomy and neurophysiology with biochemistry and molecular genetics. While a comprehensive understanding of autism will require knowledge of the cellular and molecular abnormalities involved in the disorder, this level of understanding is likely to be a long time off. Research into these areas generally requires an animal model, which does not yet exist, or autopsy material, which is difficult to obtain. Since autism does not affect longevity and longitudinal studies of disorders are fairly recent and tend to recruit younger subjects, very little autopsy material is available for neuropathological research. Because of this, in vivo neuroimaging techniques are vital to autism research. They allow us to examine the integrity of brain structures at the macroscopic level and thereby infer microscopic anomalies, and as the technology evolves, will allow us to investigate smaller and smaller structures.

Future neuroimaging studies will ask such questions as: what is the developmental time course of the process of neurological damage that leads to autistic behaviour? Since the diagnosis of autism can be made with certainty only when the child has reached the age of five years, there is a dearth of imaging data on very young autistic children. These early years, however, are precisely the period during which the most interesting anatomical and physiological developments (or maldevelopments) must be occurring. A study in progress in the Courchesne laboratory aims to fill this gap, by imaging tentatively diagnosed children very young, then confirming the diagnosis at the age of five years, an approach similar to that used by the Hashimoto laboratory. Without the proliferation of imaging technology, the luxury of over inclusive imaging followed by retrospective diagnosis would be impossible.

What brain structures are affected in autism, how much, in what subpopulations, and over what time course? While the cerebellum has received a great deal of attention in this regard, other important candidate areas have received very little study due to the fact that extensive interest in the biological bases of autism and the advent of MRI technology are both recent. Quantitative imaging studies of the parietal lobes and frontal lobes and the additional limbic structures, in particular, are attractive prospects, because of the association of these structures with attention, and executive and social function. Such quantitative techniques must be combined with longitudinal studies to elucidate the time course of abnormalities in various anatomical regions, and thereby to gain insights into which anatomical defects may be primary and which later, downstream effects. Automated analyses of MRI data, essential to such quantitative studies, currently under development.

Imaging allows us to examine macroscopic structure, to peer from the top down at the perturbed brain development that manifests as autism. Other, complementary technologies allow us to examine autistic development from the bottom up. A synthesis of both views is critical for progress toward a complete understanding of the autistic syndrome. What are the cellular and molecular mechanisms which contribute to the anatomical abnormalities seen with MRI? How might neuroanatomical and neurophysiological subtypes (cerebellar hypoplastic vs. hyperplastic, parietal-lobe damaged vs. parietal-lobe normal) relate to ætiological, biochemical, and genetic subtypes (behaviourally regressive vs. non regressive, viral vs. non viral, hyperserotonaemic, opioiduric, etc.)? Much progress has been made, but many new, more specific questions have been generated.

References

Adrien JL, Perrot A, Sauvage D, Leddet E, Larmande C, Hameury L, Barthélémy C (1992) Early symptoms in autism from family home movies. Evaluation and comparison between 1st and 2nd year of life using I.B.S.E. scale. Acta Pædopsychiatrica 55 2: 71-75

Akshoomoff NA, Courchesne E (1992) A new role for the cerebellum in cognitive operations. Behav Neurosci 106 5: 731-738

Akshoomoff NA, Courchesne E (1994) ERP evidence for a shifting attention deficit in patients with damage to the cerebellum. J Cogn Neurosci 6 4: 388-399

Allen G, Buxton RB, Wong EC, Courchesne E (submitted) Attention activates the cerebellum independently of motor involvement

American Psychiatric Association (1994) Diagnostic and statistical manual of mental disorders, 4th edition. American Psychiatric Association, Washington, DC

Attig E, Botez MI, Hublet C, Vervonck C, Jacquy J, Capon A (1991) Diaschisis cérébral croisé par lésion cérébelleuse: Rôle du cervelet dans les fonctions mentales. Rev Neurol 147 3: 200-207

Bachevalier J (1994) Medial temporal lobe structures and autism: A review of clinical and experimental findings. Neuropsychologia 32 6: 627-648

Baron-Cohen S (1989) The autistic child's theory of mind: A case of specific developmental delay. J Child Psychol Psychiat 30 2: 285-297

Baron-Cohen S, Ring H, Moriarty J, Schmitz B, Costa D, Ell P (1994) Recognition of Mental State Terms. Clinical findings in children with autism and a functional neuroimaging study of normal adults. British J Psychiat 165 5: 640-649

Bauman ML (1991) Microscopic neuroanatomic abnormalities in autism. Pediatrics 87 5: 791-796

Bauman ML, Kemper TL (1985) Histoanatomic observations of the brain in early infantile autism. Neurology 35 6: 866-874

Bauman ML, Kemper TL (1993) The Contribution of Neuropathologic Studies to the Understanding of Autism. Neurol Clinics 11 1: 175-187

Belmonte M (1997a) Shifts of Visual Spatial Attention Modulate a Steady-State Visual Evoked Potential. In preparation

Belmonte M (1997b) A Software System for Analysis of Steady-State Evoked Potentials. In preparation

Belmonte M (1997c) Abnormal Spatial Attention in Autism Demonstrated by Lack of Modulation of a Steady-State Visual Evoked Potential. In preparation

Belmonte M, Egaas B, Townsend J, Courchesne E (1995) NMR intensity of corpus callosum differs with age but not with diagnosis of autism. NeuroReport 6 9: 1253-1256

Bryson SE, Wainwright-Sharp JA, Smith IM (1990) Autism: A developmental spatial neglect syndrome? In: Enns JT (ed) The development of attention: Research and theory. Elsevier, Amsterdam, p 405

Casey BJ, Gordon CT, Mannheim GB, Rumsey JM (1993) Dysfunctional attention in autistic savants. J Clin Exp Neuropsychol 15 6: 933-946

Cook EH (1990) Autism: Review of neurochemical investigation. Synapse 6 3: 292-308

Cook EH, Charak DA, Arida J, Spohn JA, Roizen NJ, Leventhal BL (1994) Depressive and obsessive-compulsive symptoms in hyperserotonemic parents of children with autistic disorder. Psychiat Res 52 1: 25-33
Ciesielski KT, Courchesne E, Elmasian R (1990) Effects of focused selective attention tasks on event-related potentials in autistic and normal individuals. Electroencephalogr Clin Neurophysiol 75 3: 207-220 [erratum in 76 6: 566 (1990)]
Comings DE, Comings BG, Muhleman D, Dietz G, Shahbahrami B, Tast D, Knell E, Kocsis P, Baumgarten R, Kovacs BW, Levy DL, Smith M, Borison RL, Evans DD, Klein DN, MacMurray J, Tosk JM, Sverd J, Gysin R, Flanagan SD (1991) The dopamine D2 receptor locus as a modifying gene in neuropsychiatric isorders. J Am Med Ass 266 13: 1793-1800
Courchesne E, Hesselink JR, Jernigan TL, Yeung-Courchesne R (1987) Abnormal neuroanatomy in a nonretarded person with autism. Unusual Findings with Magnetic Resonance Imaging. Arch Neurol 44 3: 335-341
Courchesne E, Kilman B, Galambos R, Lincoln A (1984) Autism: processing of novel auditory information assessed by event-related brain potentials. Electroencephalogr Clin Neurophysiol 59 3: 238-248
Courchesne E, Lincoln A, Kilman B, Galambos R (1985) Event-related brain potential correlates of the processing of novel visual and auditory information in autism. J Autism Dev Disord 15 1: 55-76
Courchesne E, Lincoln A, Yeung-Courchesne R, Elmasian R, Grillon C (1989) Pathophysiologic findings in nonretarded autism and receptive developmental language disorder. J Autism Dev Disord 19 1: 1-17
Courchesne E, Press G, Yeung-Courchesne R (1993) Parietal lobe abnormalities detected with MR in patients with infantile autism. Am J Roentgenol 160 2: 387-393
Courchesne E, Saitoh O, Yeung-Courchesne R, Press G, Lincoln A, Haas R, Schreibman L (1994) Abnormality of cerebellar vermian lobules VI and VII in patients with infantile autism: Identification of hypoplastic and hyperplastic subgroups with MR imaging. Am J Roentgenol 162 1: 123-30
Courchesne E, Townsend J, Saitoh O (1994) The brain in infantile autism: Posterior fossa structures are abnormal. Neurology 44 2: 214-223
Courchesne E, Yeung-Courchesne R, Press G, Hesselink JR, Jernigan TL (1988) Hypoplasia of cerebellar vermal lobules VI and VII in autism, N Engl J Med 318 21: 1349-1354
Crepel F (1982) Regression of functional synapses in the immature mammalian cerebellum. Trends Neurosci 5: 266-269
Crispino L, Bullock TH (1984) Cerebellum mediates modality-specific modulation of sensory responses of the midbrain and forebrain in rat. Proc Nat Acad Sci 81 9: 2917-2920
Damasio A, Maurer R (1978) A neurological model for childhood autism. Arch Neurol 35 12: 777-786
Daniels WW, Warren RP, Odell JD, Maciulis A, Burger RA, Warren WL, Torres AR (1995) Increased frequency of the extended or ancestral haplotype B44-SC30-DR4 in autism. Neuropsychobiology 32 3: 120-123
Davila-Garcia MI, Azmitia EC (1989) Effects of acute and chronic administration of leu-enkephalin on cultured serotonergic neurons: Evidence for opioids as inhibitory neuronal growth factors. Dev Brain Res 49 1: 97-103
DeLong GR, Bean SC, Brown FR (1981) Acquired reversible autistic syndrome in acute encephalopathic illness in children. Arch Neurol 38 3: 191-194
DeLong GR, Nohria C (1994) Psychiatric family history and neurological disease in autistic spectrum disorders. Dev Med Child Neurol 36 5: 441-448
DeLong GR (1992) Autism, amnesia, hippocampus, and learning. Neurosci Biobehav Rev 16 1: 63-70
Deonna T (1991) Acquired epileptiform aphasia in children (Landau-Kleffner Syndrome). J Clin Neurophysiol 8: 288-298
Egaas B, Courchesne E, Saitoh O (1995) Reduced size of corpus callosum in autism. Arch Neurol 52 8: 794-801
Filipek PA (1995) Quantitative magnetic resonance imaging in autism: The cerebellar vermis. Curr Opin Neurol 8: 134-138
Filipek PA, Richelme C, Kennedy DN, Rademacher J, Pitcher DA, Zidel S, Caviness VS (1992) Morphometric analysis of the brain in developmental language disorders and autism (abstract). Ann Neurol 32: 475
Folstein S, Rutter M (1977) Infantile autism: A genetic study of 21 twin pairs. J Child Psychol Psychiat 18 4: 297-321
Gaffney GR, Tsai LY, Kuperman S, Minchin S (1987) Cerebellar structure in autism. Am J Dis Child 141 12: 1330-1332
Gao J-H, Parsons LM, Bower JM, Xiong J, Li J, Fox PT (1996) Cerebellum implicated in sensory acquisition and discrimination rather than motor control. Science 272: 545-547
Garber HJ, Ritvo ER (1992) Magnetic resonance imaging of the posterior fossa in autistic adults. Am J Psychiat 149: 245-247
George MS, Costa DC, Kouris K, Ring HA, Ell PJ (1992) Cerebral blood flow abnormalities in adults with infantile autism. J Nerv Ment Dis 180 7: 413-417
Gillberg C (1986) Onset at age 14 of a typical autistic syndrome. A case report of a girl with herpes simplex encephalitis. J Autism Dev Disord 16 3: 369-375
Gillberg C, Trygstad O, Foss I (1982) Childhood psychosis and urinary excretion of peptides and protein-associated peptide complexes. J Autism Dev Disord 12 3: 229-241
Gillberg C, Terenius L, Lonnerholm G (1985) Endorphin activity in childhood psychosis: Spinal fluid in 29 cases. Arch Gen Psychiat 42 8: 780-783
Gillberg IC (1991) Autistic syndrome with onset at age 31 years: Herpes encephalitis as a possible model for childhood autism. Dev Med Child Neurol 33 10: 920-924
Haas RH, Townsend J, Courchesne E, Lincoln AJ, Schreibman L, Yeung-Courchesne R (1996) Neurologic abnormalities in infantile autism. J Child Neurol 11: 84-92
Hallett M, Lebiedowska MK, Thomas SL, Stanhope SJ, Denckla MB, Rumsey J (1993) Locomotion of autistic adults. Arch Neurol 50 12: 1304-1308
Harter MR, Anllo-Vento L (1991) Visual-spatial attention: Preparation and selection in children and adults. In: Brunia CHM, Mulder G, Verbaten MN (eds) Event-related brain research. Elsevier, New York, p 183
Harter MR, Miller SL, Price NJ, LaLonde ME, Keyes AL (1989) Neural processes involved in directing attention. J Cogn Neurosci 1 3: 223-237
Hashimoto T, Tayama M, Miyazaki M, Murakawa K, Kuroda Y (1993) Brainstem and cerebellar vermis involvement in autistic children. J Child Neurol 8 2: 149-153
Hashimoto T, Tayama M, Murakawa K, Yoshimoto T, Miyazaki M, Harada M, Kuroda Y (1995) Development of

the brainstem and cerebellum in autistic patients. J Autism Dev Disord 25 1: 1-18

Hauser KF, Gurwell JA, Turbek CS (1994) Morphine inhibits purkinje cell survival and dendritic differentiation in organotypic cultures of the mouse cerebellum. Exp Neurol 130 1: 95-105

Heilman KM, Watson RT, Valenstein E (1985) Neglect and related disorders. In Heilman KM, Valenstein E (eds) Clinical Neuropsychology 2nd ed, New York: Oxford University Press

Heinze HJ, Luck SJ, Mangun GR, Hillyard SA (1990) Visual event-related potentials index focused attention within bilateral stimulus arrays. I. Evidence for early selection. Electroencephalogr Clin Neurophysiol 75 6: 511-527

Hetzler BF, Griffin JL (1981) Infantile autism and the temporal lobe of the brain. J Autism Dev Disord 11 3: 317-330

Holttum JR, Minshew NJ, Sanders RS, Phillips NE (1992) Magnetic resonance imaging of the posterior fossa in autism. Biol Psychiat 32: 1091-1101

Hoon AH Jr, Reiss AL (1992) The mesial-temporal lobe and autism: Case report and review. Dev Med Child Neurol 34 3: 252-259

Hughes C, Russell J, Robbins TW (1994) Evidence for executive dysfunction in autism. Neuropsychologia 32 4: 477-492

Jones V, Prior M (1985) Motor imitation abilities and neurological signs in autistic children. J Autism Dev Disord 15 1: 37-46

Kemper TL, Bauman ML (1993) The contribution of neuropathologic studies to the understanding of autism. Behav Neurol 11 1: 175-187

Kim S-G, Ugurbil K, Strick PL (1994) Activation of a cerebellar output nucleus during cognitive processing. Science 265 5174: 949-951

Kleiman MD, Neff S, Rosman NP (1992) The brain in infantile autism: Are posterior fossa structures abnormal? Neurology 42 4: 753-760

Landau WM, Kleffner FR (1957) Syndrome of acquired aphasia with convulsive disorder in children. Neurology 7: 523-530

Leiner HC, Leiner AL, Dow RS (1986) Does the cerebellum contribute to mental operations? Behav Neurosci 100 4: 443-454

Leiner HC, Leiner AL, Dow RS (1991) The Human Cerebro-Cerebellar System: Its Computing, Cogn Lang Skills Behav Brain Res 44 2: 114-128

Lovaas OI, Schreibman L, Koegel R, Rehm R (1971) Selective responding by autistic children to multiple sensory input. J Abn Psychol 77 3: 211-222

Mangun GR, Hillyard SA (1987) The spatial allocation of visual attention as indexed by event-related brain potentials. Human Factors 29 2: 195-211

Mangun GR, Hillyard SA (1988) Spatial gradients of visual attention: behavioral and electrophysiological evidence. Electroencephalogr Clin Neurophysiol 70 5: 417-428

Mangun GR, Hillyard SA (1990) Allocation of visual attention to spatial locations: Tradeoff functions for event-related brain potentials and detection performance. Percept Psychophysiology 47 6: 532-550

Marchetti B, Scifo R, Batticane N, Scapagnini U (1990) Immunological significance of opioid peptide dysfunction in infantile autism. Brain Dysfunct 3: 346-354

Martineau J, Barthélémy C, Jouve J, Muh JP, Lelord G (1992) Monoamines (serotonin and catecholamines) and their derivatives in infantile autism: Age-related changes and drug effects. Dev Med Child Neurol 34 7: 593-603

Middleton FA, Strick PL (1994) Anatomical evidence for cerebellar and basal ganglia involvement in higher cognitive function. Science 266 5184: 458-461

Mountz JM, Tolbert LC, Lill BW, Katholi CR, Liu HG (1995) Functional deficits in autistic disorder: Characterization by technetium-99m-HMPAO and SPECT. J Nucl Med 36 7: 1156-1162

Murakami J, Courchesne E, Press G, Yeung-Courchesne R, Hesselink J (1989) Reduced cerebellar hemisphere size and its relationship to vermal hypoplasia in autism. Arch Neurol 46 6: 689-694

Newman PP, Reza H (1979) Functional relationships between the hippocampus and the cerebellum: An electrophysiological study of the cat. J Physiol 287: 405-426

Novick B, Kurtzberg D, Vaughan H Jr (1979) An electrophysiologic indication of defective information storage in childhood autism. Psychiat Res 1 1: 101-108

Novick B, Vaughan H Jr, Kurtzberg D, Simson R (1980) An electrophysiologic indication of auditory processing defects in autism. Psychiat Res 3 1: 107-114

Ornitz EM (1983) The functional neuroanatomy of infantile autism. Int J Neurosci 19 1-4: 85-124

Osborne JG, Kindy MS, Hauser KF (1991) Expression of proenkephalin mRNA in developing cerebellar cortex of the rat: Expression levels coincide with maturational gradients in purkinje cells. Dev Brain Res 63 1-2: 63-69

Osborne JG, Kindy MS, Spruce BA, Hauser KF (1993) Ontogeny of proenkephalin mRNA and enkephalin peptide expression in the cerebellar cortex of the rat: Spatial and temporal patterns of expression follow maturational gradients in the external granular layer and in purkinje cells. Dev Brain Res 76 1: 1-12

Ozonoff S, Pennington BF, Rogers SJ (1991) Executive function deficits in high-functioning autistic individuals: Relationship to theory of mind. J Child Psychol Psychiat 32 7: 1081-1105

Pandya DN, Karol EA, Heilbronn D (1971) The topographical distribution of interhemispheric projections in the corpus callosum of the rhesus monkey. Brain Res 32: 31-43

Panksepp J (1979) A neurochemical theory of autism. Trends Neurosci 2: 174-177

Petersen SE, Fox PT, Posner MI, Mintun M, Raichle ME (1989) Positron emission tomographic studies of the processing of single words. J Cogn Neurosci 1 2: 153-170

Piven J, Nehme E, Simon J, Barta P, Pearlson G, Folstein SE (1992) Magnetic resonance imaging in autism: Measurement of the cerebellum, pons, and fourth ventricle. Biol Psychiat 31: 491-504

Piven J, Berthier ML, Starkstein SE, Nehme E, Pearlson G, Folstein S (1990) Magnetic resonance imaging evidence for a defect of cerebral cortical development in autism. Am J Psychicat 147 6: 734-739

Piven J, Arndt S, Bailey J, Havercamp S, Andreasen NC, Palmer P (1995) An MRI study of brain size in autism. Am J Psychicat 152 8: 1145-1149

Piven J, Arndt S (1995) The cerebellum and autism. Neurology 45: 398-399

Posner MI (1980) Orienting of attention. Quarterly J Exp Psychol 32 1: 3-25

Posner MI, Walker JA, Friedrich FJ, Rafal RD (1984) Effects of parietal injury on covert orienting of attention. J Neurosci 4 7: 1863-1874

Posner MI, Walker JA, Friedrich FJ, Rafal RD (1987) How do the parietal lobes direct covert attention? Neuropsychologia 25 1A: 135-145

Raichle ME, Fiez JA, Videen TO, MacLeod AM, Pardo JV, Fox PT, Petersen SE (1994) Practice-related changes in

human brain functional anatomy during nonmotor learning. Cerebral Cortex 4 1: 8-26
Raymond G, Bauman M, Kemper T (1989) The hippocampus in autism: Golgi analysis. Ann Neurol 26 3: 483-484
Reichelt KL, Knivsberg A-M, Lind G, Nødland M (1991) Probable etiology and possible treatment of childhood autism. Brain Dysfunct 4: 308-319
Reichelt KL, Knivsberg A-M, Nødland M, Lind G (1994) Nature and consequences of hyperpeptiduria and bovine casomorphins found in autistic syndromes. Dev Brain Dysfunct 7: 71-85
Reiss AL, Feinstein C, Rosenbaum KN (1986) Autism and genetic disorders. Schizophrenia Bull 12 4: 724-738
Ritvo ER, Freeman BJ, Scheibel AB, Duong T, Robinson H, Guthrie D, Ritvo A (1986) Lower purkinje cell counts in the cerebella of four autistic subjects: Initial findings of the UCLA-NSAC autopsy research report. Am J Psychiat 143 7: 862-866
Saitoh O, Courchesne E, Egaas B, Lincoln AJ, Schreibman L (1995) Cross-sectional area of the posterior hippocampus in autistic patients with cerebellar and corpus callosum abnormalities. Neurology 45 2: 317-324
Schaefer GB, Thompson JN, Bodensteiner JB, McConnell JM, Kimberling WJ, Gay CT, Dutton WD, Hutchings DC, Gray SB (1996) Hypoplasia of the cerebellar vermis in neurogenetic syndromes. Ann Neurol 39 3: 382-385
Sears LL, Finn PR, Steinmetz JE (1994) Abnormal classical eye-blink conditioning in autism. J Autism Dev Disord 24 6: 737-751
Shattock P, Lowdon G (1991) Proteins, peptides and autism part 2: Implications for the education and care of people with autism. Brain Dysfunct 4: 323-334
Townsend J, Courchesne E (1994) Parietal damage and narrow "spotlight" spatial attention. J Cogn Neurosci 6:3: 218-230
Townsend J, Courchesne E, Egaas, B (1996a) Slowed orienting of covert visual-spatial attention in autism: Specific deficits associated with cerebellar and parietal abnormality. Dev Psychopathol 8 3: 563-584
Townsend J, Singer-Harris N, Courchesne E (1996b) Visual attention abnormalities in autism: Delayed orienting to location. J Int Neuropsychol Soc
Vilensky JA, Damasio AR, Maurer RG (1981) Gait disturbances in patients with autistic behavior: A preliminary study. Arch Neurol 38 10: 646-649
Wainwright-Sharp JA, Bryson SE (1993) Visual orienting deficits in high-functioning people with autism. J Autism Dev Disord 23 1: 1-13
Williams K, Shattock P, Berney T (1991) Proteins, peptides and autism part 1: Urinary protein patterns in autism as revealed by sodium dodecyl sulphate-polyacrylamide gel electrophoresis and silver staining. Brain Dysfunct 4: 320-322
Williams RS, Hauser SL, Purpura DP, DeLong GR, Swisher CN (1980) Autism and mental retardation: Neuropathologic studies performed in four retarded persons with autistic behavior. Arch Neurol 37 12: 749-753
Zagon IS, Gibo DM, McLaughlin PJ (1990) Adult and developing human cerebella exhibit different profiles of opioid binding sites. Brain Res 523 1: 62-68
Zagon IS, McLaughlin PJ (1986a) Opioid antagonist (naltrexone) modulation of cerebellar maldevelopment: Histological and morphometric studies. J Neurosci 6 5: 1424-1432
Zagon IS, McLaughlin PJ (1986b) Opioid antagonist-induced modulation of cerebral and hippocampal development: Histological and morphometric studies. Dev Brain Res 28 2: 233-246
Zagon IS, McLaughlin PJ (1987) Endogenous opioid systems regulate cell proliferation in the developing rat brain. Brain Res 412 1: 68-72
Zagon IS, Rhodes RE, McLaughlin PJ (1985) Distribution of enkephalin immunoreactivity in germinative cells of developing rat cerebellum. Science 227 4690: 1049-1051
Zilbovicius M, Garreau B, Samson Y, Remy P, Barthélémy C, Syrota A, Lelord G (1995) Delayed maturation of the frontal cortex in childhood autism. Am J Psychiat 152 2: 248-252

6. Functional brain imaging studies in childhood autism

M. ZILBOVICIUS

Autism is a life-long severe developmental disorder which impairs the acquisition of some of the most important skills in life (Kanner, 1943). The major signs of the syndrome are deficits in social interaction, verbal and nonverbal communication and imaginative activity (APA, 1987; Rutter, 1978). Autism was believed to be a "psychological" disorder but over the past 20 years it has become clear that it must have a biological origin. The understanding of brain mechanisms which underlie such a severe disorder remains a major challenge for research in this field. Neuropathological studies of infantile autism are few and have revealed abnormalities in the limbic system and cerebellar circuits (Bauman and Kemper, 1988; Ritvo, 1986; Williams, 1980). Structural neuroimaging investigations, including CT and MRI, have indicated various sites of anatomical abnormalities including the cerebral cortex, ventricular system and the cerebellum of autistic adults, and relatively old autistic children (Campbell, 1982; Courchesne, 1994; Courchesne, 1988; Damasio, 1980; Gillberg and Svendsen, 1983; Hier, 1979; Piven, 1990). However, these findings are still inconsistent and none accounts fully for the clinical expression of autism. Thus, we have little evidence of structural brain abnormalities in autism, despite the various theories proposed to explain it.

The advent of functional brain imaging techniques, such as positron emission tomography (PET) and single photon emission tomography (SPECT), opened a new, promising way to study brain dysfunction in childhood autism. Both emission tomography techniques allow noninvasive, accurate measurement of cerebral glucose metabolism and/or cerebral blood flow (CBF). It has been shown that neurons increase their utilization of glucose in direct proportion to their activity. In addition, in normal conditions, the rate of glucose utilisation is coupled to CBF (Juliano and Whitsel, 1987; Sokoloff, 1977). Thus, changes in glucose metabolism and CBF reflect changes in the synaptic functional activity.

A large number of strategies can be used to study a specific brain disorder using functional brain imaging. Measurements can be performed at rest or during the performance of specific sensory, motor or cognitive task. Furthermore, functional brain imaging techniques also allow us to study in vivo the developing human brain as first demonstrated by Chugani and Phelps. Marked changes in cerebral glucose metabolic rates and in regional cerebral blood flow (rCBF) are observed during infancy and childhood, reflecting changes in synaptic density they can be used as an index of maturation of the brain (Chiron, 1992; Chugani and Phelps, 1986; Chugani, 1987). This field seems of considerable interest in the study of developmental disorders.

This review addresses the main functional brain imaging investigations performed in autistic subjects during the last 10 years. It is convenient to divise them into three different groups: measurements of resting regional cerebral glucose metabolism or cerebral blood flow, performed mainly in autistic adults; CBF measurements performed during brain activation paradigms, and longitudinal studies of brain metabolic maturation.

Resting Functional Studies

Due to technical difficulties, the first functional studies performed in autism in the late 1980s focussed on adult. They reported resting cerebral glucose utilisation (CMRglu) rates measured with PET and [18F]-fluorodeoxyglucose (FDG). Rumsey et al. (1985)

studied 10 autistic subjects aged 18 to 36 years (mean age: 26 years) and found that glucose utilisation was significantly elevated in widespread regions of the brain, but no consistent localised abnormalities were identified (Rumsey et al., 1985).

The same group performed a second analysis of the previously obtained data, adding four autistic subjects, based on data showing that the correlation coefficient between values of rCRMglu in different brain regions may provide a measure of the functional association between them. Thus, they calculated Pearson's correlation coefficients for CMRglu values obtained in 59 brain regions in autistic and control groups as an index of the functional connection between these brain regions. The autistic group showed significantly fewer positive correlations between frontal and parietal regions or between subcortical regions and the frontal and parietal lobes. It was concluded that these results were compatible with functional impairment of the interaction between frontal and parietal regions and the neostriatum and thalamus, suggesting abnormal neural connections. This impairment could reflect an anomalous brain maturational processing affecting the network which subserves attention processing, often impaired in autism (Horwitz, 1988).

On the basis of neuropathological and MRI descriptions of cerebellar abnormalities in autistic subjects, Heh et al. (1989) tested the hypothesis of cerebellar hypofunction in autistic patients. They measured CMRglu in the cerebellum of seven autistic patients (19 to 36 years old) and eight age-matched control subjects and found no cerebellar metabolic abnormalities.

Herold et al. (1988) also found no focal brain abnormalities in six young autistic men (21-25 years old), measuring CBF, oxygen and glucose consumption with PET and the oxygen 15 steady-state inhalation method.

Because the autistic behavioural syndrome is more pronounced during childhood functional brain imaging of children seems more appropriate than studies of adults. The first PET study performed in autistic children was reported by De Volder et al. (1987), but the findings were compared to these in adult controls. These workers measured the CMRglu in 14 autistic children with a wide age range (2 to 18 years) and found normal rates and regional distribution of brain glucose metabolism.

We studied 21 autistic children aged 5 to 11 years and 14 nonautistic aged-matched control children. Measuring rCBF with SPECT and xenon 133 we found no evidence of localized cortical brain dysfunction. The global and rCBF values of the autistic children were similar to those of the control group but significantly higher than those of normal young adults (Zilbovicius, 1992). These data confirm that CBF is higher in children than adults, as is cerebral glucose metabolism,. and suggest that this transient maturational high metabolic plateau is also observed in autistic children.

The lack of focal rCBF abnormalities in autistic children was confirmed by Chiron et al. (1995). Using SPECT and xenon 133 they studied 18 autistic children (from 4 to 17 years old) and 10 controls (from 4 to 16 years old) and found higher left than right rCBF in controls but not in patients with autism.

The results of all there resting functional studies performed in autistic patients must be considered in the light of some methodological limitations. The relatively poor spatial resolution (from 16 to 20 mm) of early PET and SPECT devices used in those studies precludes valid analysis of small areas of the brain that might be of crucial importance in autism. For example, rCBF or CRMglu in medial temporal structures such as the hippocampus and amygdala, which are of primary importance in the final integration of sensory information and in elaboration of behaviour, could not be measured. Thus, measurements of resting CRMglu and CBF in autistic adults and school-aged autistic children have failed to detect any consistent focal abnormalities, perhaps because any abnormalities present are too subtle to be detected by current techniques in the mature brain.

It is important to emphasise that all these studies concern the so called "nonassociated" or "idiopathic" autistic syndrome, i. e., they excluded patients with identifiable neurological syndromes, seizures or focal signs. Focal functional abnormalities have been described in other syndromes associated with autistic symptoms and in autistic patients with neurological signs. Prefrontal and temporoparietal hypoperfusion was reported in seven girls with Rett's syndrome, a condition that is still often misdiagnosed as primary autism (Nielsen, 1990). Schifter et al. (1994) had reported heterogeneous cortical metabolic abnormalities in autistic children with coexisting seizure disorders and other neurological abnormalities. Thus, a normal pattern of metabolic activity (CBF or CRMglu) in autistic children seems to indicate a nonassociated form of autism syndrome and could be of clinical value for differential diagnosis of the behavioural autistic syndrome.

Brain activation studies

One of the most exciting areas in brain imaging research is functional imaging of brain activation. Movement, sensory stimulation, and cognitive activities all lead to local changes in cerebral blood flow and metabolism which can be measured by PET. Such activation studies have produced maps of brain

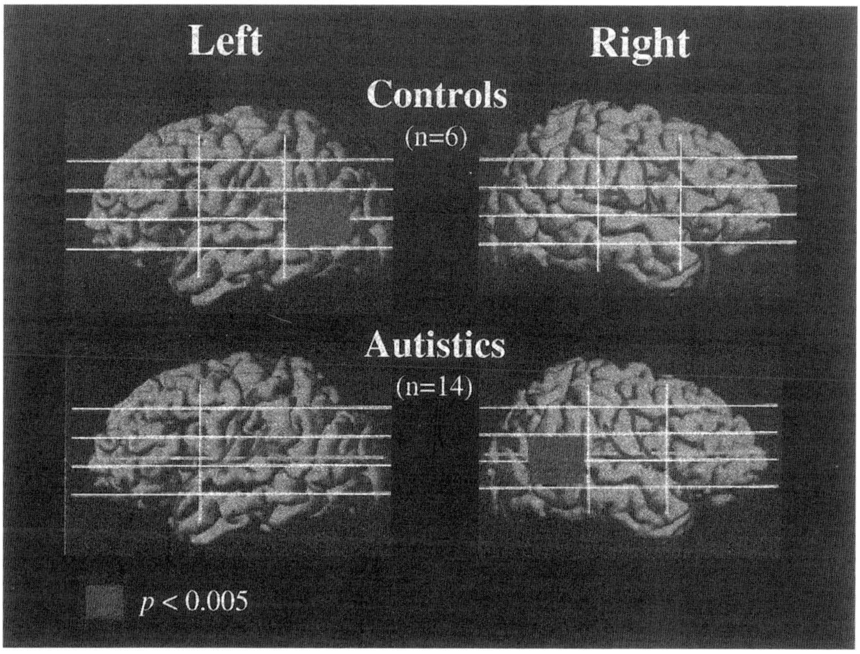

Fig. 1
A simple nonverbal auditory stimulus induced a significant rCBF increase in the left temporo-occipital cortex in control children (top) and in the right temporo-occipital cortex in autistic children (bottom).
See colour illustrations appendix

areas activated by specific physiological and psychological tasks in normal volunteers. They provide a unique context for the investigation of the pathophysiology of neurological and psychiatric diseases.

The application of activation studies to autism is still potential. To our knowledge, the only published CBF activation study was performed in our laboratory (Garreau et al., 1994). Our major objective was to look for a putative abnormal pattern of cortical activation in autistic children, to even a quite simple perceptive stimulus, which could be implicated in the genesis of the abnormal perceptive and behavioural response frequently observed in autism. A large body of evidence leads us to infer that disturbance in the perception and modulation of sensory information could be at the core of the neurobiology of autism (Ornitz, 1983). Clinically, one of the most characteristic features of autism is the abnormal response to sensory stimuli; an abnormal response to sound may be thought of as the most characteristic. Electrophysiological studies have underlined the role of sensory impairment in autism. We have used SPECT and ^{133}Xe to measure regional CBF in autistic children at rest and during simple binaural auditory stimulation. We compared 11 autistic children (aged 7 ± 2.4 years) to 5 non-autistic children (aged 8.5 ± 3.5 years). In the latter we found that the simple auditory stimulation induced a significant increase in rCBF in the left temporo-occipital cortex (+5 % ± 3 %; p = 0.004). In the autistic children there was no activation of the left hemisphere; we found an increase in rCBF in the same temporo-occipital region but in the right side (+3 % ± 4 %; p = 0.004) indicating a different pattern of cortical activation in autistic children and controls. The activation were situated in the same cortical zone, but not the same hemisphere (Fig. 1). This suggests a left hemisphere impairment for sensory information processing in autism and is in agreement with data obtained with dichotic listening tests, auditory evoked potentials and, more recently, transcranial Doppler (Bruneau et al., 1992; Dawson et al., 1986; Dawson and Lewy, 1989; Ogawa et al., 1982; Tanguay et al., 1976).

Moreover, in the light of adult data the results suggest developmental differences in patterns of cortical activation. The pattern of activation found in both autistic and control children in response to simple nonverbal auditory stimulation differs from that in adults (Mazziota et al., 1982; Petersen et al., 1988; Zatorre et al., 1992), since in the latter there is bilateral activation of the primary auditory cortex (Heschl's gyrus), and not the association cortex. We found activation of the left posterior cortex in non-autistic children, a region normally related to language processing. The activation of that region in children, who are still developing their language, could be related to ongoing "activity-dependent" shaping of language-related cortical maps. The absence of left-sided activation could be one of the neurophysiological bases of language impairment in autism.

The results of this study are preliminary but show the potential of activation studies to explore the developing brain in vivo in normal and pathological conditions.

Maturational brain studies

Metabolic maturation of the brain is a dynamic process during infancy and childhood and a knowledge of the normal pattern is essential for study of developmental brain disorders. Global metabolic changes occur over a protracted period and reflect an initial phase of rapid synaptic proliferation, during early childhood, followed by a more prolonged period of elimination and stabilisation of synapses, extending throughout later childhood. Regional changes have a different time-course: the newborn, clearly immature metabolic regional pattern rapidly evolves into a mature adult pattern by 16-24 months of age (Chugani and Phelps, 1986; Chugani et al., 1987). These rapid changes in regional metabolic pattern occur during the first year of life according to a precise time-table, which may reflect the may indicate the succesive "turning-on" of the phase of rapid synaptic proliferation in different cortical areas. It is of interest that metabolic studies have shown that the last cortical area to undergo maturation is the frontal cortex, which has been the focus of much interest in autism research.

Based on these data, longitudinal functional studies during early childhood appear appropriate for detecting transient postnatal brain developmental abnormalities in autistic children. We investigated the metabolic maturation of the frontal cortex in preschool autistic children by performing a longitudinal rCBF study in five children with primary autism. rCBF measurements were performed: at the age of 2 to 4 years (41 ± 7.8 months old), and three years later (6.6 ± 0.6 years). At each stage, the children were compared to an age-matched group of 5 non-autistic children with normal development. In the first examination autistic children had significantly lower frontal CBF than that control children (0.86 ± 0.03 vs. 0.96 ± 0.07; $p < 0.02$), but posterior and mean cortical CBF was within the normal range. When we compared the autistic children rCBF with that of 36 control children (aged from 2 days to 12 years), we found that their frontal perfusion was more like that of much younger normal children (19 ± 13 months old). Three years later the frontal CBF had increased, and the same autistic children now showed normal frontal CBF for their age (0.98 ± 0.05 vs. 0.97 ± 0.09) (Fig. 2). Thus, transient frontal hypoperfusion, resembling that in younger normal children was found in 2-4 year old autistic children, (Zilbovicius et al., 1995).

These findings suggest delayed postnatal metabolic maturation of the frontal lobes in children with primary autism. The normal values found at the second examination were consistent with previous report of normal CBF in autistic children older than 5 years. Thus, the maturational CBF increase observed during the first two years of life in normal children, was observed in autistic children between 3 to 5 years.

In autistic children the delayed CBF maturation of the frontal lobe is highly consistent with several key

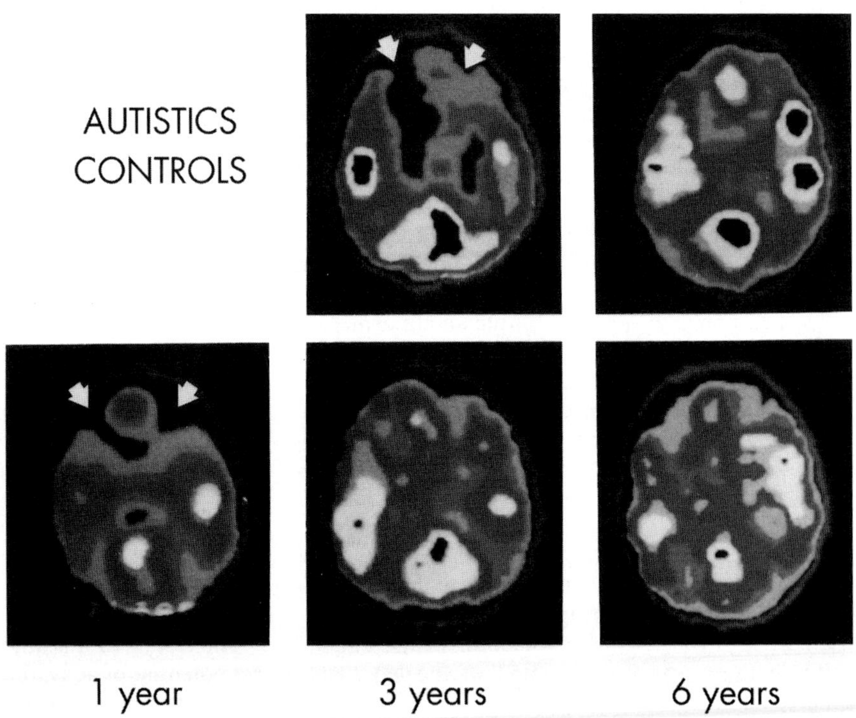

Fig. 2
SPECT rCBF images illustrating transient frontal hypoperfusion observed in autistic children.
(Top): An autistic child examined at 3 years and at 6 years. At the first examination we observed clear-cut bilateral frontal hypoperfusion (white arrows), while the later examination was a normal.
(Bottom): Three normal children's SPECT images obtained at different stages of development, indicating that frontal hypoperfusion is present at the age of one year (white arrows) but that the frontal lobes show a normal perfusion pattern by the age of three years.
See colour illustrations appendix

abnormalities in cognitive development. For example, Adrien et al. (1993, 1994) showed that Piaget's classical object permanence task is performed by four year old autistic children at the same level or worse than normal 16 month old children. As demonstrated by Diamond and Goldman-Rakic (Diamond and Goldman-Rakic, 1989; Diamond, 1990), improved performance on this task provides an index of maturation of frontal cortex function. High-functioning autistic children have also been shown to perform poorly on executive tasks closely linked to the frontal lobes (Ozonoff et al., 1991; Hughes et al., 1994). The prefrontal cortex is probably also necessary for the formation of second-order cognitive representations of the world, which are dramatically impaired in autistic children, leading to a severe abnormality in the development of the "theory of mind" (Baron-Cohen, 1989; Frith et al., 1991). Finally, adults with histories of infantile autism show dramatic deficits on problem-solving tasks such as the Wisconsin card sorting test, indicating a residual frontal lobe deficit (Rumsey and Hamburger, 1988).

The delayed metabolic maturation of the frontal lobes constitutes an important link between cognitive deficits and brain dysfunction in childhood autism. Longitudinal rCBF studies with high resolution functional brain imaging facilities in a large population of autistic children will be helpful for more accurate identification of the temporal and spatial components of frontal maturational dysfunction.

Conclusions

Three main points summarise the data obtained from functional brain imaging in autism.

First, resting metabolic and CBF studies have failed to detect consistent focal brain abnormalities in autistic adults and school-aged children. This suggest that the autistic syndrome is not the consequence of a single abnormality of an isolated region of the brain. The application of the lesional neurological model thus seems inappropriate for neurobiological research into autism.

Second, autistic children have abnormal patterns of cortical activation in response to auditory stimuli. In adults a decreased number of metabolic correlations between different cortical regions was found at rest.

Third, delayed metabolic maturation of the frontal lobes was found in young autistic children, which may constitute an important link between cognitive deficits and brain dysfunction in childhood autism.

Taken together, these findings suggest abnormal cortical connectivity and/or activation in autism associated with abnormal maturational brain processing. Since the late phase of cortical maturation is thought to reflect selection and elimination of synapses, in part depending on neural activity and occurring during critical periods, it is conceivable that postnatal shaping of neural connections is disturbed in many parts of the brain of autistic children. We might speculate that autism is the consequence of a failure of regulation of neuronal maturation in cortical or subcortical information processing regions, leading to disruption of normal synaptogenesis and circuit formation.

Other aspects of the brain maturational processing need to be investigated in autism, in particular neurochemical development. Functional brain imaging allows in vivo study of the main neurotransmitter systems, such as the dopaminergic, GABAergic, and serotononergic. It should be useful for assessing the maturational changes in these system during normal development and their putative abnormalities in childhood autism.

References

Adrien JL, Martineau J, Barthelemy C, Bruneau N, Garreau B, Sauvage D (1994) Disorders of regulation of cognitive activity in autistic children. J Autism Dev Disord 25: 249-263

Adrien JL, Tanguay P, Barthelemy C, Martineau J, Perrot A, Hameury L, Sauvage D (1993) Autistic children and the object permance task. Acta Paedopsychiatrica 56: 25-29

APA (1987) Diagnostic and statistical manual of mental disorders. DSM-III-R. 3 rd edn Revised. APA, Washington DC

Baron-Cohen S (1989) The autistic child's theory of mind: a case of specific developmental delay. J Child Psychol Psychiat 30: 285-297

Bauman ML, Kemper TL (1988) Limbic and cerebellar abnormalities: consistent findings in infantile autism. J Neuropathol Exp Neurol 47: 369

Bruneau N, Dourneau MC, Garreau B, Pourcelot L, Lelord G (1992) Blood flow responses to auditory stimulations in normal mentally retarded and autistic children. A preliminary transcranial doppler ultrasonographic study of the middle cerebral arteries. Biol Psychiat 32: 691-699

Campbell M, Anderson LT, Small AM, Perry R, Green WH, Caplan R (1982) The effects of haloperidol on learning and behavior in autistic children. J Autism Dev Disord 12: 167-175

Chiron C, Leboyer M, Leon F, Jambaqué I, Nuttin C, Syrota A (1995) SPECT of the brain in childhood autism: evidence for a lack of normal hemispheric asymetry. Dev Med Child Neurol 37: 849-860

Chiron C, Raynaud C, Maziere B, Zilbovicius M, Laflame L, Masure MC, Dulac O, Bourguignon M, Syrota A (1992) Changes in regional cerebral blood flow during brain maturation in children and adolescents. J Nucl Med 33: 696-703

Chugani HT, Phelps ME (1986) Maturational changes in cerebral function in infants determined by 18FDG positron emission tomography. Science 231: 840-843

Chugani HT, Phelps ME, Mazziota JC (1987) Positron emission tomography study of functional development. Ann Neurol 22: 487-497

Courchesne E, Townsend JP, Saitoh O (1994) The brain in infantile autism: posterior fossa structures are abnormal. Neurology 44: 214-223

Courchesne E, Yeung-Courchesne R, Press GA, Hesselink JR, Jernigan TL (1988) Hypoplasia of cerebellar vermal lobules VI and VII in autism. N Eng J Med 318: 1349-1354

Damasio H, Maurer RG, Damasio AR, Chui HC (1980) Computerized tomography scan findings in patients with autistic behavior. Arch Neurol 37: 504-510

Dawson G, Finley C, Phillips S, Galpert L (1986) Hemispheric specialization and the language abilities of autistic children. Child Dev 57: 1440-1453

Dawson G, Lewy A (1989) Reciprocal subcortical-cortical influences in autism: the role of attentional mechanism. In: G Dawson (ed)Autism: nature, diagnosis and treatment. Guilford Press, New York, p 144-173

De Volder A, Bol A, Michel C, Congneau M, Goffinet A (1987) Brain glucose metabolism in children with the autistic syndrome: positron tomography analysis. Brain Dev 9: 581-587

Diamond A (1990) Developmental time course in human infants and infant monkeys and the neural bases of inhibitory control in reaching. Ann N Y Acad Sci 608: 637-669

Diamond A, Goldman-Rakic PS (1989) Comparison of human infants and rhesus monkeys on Piaget's AB task evidence for depence on dorsolateral prefrontal cortex. Exp Brain Res 74: 24-40

Frith U, Morton J, Leslie AM (1991) The cognitive basis of a biological disorder: autism. Trends Neurosci 14: 433-438

Garreau B, Zilbovicius M, Guerin P, Samson Y, Syrota A, Lelord G (1994) Effects of auditory stimulation on regional cerebral blood flow in autistic children. Dev Brain Dysfunc 7: 119-128

Gillberg C, Svendsen P (1983) Childhood psychosis and computed tomographic brain scan findings. J Autism Dev Disord 13: 19-32

Heh CWC, Smith R, Wu J, Hazlett E, Russell A, Asarnow R, Tanguay P, Buchsbaum MS (1989) Positron emission tomography of the cerebellum in autism. Am J Psychiat 146: 242-245

Herold S, Frackowiak RSJ, LeCouteur A, Rutter M, Howlin P (1988) Cerebral blood Flow and metabolism of oxygen and glucose in young autistic adults. Psychol Med 18: 823-831

Hier DB, LeMay M, Rosenberger PB (1979) Autism and unfavorable left-right asymmetries of brain. J Autism Dev Disord 9: 153-159

Horwitz B, Rumsey JM, Grady CL, Rapoport SI (1988) The cerebral metabolic landscape in autism: intercorrelations of regional glucose utilization. Arch Neurol 45: 749-755

Hughes C, Russell J, Robbins TW (1994) Evidence for executive dysfunction in autism. Neuropsychologia 32: 477-492

Juliano SL, Whitsel BL (1987) A combined 2-deoxyglucose and neurophysiological study of primate somatosensory cortex. J Comp Neurol 263: 514-525

Kanner L (1943) Autistic disturbances of affective contact. Nerv Child 2: 217-250

Mazziota JC, Phelps ME, Carson RE, Kuhl DE (1982) Tomographic mapping of human cerebral metabolism auditory stimulation. Neurology 32: 921-937

Nielsen JB, Friberg L, Lou H, Lansen NA, Sam ILK (1990) Immature pattern of brain activity in Rett syndrome. Arch Neurol 47: 982-986

Ogawa T, Sugiyama A, Ishiwa S, Suzuki M, Ishihara T, Sako K (1982) Ontogenic development of EEG asymetry in early infantile autism. Brain Dev 4: 439-449

Ornitz EM (1983) The functional neuroanatomy of infantile autisme. Int J Neurosci 19: 85-124

Ozonoff EM, Pennington BF, Rogers SF (1991) Executive function deficits in high-functioning autistic individuals: relationship to theory of mind. J Child Psychol Psychiat 32: 1081-1105

Petersen SE, Fox T, Posner MI, Mintun M, Raichle ME (1988) Positron emission tomographic studies of the cortical anatomy of single word processing. Nature 331: 585-589

Piven J, Berthier M, Starkstein S, Nehme E, Pearlson G, Folstein S (1990) magnetic resonance imaging evidence for a defect of cerebral cortical development in autism. Am J Psychiat 147: 734-739

Ritvo ER, Freeman BJ, Scheibel AB (1986) Lower Purkinje cell counts in the cerebella of four autistic subjects: ini-

tial findings of the UCLA-NSAC autopsy research report. Am J Psychiat 143: 862-866
Rumsey JM, Duara R, Grady C, Rapoport LJ, Margolin RA, Rapoport ST, Cutler NR (1985) Brain metabolism in autism: Resting cerebral glucose utilization rates as measured with positron emission tomography. Arch Gen Psychiat 42: 448-455
Rumsey JM, Hamburger SD (1988) Neuropsychological findings in high-functionning men with infantile autism: residual state. J Clin Exp Neurol 10: 201-221
Rutter M (1978) Diagnosis and definition. In: Autism: a Reappraisal of Concepts and Treatment. Rutter M, Schopler E (eds). Plenun, New York p 1-25
Schifter T, Hoffman JM, Hatten P, Hanson MW, Coleman RE, DeLong GR (1994) Neuroimaging in infantile autism. J Child Neurol 9: 155-161
Sokoloff L, Reivich M, Kennedy C, Des Rosiers MH, Patlak CS, Petitgrew KD, Sakurada O, Shinohada M (1977) 14C-deoxyglucose method for measurement of local cerebral glucose utilisation: theory, procedure, normal values in the conscious and anestetized albino rat. J Neurochem 28: 897-916
Tanguay PE (1976) Clinical and electrophysiological research. In: Autism: Diagnosis, research, management. Ritvo E (ed). Spectrum, New York, p 75-84
Williams RS, Hauser SL, Purpura DP, DeLong R, Swisher CN (1980) Autism and mental retardation: neuropathologic studies performed in four retarded persons with autistic behavior. Arch Neurol 37: 749-753
Zatorre R, Evans AC, Meyer E, Gjedde A (1992) Lateralization of phonetic and pitch discrimination in speech processing. Science 256: 846-849
Zilbovicius M, Garreau B, Tzourio N, Mazoyer B, Bruck B, Martinot JL, Raynaud C, Samson Y, Syrota A, Lelord G (1992) Regional cerebral blood flow in childhood autism: a SPECT study. Am J Psychiat 149: 924-930
Zilbovicius M, Garreau B, Samson Y, Remy P, Barthélémy C, Syrota A, Lelord G (1995) Delayed frontal cortex maturation in childhood autism. Am J Psychiat 152: 248-252

7. ^{31}P Magnetic resonance spectroscopy and its application to autism and brain development

N.J. MINSHEW, J.W. PETTEGREW

Magnetic resonance spectroscopy (MRS) is a powerful non invasive technique for investigating the molecular metabolic underpinning of brain disorders which involve abnormalities in the development, remodeling, or turnover of neuronal membranes. MRS of the naturally-occurring phosphorus isotope (^{31}P) is ideally suited to the study of such disorders, because of its capacity for directly measuring brain membrane production and degradation, and the bioenergetics that support normal neuronal function. MRS furthermore relies on naturally occurring isotopes and the same nuclear magnetic resonance principles as magnetic resonance imaging (MRI), making repeated studies and studies of children both possible and safe.

Recognition of the unique and important capabilities of MRS for delineating the pathophysiological mechanisms of brain disorders has been limited to date, largely as a result of the focus in medicine on imaging. The addition of MRS to the armamentarium of research imaging tools results in an exceedingly powerful and complementary array of non invasive method for examining disease processes at the gross structural level with volumetric MRI, at the neural systems level with functional MRI (fMRI) and at the molecular metabolic level with MRS. Among research imaging techniques, MRS is unique in assaying brain membrane synthesis and turnover, and in directly measuring levels of phosphocreatine (PCr), adenosine triphosphate (ATP), adenosine diphosphate (ADP), and inorganic orthophosphate (Pi), a final product of energy consumption. MRS also provides an accurate measure of intracellular brain pH. However, in contrast to other imaging techniques such as positron emission tomography (PET) or single photon emission tomography (SPECT), which MRS directly measures steady-state levels of energy metabolites and not their rate of consumption. Thus, it provides information about bioenergetics fundamentally different from that provided by PET and SPECT, and findings across techniques may diverge.

MRS is a method which encompasses a wide range of approaches to the definition of the molecular and metabolic underpinnings of brain disorders. MRS can readily be applied to the study of the living brain in human subjects. However, the investigation of a disease process can also be extended to higher resolution laboratory conditions, substantially improving the analytical sensitivity of this technique. The application of these methods to the study of brain tissue, brain slices, and animal models provides important amplification of *in vivo* findings. In addition, MRS of molecules in solution and solids can be used to address key questions about physico chemical relationships relevant to molecular and metabolic dynamics *in vivo*.

^{31}P Magnetic Resonance Spectroscopy and Brain Development

^{31}P magnetic resonance spectroscopy is particularly suited to the study of developmental disorders of neuronal organisation which alter the synthesis or degradation of brain membranes. Neuronal organisation encompasses the events in brain development which result in the intricate neural circuitry characteristic of the human brain (Volpe, 1995). Neuronal organisation begins in approximately the sixth month of gestation and continues for many years postnatally. The timing of the organisational events varies with the brain region, being relatively rapid in the hippocampus and following a more prolonged course in the neocortex. The organisation of the late maturing frontal lobe circuitry, for example, extends well into the second decade of life.

The processes involved in the development of the elaborate circuitry of the human brain include the attainment of alignment, orientation, and layering of the cortical neurons; elaboration of dendritic and axonal ramifications; establishment of synaptic contacts; cell death and selective elimination of neuronal processes; and proliferation and differentiation of glia (Volpe, 1995). There has been no neuropathological evidence in autism to suggest primary abnormalities in the alignment, orientation or layering of cortical neurons, or in myelination of neurons. Rather, the neuropathological and imaging evidence has implicated abnormalities in those events related to elaboration of dendritic and axonal ramifications in the hippocampus (decreased), establishment of synaptic contacts (decreased intra cortical and cortico subcortical), selective elimination of neuronal processes in the cerebral cortex (decreased pruning), and selective cell death in the cerebellum (increased). It is these organisational events that ^{31}P MRS has the potential for monitoring.

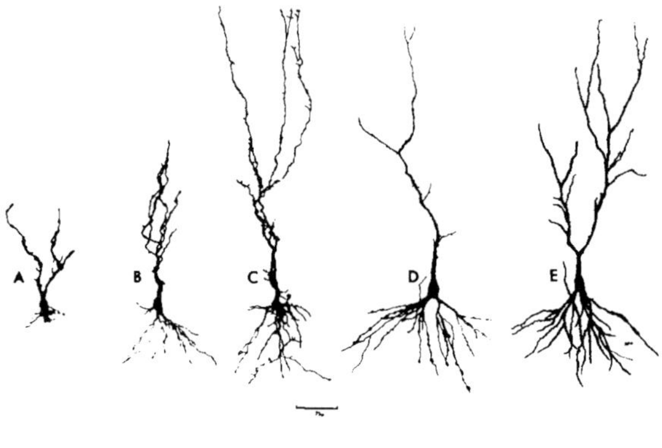

Fig. 1. Development of dendritic spines on apical dendritic shafts of layer V pyramidal neurons. Rapid Golgi preparations. 1: fetus, 18 weeks conceptual age. Filopodia and growth cones are evident along with some thin spines. 2: fetus, 22 weeks conceptual age. An increase in long, thin spines is seen at this stage. 3: 33 weeks conceptual age. There is a rapid development of long, thin spines and a few mushroom-shaped and stubby spines. 4: 6 months postnatal. Few thin spines are noted. The vast majority of spines have stubby necks and many mushroom-shaped spines are evident. 5: 7 years (accident case). Most spines are stubby and mushroom-shaped. Little change occurs in the characteristics of dendritic spines between 6 months and 7 years. (Reprinted with permission from: Dr. Dominick Purpura).

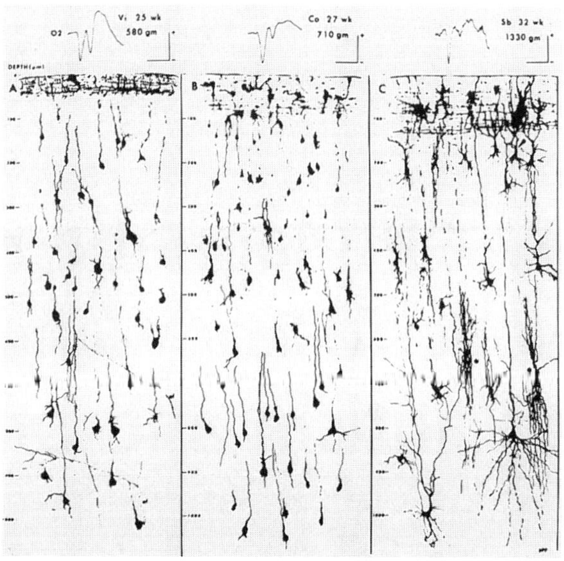

Fig. 2. Camera lucida composite drawings of neurons in visual (calcarine) cortex of human infants of indicated gestational ages. Note the appearance and elaboration of basilar dendrites and the tangential spread of apical dendrites, as well as the accompanying maturation of the visual evoked response (top). (Reprinted with permission from: Dr. Dominick Purpura).

The histological manifestations of neuronal organisation events in the hippocampus and cerebral cortex are shown in Fig. 1-5. Figure 1 demonstrates the normal course of dendritic development in pyramidal neurons of the hippocampus between 18 and 34 weeks of conceptual age (Purpura, 1979). By 18 weeks (Fig. 1A), the neurons exhibit apical dendrites, many varicosities and irregularities and growth processes typical of rapidly developing neural elements; in contrast, basilar dendrites are thin and undeveloped (Purpura, 1979). During the next 8 weeks (Fig. 1B-D), the apical dendrites increase in length and develop basic branching patterns and basilar dendrites become more prominent and develop the characteristics previously exhibited by the apical dendrites. By 32-34 weeks (Fig. 1E), the basilar and apical dendrites are both relatively well developed but further increases in length and additional branching of distal segments occur throughout the first postnatal year. A similar prenatal pattern of dendritic development has been documented in the neurons of visual cortex. Figure 2 demonstrates the appearance and elaboration of basilar dendrites and the tangential spread of apical dendrites in neurons of visual cortex between 25 and 32 weeks of gestation and Figure 3 depicts the neurons in the cortex of a 6 year old child demonstrating the continuation of this developmental process in the more abundant and complex horizontal and tangential dendritic branches (Huttenlocher, 1975; Purpura, 1979; Volpe 1995). Figure 4 demonstrates the growth in dendritic

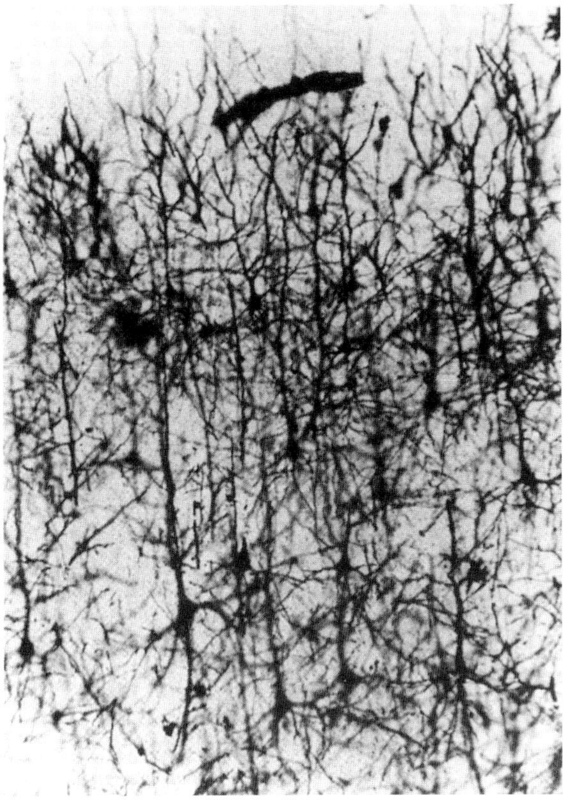

Fig. 3. Middle frontal gyrus from a 6-year-old child without known neurological disease. Golgi-Cox method, X 80. (Reprinted with permission from: Dr. Peter Huttenlocher).

spines on cortical neurons in the 18 week fetus, 26 week fetus, 33 week premature infant, 6 month old infant, and 7 year old child. Development is associated initially with the appearance of long, thin spines and a few stubby and mushroom-shaped spines. With further development, the latter two types of spines become prominent. Figure 5, comparing the cortex at birth, six, and fourteen years old provides evidence of the impact of regressive events during adolescence. The density of the dendritic arbor is less at 14 years of age, reflecting the consequences of normal pruning which eliminates neuronal processes that failed to make functional connections or made inappropriate connections.

Physicochemical basis of NMR spectroscopy

The principles of nuclear magnetic resonance have been widely discussed in connection with MRI and will not be reviewed here. Detailed descriptions of the fundamentals of nuclear magnetic spectroscopy are provided elsewhere (McClure et al., 1996; Minshew and Pettegrew, 1996; Pettegrew et al., 1993; Silverstein et al., 1991). A few essential principles related to key methodological considerations will be briefly described here.

Chemical shift

The basis of the analytical capabilities of MRS is the phenomenon of chemical shift, the shift in resonance frequency that results from the influence of adjacent nuclei in the molecule. When atomic nuclei are covalently bonded in molecules, the electron cloud distribution surrounding each nucleus is altered as a result of interactions with the electron clouds of neighbouring nuclei in the molecule. Thus, for example, the electron clouds surrounding each of the three phosphorus nuclei in ATP are different. In the presence of an externally-applied magnetic field, the electron cloud of the nucleus produces a magnetic field opposite to the main magnetic field, thereby decreasing the actual magnetic field experienced by the nucleus and altering its resonance frequency. This alteration in the resonance frequency of a nucleus as a result of the influence of neighbouring atoms in the molecule is referred to as chemical shift. The strength of the secondary magnetic field produced

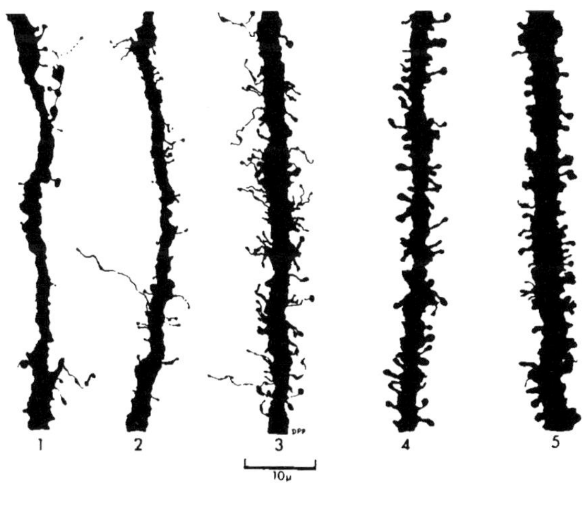

Fig. 4. Camera lucida drawings of proximal apical dendritic segments of motor cortex pyramidal neurons during development. 1. 18-week-old fetus; 2, 26-week-old fetus; 3. 33-week-old preterm infant; 4. 6-month-old infant; 5. 7-year-old child. Early phase of dendritic spine differentiation in proximal apical segments is associated with the development of long, thin spines and relatively few stubby and mushroom-shaped spines. The latter two types are prominent in the postnatal period and early childhood. (Reprinted with permission from: Dr. Dominick Purpura).

by the electron cloud and, thus, the magnitude of the chemical shift are proportional to the field strength of the externally applied magnet. Chemical shift dispersion, or the separation between the resonance peaks in a spectrum, therefore, increases with magnetic field strength.

Chemical shifts are one of the primary spectral characteristics used for identifying the origin of MRS resonances in a spectrum. Chemical shifts are expressed as the difference between the resonance position of the nucleus and the resonance position in the same spectrum of an arbitrarily chosen reference nucleus. Chemical shifts are usually reported in accordance with the International Union of Pure and Applied Chemistry convention in units of parts per million or ppm, which are independent of field strength. PPM values are obtained by dividing resonance frequency by applied frequency and multiplying by 10^6. Chemical shifts can also be reported in terms of resonance frequency (Hz) rather than ppm units, but then the applied field strength must also be specified, since chemical shift varies as a function of field strength. Chemical shifts are designated relative to a standard reference frequency. For ^{31}P NMR of the brain, the glycerol-3-phosphorylcholine signal is set at -0.13 ppm. Resonances upfield from the designated 0 ppm position have positive chemical numbers and those downfield negative.

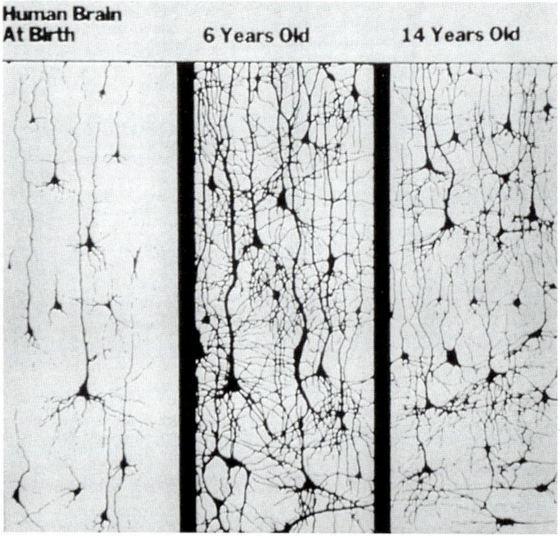

Fig. 5. This series of photomicrographs shows the density of neuronl connections at birth, at 6 years old, and at 14 years old. Note that the density is actually lower in the 14-year-old, as a result of the normal "pruning" process that removes "excess" connections and leaves in place those that become functional circuits.

The ^{31}P MRS spectrum of mammalian brain

In vitro ^{31}P MRS spectrum

In vitro studies of brain tissue provide the optimal conditions for MRS and for peak identification. Sample preparation with perchloric acid extraction to remove line broadening cations, much higher field strength, and the superior field homogeneity of smaller bore laboratory magnets greatly improve spectral resolution over *in vivo* conditions. Field strength generally increases both chemical shift dispersion and the proportion of nuclei in the excited state, thereby improving signal strength and peak resolution. For example, increasing field strength from 1.5T to 3.0T increases signal strength for ^{31}P MRS three-fold, and from 1.5T to 10T, signal strength is increased 17-fold. A number of chemical procedures also can be employed *in vitro* to improve peak resolution further and aid in peak identification. For example, perchloric acid extraction of brain tissue samples removes cations which make a significant contribution to line broadening of resonances. Also, sample pH can be manipulated to achieve optimal separation of peaks and this can aid in identifying resonances containing acidic or basic functional groups; the identity of a peak can be confirmed by adding a known compound to the mixture. Various NMR properties also can be used to characterise the chemical origin of resonances.

Composition of the *in vitro* spectrum

A ^{31}P MRS *in vitro* spectrum at 11.7T of a perchloric acid extract of freeze-clamped rat brain is shown in Figure 6. The identities of the major peaks in the *in vitro* ^{31}P MRS spectrum have been well documented (Glonek et al., 1982; Klunk et al., 1994). The readily identifiable peaks in this spectrum include: 1. the phosphomonoesters (PME): a-glycerol phosphate (a-GP, 4.35d), inositol phosphate (IP, 4.05d), phosphoethanolamine (PE, 3.94d), and phosphocholine (PC, 3.43d); 2. inorganic orthophosphate (Pi, 2.66d); 3. the phosphodiesters (PDE): glycerol 3-phosphoethanolamine (GPE, 0.66d) and glycerol 3-phosphocholine (PGC, -0.13d); 4. phosphocreatine (PCr,-3.12d); 5. the nucleotide triphosphates, predominantly adenosine triphosphate (ATP, g -5.80d, a -10.92d, b -21.7d); 6. the nucleotide diphosphates, predominantly 5'-adenosine diphosphate (ADP, b -6.11d, a -10.61d); 7. dinucleotides, such as nicotin-

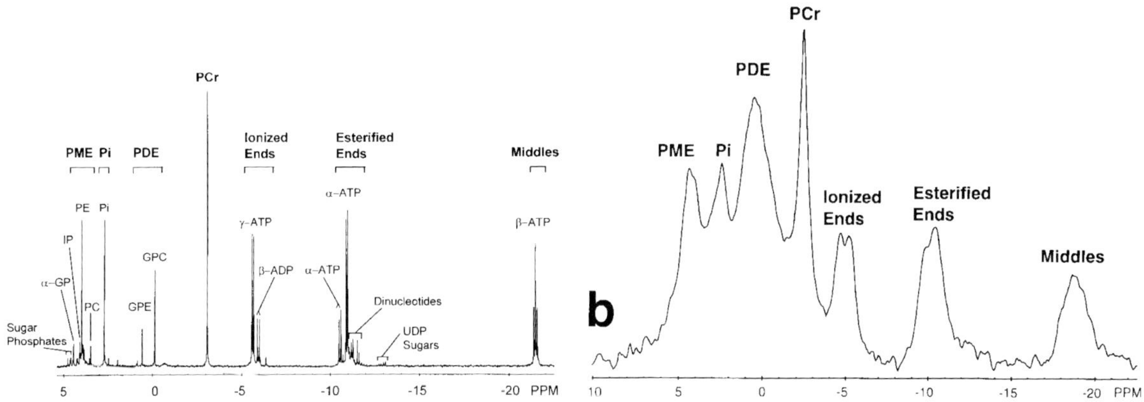

Fig. 7. Comparison of (A) an *in vitro* ^{31}P MRS spectrum of perchloric acid extract of freeze clamped rat brain tissue at 11.7 T with (B) an *in vivo* ^{31}P MRS of the dorsal prefrontal cortex of a human subject demonstrating the correspondence between the peak composition of the *in vitro* and *in vivo* spectra. In the *in vivo* spectrum is composed of seven peaks from left to right representing the levels of the phosphomonoesters (PME), inorganic orthophosphate (Pi), phosphodiesters (PDE), phosphocreatine (PCr), ionized ends (g-ATP and b-ADP), esterified ends (a-ATP and a-ADP), and middles (b-ATP). In the *in vitro* spectrum, the seven peaks in the *in vivo* spectrum are seen to be composed of several individually discernable peaks; thus the PME resonance is discernable in the *in vitro* spectrum as peaks for inositol phosphate (IP), phosphoethanolamine (PE), and phosphocholine (PC).

amide adenine dinucleotide (NAD, -11.37d); and 8. a complex resonance band centered around -12.89d composed of nucleoside diphospho- derivatives such as uridine diphosphosugars, and cytidine diphospho- derivatives, such as cytidine diphosphocholine and cytidine diphosphoethanolamine. To obtain reliable measures of the unstable high-energy phosphate metabolites (e.g., PCr, ATP, ADP), the PCA extraction is carried out rat brain tissue freeze-clamped with liquid nitrogen at the time of harvesting. Identification of the peaks contained in the *in vitro* spectrum was accomplished with various physico chemical methods and validated with classical chemical assays; these analyses and the *in vitro* spectrum provide a foundation for the identification of the peaks in the *in vivo* spectrum.

Quantitation of the *in vitro* spectrum

The quantitation of the metabolite levels from the *in vitro* ^{31}P MRS spectrum can be accomplished by adding a known amount of an internal standard to the weighed tissue at the time of tissue preparation. The metabolite levels are then reported in absolute units of mmol/g of tissue. Alternatively, the metabolites can be used as their own internal standard, in which case the data are expressed as mole % of the total phosphorus signal. The advantage of the latter method is that it is independent of tissue volume and thus allows direct comparisons across *in vitro* and *in vivo* samples regardless of tissue volume. This advantage becomes key in the case of *in vivo* studies, where variations in brain volume become a major consideration. One potential limitation of the mole % method of quantitation was the possibility that a substantial reduction in the concentration of a major component in the sample may result in a false increase in the levels of the other components. This issue was directly investigated in an empirical experiment, which demonstrated that this does not occur (Klunk et al., 1994).

In vivo ^{31}P spectrum at 1.5 T

The *in vivo* ^{31}P spectrum of the human brain (Fig. 7) is considerably less well resolved than that *in vitro*. The lower resolution of the *in vivo* spectrum is due in part to the lower magnetic field strength involved in *in vivo* studies. Power deposition in the brain increases with field strength, limiting the highest practical field strength for *in vivo* MRS in humans to 4.0 T. The resonance peaks in the *in vivo* spectrum also are broadened by the effect of the living tissue environment on the T2 relaxation of molecules (Bolinger and Lenkinski, 1992). Additional factors contributing to line-broadening in the *in vivo* spectrum include field inhomogeneity within the tissue sample and chemical exchange (complexation with and dissociation from) cations, which results in different local magnetic field environments for the excited state nucleus. Thus, increasing field strength for MRS of humans from 1.5 T to 4.0 T would improve spectral resolution to some extent, but will not yield the well resolved spectra characteristic of *in vitro* MRS of perchloric acid extracts of brain tissue, because of the tissue and field inhomogeneity factors. Despite loss of detail, it was established many years ago that *in vivo* MRS produces meaningful data which are both reliable and valid (Ackerman et al., 1980).

Composition of the *in vivo* spectrum

The *in vivo* ^{31}P MRS spectrum of human brain at 1.5 T (Fig. 7) yields quantifiable spectral peaks for the following components: the phosphomonoesters (PME), inorganic orthophosphate (Pi), phosphocreatine (PCr), phosphodiesters (PDE), and three polyphosphate peaks that represent the a, b, and g phosphates of the nucleotide triphosphates and the a and b phosphates of the nucleotide diphosphates. In addition, intracellular pH can be determined by the chemical shift difference between the PCr and Pi resonances (Petroff et al., 1985). Identification of the origin of *in vivo* resonance signals requires detailed knowledge of *in vitro* spectra of brain extracts under conditions as close as possible to those *in vivo*. Peak identity in the *in vivo* spectrum is confirmed by comparison with the *in vitro* spectrum, as demonstrated in Figure 7.

Quantitation of the *in vivo* spectrum

Because the resonance peaks in the *in vivo* spectrum are broad and overlapping, the areas under them are quantified with a nonlinear curve fitting of Lorentizian peaks to the experimental data (fig. 8) using curve-fitting software programs. The test-retest and interrater reliability for these procedures in our laboratories have been ≥ 95 %, and *in vivo* values has been demonstrated to be highly comparable to previously published *in vitro* MRS data and determination with classical analytical methods (Glonek et al., 1982; Klunk et al., 1994; Pettegrew et al., 1984; Pettegrew et al., 1994).

Ideally, quantitation of the *in vivo* spectrum would be based on a comparison of sample signal to a reliable internal standard. However, no such standard exists for *in vivo* MRS. To express *in vivo* data in absolute units of mmole/g, external standards have been attached to the head and measured simultaneously (Bottomley et al., 1988; 1992) or placed in

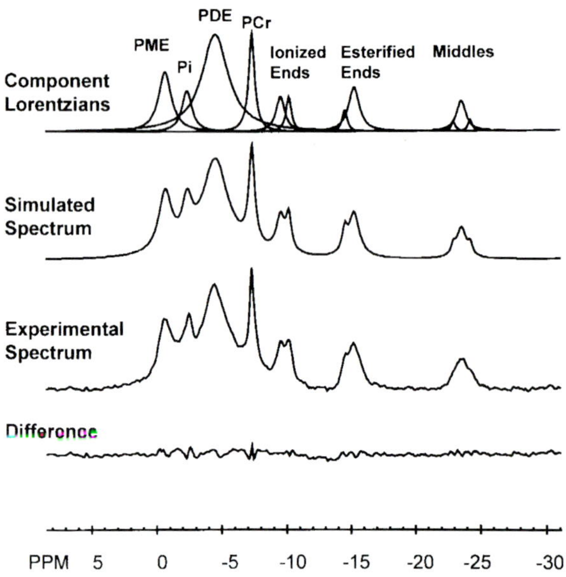

Fig. 8. Quantitation of the *in vivo* ^{31}P MRS spectrum from dorsal prefrontal cortex of human subject. The experimental spectrum is shown at the top after baseline correction. This spectrum is then decomposed into the component Lorentzian peaks at the bottom. Addition of the Lorentzian peaks yields the simulated spectrum. Subtraction of the simulated spectrum from the experimental spectrum produces the difference tracing at the bottom. The goodness of fit to the experimental data is controlled by ensuring that the difference between the experimental and simulated spectra is negligible.

phantoms and measured separately (Gruetter et al., 1992). Another method obtains estimates of absolute concentration by assuming a known, unchanging concentration of one metabolite such as creatine; this method expresses data as a molar ratio despite the use of absolute units (Frahn et al., 1989; Sappey-Marinier et al., 1992). Each such method introduces its own source of errors. Because it is independent of tissue volume, we have used the relative mole % method in which tissue metabolites serve as their own internal reference (Pettegrew et al., 1991; Klunk et al., 1994).

Spatial localization for *in vivo* MRS

For *in vitro* studies, the sample is analysed as a whole. *In vivo* studies, however, use spatial localisation methods to obtain signal from subregions of the brain. Two methods have been used. The surface coil method, used in the studies described below, involves two concentric coils, a transmitter and a smaller inner receiver coil, positioned on the surface of the head. Pulse parameters are adjusted so that brain receives a 90° pulse, while skin and muscle on the surface of the head receive a 180° or null pulse to eliminate contributions from them. The skull does not contribute to the signal under *in vivo* conditions, because of the extremely long relaxation times associated with the immobilization of phosphates in bone. The resulting radiofrequency field is conical, with its base at the surface of the scalp and depth equal to the radius of the coil. The localisation of the signal from the brain is confirmed by collecting an image with the coil used to produce the MRS signal. Thus, in the depth-pulse localisation method, variation in radiofrequency flip angle, depth of tissue penetration, and size of the surface coil are used to localise the volume of brain tissue of interest. This method can be used for studying 15-20cc of brain tissue close to the surface of the skull in regions without significant intervening non-neural tissue, which essentially confines this method to the study of the frontal lobes, as other regions have significant intervening blood or muscle between scalp and brain. The major advantages of this method are the high quality of the spectra with regard to signal to noise and the absence of a delay in acquisition of the MRS signal following the simple pulse sequence, which ensures that all of the initial signal from the phospholipid components can be recorded. Other methods using complex pulse sequences are also in use, and have been recently refined so that the loss of phospholipid signal associated with the earlier methods has been largely eliminated (Lim et al., 1994). The latest methods allow the simultaneous collection of spectra from multiple locations within a 35 mm slice of brain tissue.

Chemical contributions to the ^{31}P MRS spectrum

High-energy phosphate resonances

The resonances related to bioenergetics (Pi, PCr, and the three nucleoside phosphate resonances) are derived from small molecules. The simplest cases are Pi, which is solely derived from inorganic phosphate (mainly $H_2PO_4^{-1}$ and HPO_4^{-2} at physiological pH), and PCr, which is derived solely from phosphocreatine. The nucleoside phosphates include contributions from adenosine, cytosine, guanosine, and uridine mono-, di-, and tri- phosphates (NMP, NDP, and NTP, respectively), but the adenosine compounds are the predominant species. The ionised ends resonance (-5 to -8 ppm) is made up of the terminal, b-phosphate of NDP s and the terminal, g-phosphates of NTP s, thus mainly representing ADP and ATP. The esterified ends resonance (-8 to -14 ppm) is made up of the nucleoside-coupled a-phosphates of NDP s and NTP s, again mainly representing ADP and ATP but also a minor contribution from dinucleotides such as NADP and NADPH and UDP-sugars. The middles resonance (-18 to -23 ppm) is the simplest of the nucleoside resonances, being composed only of the middle, b-phosphate of NTP s, mainly ATP. The linewidth of these nucleoside resonances is increased by increased intracellular levels of free Ca^{2+} or Mg^{2+}, which form complexes with the nucleoside phosphates producing the phenomenon of chemical exchange line broadening (Pettegrew et al., 1988).

In vivo ^{31}P MRS also provides a direct assessment of intra cellular pH, which is determined from the difference between the chemical shifts of PCr and Pi (Petroff et al., 1985) or between the ionised and esterified ends (Pettegrew et al., 1988). *In vivo* measurement of brain pH is important as it provides information on: physiochemical buffering capacity; consumption and production of metabolic acids such as lactic acid, and transmembrane fluxes of H^+ and HCO_3^-. Intracellular brain pH is also important because of its influence on enzymes and metabolic processes such as creatine kinase, phosphofructokinase, redox ratios, and oxyhaemoglobin dissociation (Siesjo, 1978).

Phospholipid resonances

The resonances related to phospholipid membrane metabolism are no less complex. The PME resonance represents both small, rapidly tumbling molecules, which give narrow linewidths, and large, slowly moving macromolecules, which give broad linewidths. The small molecules include: phosphoethanolamine (PE), phosphocholine (PC), inositol-1-phosphate (IP), and small amounts of phosphoserine (PS), NMP phosphates such as AMP, sugar phosphates such as glucose-6-phosphate, and a-glycerol-phosphate (a-GP). The macromolecules are mainly comprised of relatively mobile proteins containing phosphorylated serine and threonine residues. The macromolecular component appears to be relatively small, as at least (two thirds) of the total *in vivo* PME concentration, reported to be approximately 3 mmoles/g (Bottomley et al., 1992, Klausner et al., 1992), is accounted for by the small water-soluble metabolites. Phosphoethanolamine alone contributes about 1 mmole/g.

The PDE also have small and large molecular components. The small molecules are mainly glycerophosphocholine (GPC) and glycerophosphoethanolamine (GPE), which give relatively narrow linewidths. The large molecules are choline, ethanolamine, and serine phospholipids in small, mobile structures, such as synaptic vesicles, and phospholipid vesicles, such as those in endoplasmic reticulum and Golgi (Kilby et al., 1991; Murphy et al., 1992; Pettegrew et al., 1994) which give the broad linewidth components. In practice, the broadest components due to membrane bilayers are typically not observed due to choice of spectral acquisition parameters, or are removed by processing the spectral baseline. Phospholipids in myelin, or even external cell membranes and large organelle membranes, also are too immobile to be recorded with *in vivo* ^{31}P MRS (Kilby et al, 1991). Thus, as typically applied, the PDE peak of the *in vivo* ^{31}P MRS measures GPE, GPC, and mobile vesicular phospholipids (Pettegrew et al., 1994). The mobile vesicular phospholipid contribution appears to predominate as the concentration of GPE plus GPC approaches 3 mmole/g brain in water-soluble extracts and the total PDE peak has been estimated to be on the order of 15 mmole/g *in vivo* (Bottomley et al., 1992; Klausner et al., 1992).

In summary *in vivo* ^{31}P MRS, the PME peak predominantly indicates levels of small, water-soluble precursors of phospholipid membrane synthesis, such as a-GP, IP, PE and PC. The PDE peak gives information on both small water-soluble phospholipid membrane breakdown products (GPE and GPC) and mobile phospholipid vesicles such as synaptic vesicles. The Pi peak constitutes the final end-product of all of the phosphorus metabolites. The PCr peak specifically measures the level of this one high-energy metabolite. PCr is the most metabolically labile of the high-energy compounds, falling prior to ATP in situations of rapid energy consumption. The nucleoside phosphate resonances (ionised ends, esterified ends, and middles) mainly represent levels of ATP and ADP. Changes in the ionised and/or esterified ends without a similar change in the middles resonance, suggest a change in ADP more than ATP. Changes in the middles resonance, mainly indicative of changes in ATP levels.

Metabolic information

From a metabolic perspective, the PCr, ATP, ADP, Pi and brain pH values provide steady state information about the energy status of the brain. The phosphomonoesters (aGP, IP, PE, and PC) are the building blocks of membrane phospholipids and the relative concentrations of these metabolites are a measure of the active synthesis of membranes (Vance, 1991). Sources of PME include: phosphorylation of their respective bases by kinases; phospholipase C cleavage of their respective phospholipids; and phosphodiesterase cleavage of their respective PDE. The phosphodiesters (GPE, GPC) are the major catabolic products of membrane phospholipid degradation (Carlsson 1988; Vance 1991). They are the products of phospholipase A1 and A2 activity toward their phospholipids and are converted to their respective PME by PDE phosphodiesterase activity.

^{31}P MRS studies of normal brain development, maturation, and senescence in an animal model

Histological, Neurochemical and Neurophysiological Events in rat brain development

The capacity of ^{31}P MRS for monitoring changes in brain membranes and bioenergetics occurring with brain development and ageing was initially investigated in an animal model. This was accomplished by assaying perchloric acid extracts of the brain from Fisher 344 rats ranging in age from newborn (12 hours) through senescence (12 to 24 months of age in the rat) (Pettegrew et al., 1990). Brain development and maturation in the rat have been divided arbitrarily into five periods summarised in Table 1 (McIlwain and Bachelard, 1985). Period I is the period of cellular division and extends up to birth, at which point the rat brain has no recordable electrical activity and has attained 15 % of its adult weight. From birth to 10 days of age (Period II), there is growth in the size of individual cells, rapid outgrowth of axons, and rapid development of dendritic connections. These changes are associated with a rapid increase in brain lipid content, which peaks at about 10 days of age. Naturally occurring cell death also begins during Period II and continues through Period III (Clarke, 1985; Cowan et al., 1984; Oppenheim 1985; Pittman and Oppenheim, 1979). From 10-20 days (Period III), neuronal cell volume, synaptic density, and the number of nerve terminals rapidly increase. Simultaneously, intracellular K^+ space increases and the extracellular Na^+ and Cl^- space decreases. These changes are associated with the appearance of electrical activity on the electroencephalogram. Neurochemical correlates of the structural and neurophysiological developments in periods II and III are manifest in a steady increase after birth in adenosine triphosphatase activity including Na^+-K^+ ATPase, and increases in the rates of glucose uptake, glycolysis, and oxidative phosphorylation, which reach adults levels during Period III. Periods II and III, or birth to approximately one month of age in the rat, are therefore a time of active neuronal growth, synaptogenesis, and neuronal organisation. As in humans, naturally-occurring cell death is also an integral part of the developmental process in the rat. Period IV in rat brain development begins at approximately 20 days of age and is associated with active myelination but little further growth in brain size. During this phase, creatine phosphokinase activity reaches maximum levels. Senescence in the rat (Period V) is thought to develop after 12 months and certainly by 24 months of age.

Table 1
^{31}P magnetic resonance spectroscopy (MRS) of brain development and ageing in the rat

Period	Age	Anatomical event	MRS findings: Phospholipid metabolism	MRS findings: PCr[a]
II	Birth-10 days	Neuronal organisation • Rapid increase in brain lipid content • Synaptogenesis • Programmed cell death starts	PME levels high PDE levels low PME/PDE > 150	• PCr levels low • P_i levels high • PCr/P_i ratio low
III	10-20 Days	Neuronal organisation • Synaptogenesis • EEG activity appears • Programmed cell death continues	PME levels decreasing PDE levels increasing	• Rapid increase in PCr and PCRP_i ratio • Rapid decrease in P_i level, which correlates with development of glycolytic and oxidative pathways • Increase in Na^+-K^+-ATPase and EEG activity
IV	20 Days-12 months	Myelination	PME/PDE ≈ 1-2	• Slight increase in PCr and P_i • PCr/P_i: no change
V	> 12 months	Aging and senescence	PME/PDE < 1	• Slight increase in PCr and P_i • Slight increase in PCr/P_i suggesting decrease in PCr utilisation

[a] There were no changes in adenosine triphosphate with age.
PCr phosphocreatine; *PME* phosphomonoester; *PDE* phosphodiester; P_i inorganic orthophosphate; *ATPase* adenosine triphosphatase; *EEG* electroencephalogram

The brains collected from rats from birth to senescence were freeze clamped to preserve the high-energy metabolites, subjected to perchloric acid extraction, and analysed with ^{31}P MRS at 4.7 T to obtain mole % values for PCr, Pi, ATP, a-glycerol phosphate (a-GP), phosphocholine (PC), phosphoserine (PS), phosphoethanolamine (PE), glycerophosphocholine (GPC), and glycerophosphoethanolamine (GPE). Striking changes were observed with development in the levels of the phosphomonoesters, phosphodiesters, phosphocreatine, and inorganic orthophosphate (Table 1).

Changes in phospholipid metabolism with brain development and maturation

The phosphomonoesters (a-GP, PE, PC, PS), particularly PE and PS, were high in the immature brain at birth and rapidly decreased from the newborn period to three months of age ($p = 0.0001$) (Fig. 9). Thereafter, changes in the phosphomonoesters were relatively slight. Between three months and 12 months, the levels of a-GP and PC remained relatively constant and the levels of PE+PS increased slightly ($0.01 < p < 0.05$). From 12 to 24 months, the levels of PC decreased slightly ($0.001 < p < 0.01$). In contrast, the levels of the phosphodiesters (GPE, GPC) were very low or undetectable in the newborn period and then exhibited a rapid increase up until 3

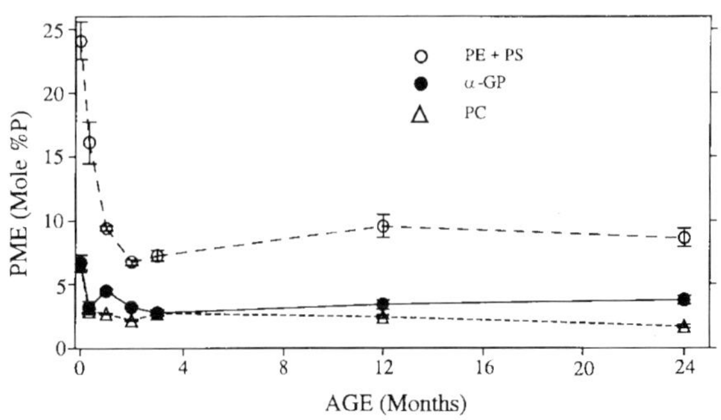

Fig. 9. Levels of the phosphomonoesters in rat brain as a function of postnatal age as determined by *in vitro* ^{31}P MRS at 11.7 T following freeze clamping and perchloric acid extraction. Reproduced with permission from the *Journal of Neuropathology and Experimental Neurology*, 1990, 237-249.

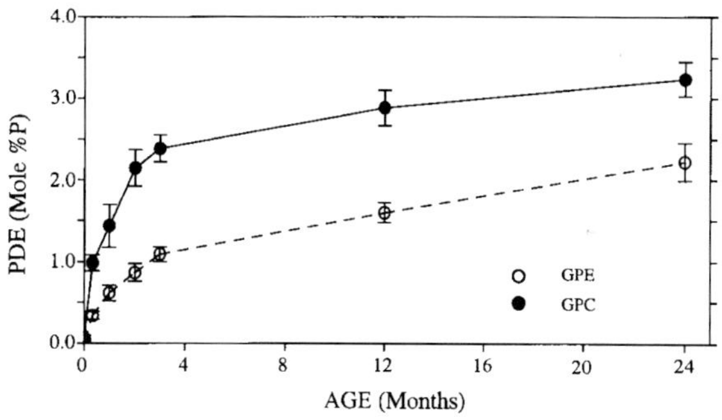

Fig. 10. Levels of the phosphodiesters in rat brain as a function of postnatal age as determined by *in vitro* ^{31}P MRS at 11.7 T following freeze clamping and perchloric acid extraction. Reproduced with permission from the *Journal of Neuropathology and Experimental Neurology*, 1990, 237-249.

months of age ($p = 0.0001$) (Fig. 10). Thereafter they rose at a slower rate, up to 24 months of age.

The PME/PDE ratio, an estimate of membrane phospholipid anabolic/catabolic rate, was high in the newborn period. It rapidly decreased up to three months of age ($p < 0.0001$), and then remained relatively constant up to 12 months of age. After 12 months, the PME/PDE ratio decreased slightly. ($0.01 < p < 0.05$). These results are indicative of very high phospholipid anabolic activity without appreciable catabolic activity from 12 hours to 10 days of age in the rat brain. This metabolic profile coincides with the histological increase in the size of neuronal cells, the rapid outgrowth of axons, and the rapid development of dendritic connections observed in Period II of rat brain development. After 10 days of age, there was a rapid decrease in PDE, the catabolic breakdown products of membrane phospholipids, and a decrease in the PME, the anabolic precursors, but the PME/PDE ratio remained high (< 10). The increasing PDE levels between 10 and 30 days of age coincide with the naturally occurring cell death and pruning of neuritic connections. Between one and three months of age, the PME continued to decrease and the PDE to increase, although not as rapidly as before. The PME/PDE ratio fell from 10 to 1, indicating a progressive decline in membrane accumulation. After three months of age, the turnover rate of phospholipids (PME/PDE) remained relatively stable until 12 months of age. Between 12 and 24 months of age, the PME/PDE ratio declined further ($0.01 < p < 0.05$), suggesting that membrane catabolism was proceeding slightly faster than membrane anabolism during senescence in the rat.

These findings provide evidence of the capacity for ^{31}P MRS to monitor important membrane events related to neuronal development, maturation, and senescence.

Changes in bioenergetics with brain development and maturation

There were no changes in ATP or ADP levels with brain development, maturation, or ageing, indicating that the brain maintained very stable levels of these energy metabolites. In contrast, the level of PCr, the most labile of the high energy phosphates, was quite low in the newborn period and decreased further until five days of age (Fig. 11). After five days of age, PCr levels rose rapidly up to one month, followed by less rapid increases between one and three months of age ($p = 0.0001$). After three months of age, the PCr levels exhibited slight but steady increases up through 24 months of age. In contrast, the levels of Pi were relatively high in the newborn period, decreased up to five days of age, and increased up to ten days of age. After ten days of age, the Pi levels dropped rapidly until three months of age ($0.01 < p < 0.05$). From three months to 12 months, the Pi levels increased slightly followed by more rapid increases from 12 to 24 months.

The PCr/Pi ratio, an index of energy utilisation, was quite low in the newborn period until five days of age, and then increased rapidly up to three months of age ($p = 0.0001$). After this, the PCr/Pi ratio remained constant to 24 months of age. The rapid increase in the PCr/Pi ratio up to one month of age correlates with the development of the glycolytic and oxidative pathways, increasing Na^+-K^+ ATPase activity, and the onset of electroencephalographic activity. The slight increase in the PCr/Pi ratio after 12 months of age is consistent with the decreased utilisation of PCr with senescence.

These findings provide evidence of the capacity for ^{31}P MRS to monitor biologically significant changes in bioenergetics with brain development and senescence.

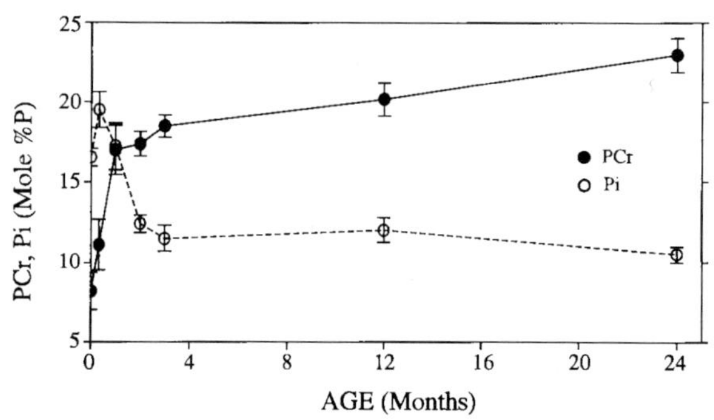

Fig. 11. Levels of phosphocreatine and inorganic orthophosphate in rat brain as a function of postnatal age as determined by *in vitro* ^{31}P MRS at 11.7 T following freeze clamping and perchloric acid extraction. Reproduced with permission from the *Journal of Neuropathology and Experimental Neurology*, 1990, 237-249.

In vivo studies of brain maturation in normal infants, adolescents, and adults

Buchli et al. (1994) conducted an *in vivo* study of 16 term neonates, 17 infants, and 28 healthy adults using a volume-selective pulse sequence (ISIS) to localise 125, 216, and 343 cm^3 brain tissue respectively in the three age groups. This volume contained approximately 45 % parietal lobes, 15 % frontal lobes, 10 % occipital lobes, and 20 % basal ganglia in all three groups. This study showed higher PME and lower PDE levels in the neonates than the adults. In addition, the concentrations of PDE, PCr, Pi, and ATP increased by factors of 3.5, 2.4, 1.9, and 1.8 respectively from birth to adulthood. The intracellular pH declined from 7.11 to 7.02 during brain development. There was also linewidth broadening and a change in the chemical shift of the PME from neonates to adults, suggesting a change in the chemical composition of PME with age.

In vivo ^{31}P MRS of dorsal prefrontal cortex has been completed with the depth pulse localisation method in 100 normal individuals between 10 and 45 years of age, recruited as control subjects for studies in autism, Down syndrome, and schizophrenia (Pettegrew et al, unpublished data). Control subjects were recruited from community volunteers in response to advertisements and were required to have a normal medical, neurological and psychiatric examination as well as a negative past and family history of developmental, neurological, and psychiatric disorders.

During late childhood and adolescence, these subjects exhibited an exponential decrease in the levels of PME and in the oxidative metabolic rate (V/Vmax calculated from the ratio of Pi/PCr) and an exponential increase in the levels of PCr in the prefrontal cortex. These changes in the brain levels of PME and PCR between 10 and 20 years of age were thought to reflect the normal process of synaptic pruning of the prefrontal cortex.

These MRS findings in normal human subjects are consistent with the developmental patterns previously documented in the *in vitro* ^{31}P MRS study of brain development in the rat.

In vivo ^{31}P MRS studies in adolescents and adults with autism

Autism is now widely viewed as a disorder of neuronal organisation, and is thought to involve abnormalities in dendritic tree development, the development of brain connections at the neural systems level, and synaptic pruning. The initial MRS study of the brain in autism focused on the frontal lobes and included correlations with neuropsychological indices of the deficits. The following are the evidence for the involvement in autism of the frontal lobes, brain membrane development and selective pruning, and abnormalities in neurophysiological function relevant to the MRS studies.

Evidence for neurophysiologic and frontal systems abnormalities in autism

Evoked potential studies in autism over the past 10 to 15 years have uniformly implicated late information processing, providing evidence of bilaterally symmetrical neurophysiological abnormalities in late, endogenous potentials thought to be related to the function of parietal and frontal cortex. Early and midlatency potentials, including the N100 and N200, have been normal. Thus, the neurophysiology of autism has been characterised by abnormalities in late endogenous components, defining autism neurophysiologically as a disorder of late information processing.

This neurophysiological profile has been replicated recently with oculomotor physiology, a method which has the added advantage of well established localisation of the parameters. Cortically controlled eye movement tasks analogous to those employed by Goldman-Rakic (1987) to investigate neocortical circuitry in non human primates have provided evidence of major alterations in the localised circuitry of dorsal prefrontal cortex and working memory in autism (Minshew et al., 1995). Impairments were indicative of neocortex as the primary source of dysfunction in the affected neural systems, and were not consistent with a subcortical origin. Studies of basic ocular motor and oculovestibular function in autism have provided evidence of intact function of subcortical pathways. Thus, eye-movement methods have provided evidence of primary dysfunction in neocortical systems with neocortex as the primary dysfunctional component.

Neuropsychological profile: evidence of a complex information processing disorder

Investigations of the neuropsychological profile in autism have provided evidence of a generalised abnormality in higher-order cognitive abilities with the exception of visuo spatial abilities. Specifically, deficits have been documented in complex abilities in the reasoning, memory, language and motor domains with preservation of simpler abilities within these same domains (Minshew et al., in press). The auditory and visual domains were equally effected. Information acquisition abilities, such as sensory perception and attention, were intact. Notable also was the sparing of information processing in the visuo spatial domain.

This pattern of deficits and intact abilities is not readily explicable in terms of a single common clinical deficit, but rather suggests that the deficits are unified at the clinical level by dependence on the processing of complex information and at the neurobiological level by dependence on a common type of dendritic architecture specialised for the analysis of the most complex information. Within this framework, neuropsychological deficits are characterised across age and autism severity in terms of high information-processing load relative to general intellectual level and task dependence on association cortex.

Structural brain abnormalities in autism: too much, too little, unconnected

Neuropathological studies in autism have reported an increase in brain weight, on the one hand, and, on the other hand, a truncation in dendritic tree development in limbic system neurons and reduced Purkinje and granule cell populations in the cerebellum (Bauman and Kemper, 1994). Volumetric MRI measurements of the brain in autism have provided evidence of an increase in the size of the supratentorial brain involving cortical grey and white matter in the occipital, parietal and temporal lobes but not the frontal lobes (Piven et al., 1995; 1996). These imaging findings are consistent with the increase in brain weight observed neuropathologically and the increased head circumference reported clinically (Bailey et al., 1993). Thus, data on brain structure in autism have provided evidence of both an increase in brain tissue involving the cerebral cortex and its white matter projections, but a decrease in the neural connections achieved with the limbic system and cerebellum. This constellation of findings suggest that there has been a disruption in the dynamics of brain development, which normally consist of successive waves of growth and selective pruning.

The pathophysiological bridge between the structural and functional alterations in neocortical systems and the histological abnormalities in limbic system and cerebellum is suggested by PET findings. Horwitz et al. (1988) reported evidence of a widespread decrease in the functional metabolic correlations of frontal and parietal cortex both intracortically with association regions as well as with limbic and subcortical structures. In a more recent study of blood flow, Zilbovicius et al. (1993) reported evidence of delayed maturation of blood flow to the frontal lobes of preschool autistic children which correlated with performance deficits on frontal lobe tasks.

This constellation of neuroanatomical findings in autism suggests that brain development is interrupted at a stage of overgrowth and underpruning of neocortex and its projections and failure of neocortex to attain normal connectivity with limbic and cerebellar structures, resulting in truncation of dendritic tree development in the limbic system and cell loss in cerebellum. The development and remodelling of neocortex is insufficient to support the emergence of brain organisation at the neural systems level. In high-functioning autistic individuals, the impact of this block in development is particularly apparent in the highest order neural systems, e.g., frontal systems.

In vivo ^{31}P MRS of frontal cortex in autism

A ^{31}P MRS study in autism was undertaken to investigate *in vivo* brain membrane phospholipid and energy metabolism in autism and its relationship to the pathophysiology (Minshew et al., 1993). Phospholipid metabolism is of obvious interest, because of the well-documented evidence of abnormalities in development of the dendritic tree of both cortical and limbic neurons. Brain bioenergetics has received relatively little attention in autism, because of the lack of evidence for primary energy failure. However, recent PET and evoked potential mapping studies in normal individuals have provided evidence that brain activation and bioenergetics also may reflect alterations in neurophysiological function. Specifically, mapping studies with cognitive evoked potentials and positron emission tomography in normal individuals have demonstrated less efficient brain function, i.e., activation of more neural circuits, with incorrect answers, decreasing IQ, and new task learning (Gevins et al., 1983, 1987, 1989; Haier et al., 1992; Squire et al., 1992), suggesting a relationship between brain bioenergetics and neurophysiological function. Such a relationship was actually suggested in autism in the first P300 studies, which concluded that the neurophysiological alterations in autism reflect the reliance by brain on less efficient, alternative neural pathways for the processing of information (Novick et al., 1979, 1980).

In our study, ^{31}P MRS of the dorsal prefrontal cortex was completed in 11 rigorously diagnosed high-functioning autistic adolescents and young adults and 11 normal control subjects individually matched on age, IQ, sex, and race, and group matched for family socioeconomic level (Minshew et al., 1993). MRS was performed using the depth pulse localization method (Minshew et al., 1993; Pettegrew et al., 1991a, 1991b, 1994). The MRS phospholipid and energy metabolite levels were then compared with indices of the severity and deficits in autism. Specifically, IQ scores (FSIQ and VIQ) and language (composite score, test of language competence) ability were used as overall indicators of relative autism severity (Venter et al., 1992). The perseverative error score from the Wisconsin card sorting test, delayed recall score from the California verbal learning test, making inferences subtest score from the test of language competence and token test score were used as indicators of the reasoning, complex memory, and higher order language deficits in autism.

Analysis of these data revealed intergroup differences for two metabolites and a consistent pattern of metabolic correlations with PME, PDE and PCr across test scores in the autistic subjects but not the controls. Decreased levels of PCr and esterified ends (aATP + aADP + dinucleotides + cytidine diphosphocholine and cytidine diphosphoethanolamine + uridine diphosphosugars) were found in the autistic group. In the absence of alterations in brain pH which would alter the kinetics of the creatine kinase enzyme, this decrease in PCr levels suggests increased utilisation of PCr to maintain ATP levels, or a hypermetabolic state. The esterified-ends resonance region contains contributions related to bioenergetics, lipid and protein glycosylation, and membrane biosynthesis. In the absence of alterations in the other resonances to which ATP and ADP contribute, the reduction in the esterified ends resonance is more likely to be related to alterations in membrane biosynthesis rather than to bioenergetics. The most significant findings of the study, however, pertained to the pattern of clinico-metabolic correlations. In the autistic group, there was a consistent pattern of significant correlations between PME (phosphomonoesters, membrane building blocks), PDE (phosphodiesters, membrane degradation products), and PCr levels across all clinical parameters. Specifically, as performance on these instruments declined in the autistic subjects, PCr and PME levels fell and PDE levels rose (Table 2, fig. 12A-E). This pattern of correlations was not present in the control group. In addition, no significant clinico metabolic correlations were found with age in either subject group or with IQ in the control group, suggesting that these findings were not the consequence of age or IQ effects.

The positive correlation between falling PCr levels and declining test performance in autism is consistent with a hypermetabolic state. It is noteworthy that the cognitive evoked potential abnormalities in autism have been most prominent in frontal cortex in autistic subjects with comparable age, IQ and sex to the declining subjects in this study. In view of the PET and cognitive evoked potential mapping data in normal individuals suggesting increasing activation of neural circuitry with declining performance, it is possible that the hypermetabolic state demonstrated in this study is a reflection of the neurophysiological abnormalities documented in autism.

The phospholipid correlations (¯PME–PDE) in the autistic subjects with declining test performance are consistent with undersynthesis and enhanced degradation of brain membranes. This clinico-metabolic pattern in the frontal cortex of these high functioning autistic subjects is furthermore consistent with the predominance of neuropsychologic findings related to frontal lobe dysfunction in these individuals, the truncation in dendritic tree development in limbic structures with extensive frontal connections, and the postero anterior maturation of cortex during

Table 2
Significant clinical-metabolic correlations

		PCr		PME		PDE	
		Autistic	Control	Autistic	Control	Autistic	Control
Full Scale IQ	*(r)*	0.92	−0.31	0.44	0.22	−0.76	−0.11
	(p)	0.0001	NS	NS	NS	0.01	NS
Verbal IQ	*(r)*	0.81	−0.26	0.70	0.40	−0.82	0.14
	(p)	0.002	NS	0.02	NS	0.002	NS
WCST	*(r)*	−0.83	−0.18	−0.24	0.14	−0.81	−0.13
	(p)	0.01	NS	NS	NS	0.01	NS
CVLT	*(r)*	0.79	−0.33	0.33	0.02	−0.65	−0.04
Delayed free recall	*(p)*	0.004	NS	NS	NS	0.03	NS
Token test	*(r)*	0.49	0.31	0.79	0.33	0.75	0.58
	(p)	NS	NS	0.003	NS	0.008	NS
TOLC	*(r)*	0.35	−0.09	−0.65	0.27	0.57	0.00
composite	*(p)*	NS	NS	0.03	NS	NS	NS

WCST Wisconsin Card Sort; *CVLT* California Verbal Learning Test; *TOLC* Test of Language Competence

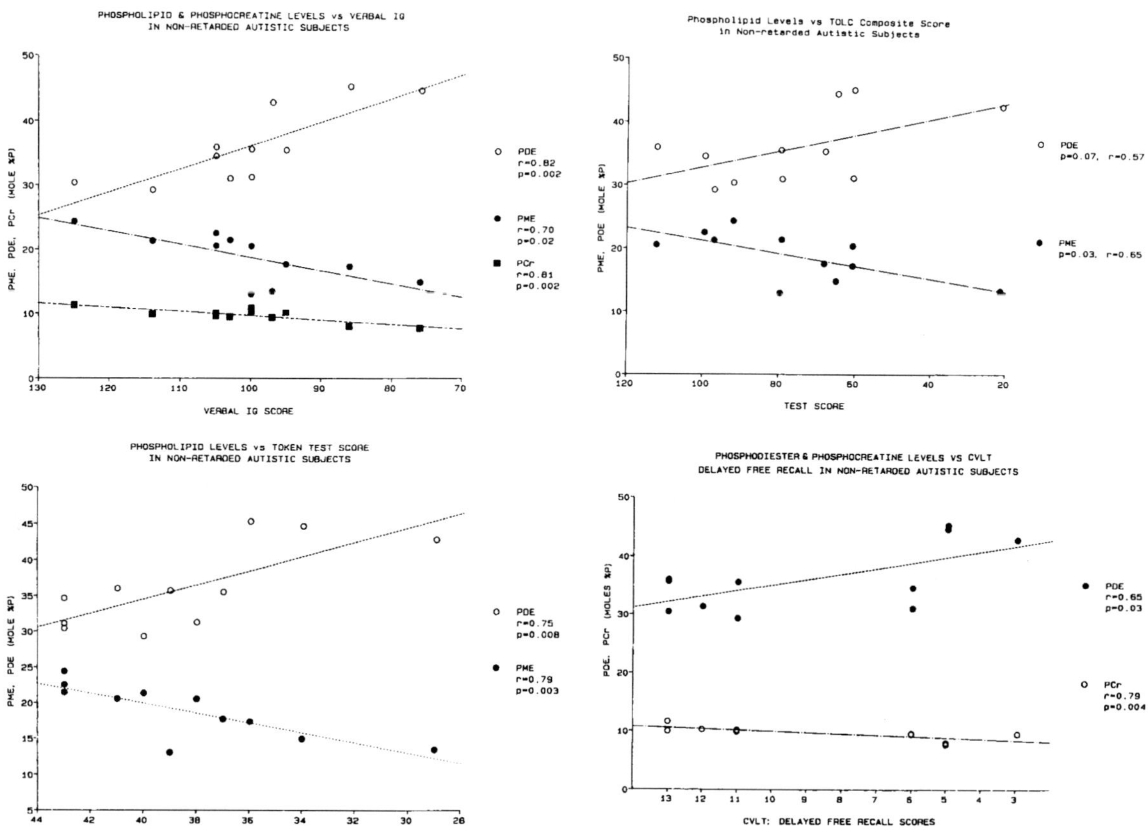

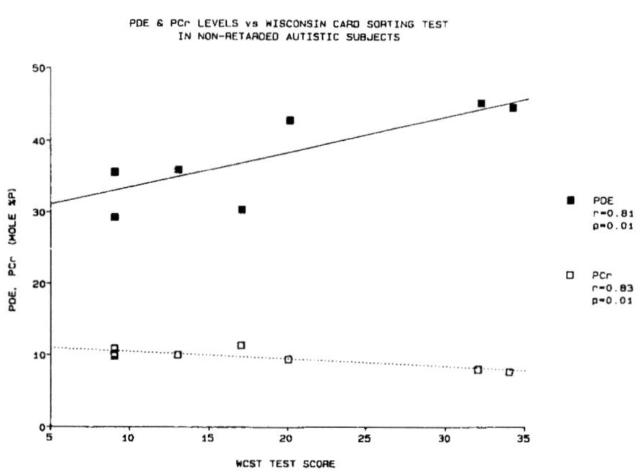

Fig. 12. Correlations between frontal cortex levels of phosphomonoesters (PME), phosphodiesters (PDE), and phosphocreatine (PCr) determined by *in vivo* ^{31}P MRS and subject: a) Verbal IQ score; b) composite score from the test of language competence; c) Token test score; d) delayed free recall score from the California verbal learning test; and d) perseverative error score from the Wisconsin card sorting test. Reproduced from *Biological Psychiatry*, 1993.

development, which would leave frontal lobe and higher order processing systems most vulnerable to developmental pathology. The presence of evidence for enhanced degradation or turnover of brain membranes in autism has additional clinical significance, in that approximately one-third of autistic children present with regression and loss of previously acquired milestones and a minority of older autistic children experience a significant regression in later life. Consistent with MRS evidence of increased brain membrane turnover, Ahlsen et al. (1993) recently reported increased CSF ganglioside levels in autistic and autistic-like children. As gangliosides are considered synaptic markers, an increase in their levels suggests increased turnover of synaptic membranes in autism. They also found a three fold increase in glial fibrillary acidic protein (GAP) in the CSF in autism. In the absence of gliosis (Bauman and Kemper 1985; Bauman 1991), the increase in GAP levels also may reflect increased turnover of synaptic membranes, since all synapses are insulated with astrocytic processes.

In summary, this pilot study provides preliminary evidence of alterations in brain energy and phospholipid metabolism that correlate with clinical deficits in autism. These findings are consistent with a hypermetabolic energy state and undersynthesis and enhanced degradation of brain membranes, and may relate to the neurophysiologic and neuropathologic abnormalities in autism.

Metabolic correlations in autism as a function of information-processing load

To investigate the potential validity of the complex information processing model of this clinical syndrome, a comparison was made between the brain membrane metabolite levels (PME, PDE) and neuropsychological variables with high or low demands for on-line information processing for subjects of this age and IQ level. A recent analysis of data from 8 autistic subjects investigated the dissociation between high and low information processing load tasks on a neuropsychological battery in relation to MRS phospholipid metabolites. As previously discussed, neuropsychological data in 85 high-functioning autistic and 65 matched normal control subjects revealed a dissociation between complex and simple tasks with a generalised pattern of deficits in complex cognitive abilities across domains and sensory modalities and intact or superior performance on simpler tasks in the same domains. To further explore the significance of this neuropsychological dissociation in relation to the pathophysiology of autism, we defined two sets of variables,- one reflecting high and the second low information processing demand relative to general level of intellectual function. High information processing load variables included: perseverative error score from the Wisconsin card sorting test; total number of moves and total number of problems solved from the Tower of Hanoi; logical memory score from the Weschler memory scale; delayed recall score for the Rey-Osterrieth figure; and making Inferences subtest score from the test of language competence. Low information-processing load variables were chosen to reflect simpler, more automatic skills in these same functional domains. These variables included: Trails A score; total error score from the letter cancellation test; and the reading decoding and spelling scores from the Kaufman test of educational achievement. The correlations between scores on these instruments and PME and PDE levels in the frontal lobes of these subjects are given in Table 3.

Preliminary analyses of these clinico metabolic correlations revealed significant and consistent correlations with PME and PDE for the high information processing load variables, but also equal and opposite correlations with the low information processing variables. In this slightly younger group of autistic subjects, PME and PDE levels increased with increasing severity of the deficits, suggesting increasing production and also turnover of brain membranes. This pattern is consistent with the increases in head circumference, and grey and white matter on MRI on the one hand, brain weight at autopsy, and the CSF evidence of increased turnover of synaptic membranes. The relationship between performance on low information processing load variables and the PME-PDE levels is in the opposite direction of the PME-PDE correlations with the high information processing load variables. This inverse relationship of high and low information-processing variables to PME-PDE levels mirrors what is observed clinically, which is a trade-off with developmental progress between the loss of excellence in savant type simple skills, such as hyperlexia or incidental memory for details, and small gains in language comprehension and reasoning. We have speculated that this trade-off reflects a neurobiological relationship during information processing in which a "figure-ground transformation" of incoming environmental stimuli normally results in the emergence of a concept by

Table 3
Neuropsychologic al correlations with PME and PDE levels

High information-processing load variables	**Neuropsychological Test Score Format**[a]	**PME**[b]	**PDE**[c]
Wisconsin Card Sorting Test, perseverative errors	↓	.69	.47
Tower of Hanoi: total nummber of moves	↓	.81	.49
Tower of Hanoi: total number solved	↑	-.87	-.45
Test of Language Competence, making inferences	↑	-.41	-.40
WMS-R, Logical Memory [story recall]	↑	-.42	-.06
Rey-Osterrieth Figure, delayed recall	↑	-.42	.12
Low information-processing load variables			
Trails A, seconds	↓	-.03	.10
Letter cancellation, errors	↓	-.02	.16
K-TEA: Reading decoding	↑	.53	-.26
K-TEA: Spelling	↑	.49	.06
WMS-R, Visual reproduction	↑	.44	-.28

[a] ↓ higher scores are associated with poorer performance; ↑ higher scores reflect better performance
[b] PME (phosphomonoesters) are the synthetic building blocks for brain membranes
[c] PDE (phosphodiesters) are the membrane degradation products

suppressing some details. In autism, we suggest that abnormal information processing disturbs the "figure-ground" process, leaving these individuals with both an unusual clarity of memory for details and at the same time a poverty of concepts.

Summary

The initial studies presented in this chapter demonstrate the potential of ^{31}P MRS for monitoring *in vivo* neuronal membrane organisation events and energy metabolism during normal brain development, maturation, and aging, and for detecting pathological states involving alterations in these metabolic profiles. MRS also may capture the metabolic consequences of neurophysiological alterations involving neural circuitry.

Acknowledgements. The careful and dedicated technical assistance of Evelyn J. Herbert is acknowledged and appreciated. This work was supported by NINDS grant NS33355 to Nancy J. Minshew.

References

Ackerman JJ, Grove TH, Wong GG (1980) Mapping of metabolites in whole animals by 31P NMR using surface coils. Nature 283: 167-170

Ahlsen G, Rosengren L, Belfrage M (1993) Glial fibrillary acidic protein in the cerebrospinal fluid of children with autism and other neuropsychiatric disorders. Biol Psychiat 33: 734-743

Bailey A, Luthert P, Bolton P, LeCouteur A, Rutter M (1993) Autism and megalencephaly. Lancet 34: 1225-1226

Bauman ML (1991) Microscopic neuroanatomic abnormalities in autism. Supplement to Pediatrics 87(5): 791-796

Bauman M L, Kemper T L (1994) Neuroanatomic observations of the brain in autism. In: Bauman ML, Kemper TL (eds) The Neurobiology of Autism. Johns Hopkins Press,Baltimore, p 119-145

Bauman ML, Kemper TL (1985). Histoanatomic observations of the brain in early infantile autism. Neurology 35: 866-874

Bolinger L, Le nkinski RE (1992) Localization in clinical NMR spectroscopy. In: Berliner LJ, Reuben J (eds) Biological Magnetic Resonance 11 In vivo spectroscopy. Plenum Press,New York, p 1-53

Bottomley PA, Cousins JP, Pendrey DL (1992) Alzheimer dementia: Quantification of energy metabolism and mobile phosphoesters with P-31 NMR spectroscopy. Radiology 183: 695-699

Bottomley PA, Charles HC, Roemer PB, Flamig D, Engeseth H, Edelstein WA, Mueller OM (1988) Human *in vivo* phosphate metabolite imaging with ^{31}P NMR. Magn Reson Med 7: 319-336

Buchli R, Martin E, Boesiger P, Rumpel H (1994) Developmental changes of phosphorus metabolite concentrations in the human brain: A ^{31}P magnetic resonance spectroscopy study *in vivo*. Pediatr Res 35: 431-435

Carlsson A (1988) The current status of the dopamine hypothesis of schizophrenia. Neuropsychopharmacology 1: 179-186

Clarke PG (1985). Neuronal death in the development of the vertebrate nervous system. Trends Neurosci 8: 345-349

Cowan WM, Fawcett JW, OLeary DDl (1984) Regressive events in neurogenesis. Science 225: 1258-1265

Frahm J, Bruhn H, Gyngell ML, Merboldt KD, Hanicke W, Sauter R (1989) Localized proton NMR spectroscopy in different regions of the human brain *in vivo*. Relaxation times and concentrations of cerebral metabolites. Magn Reson Med 11: 47-63

Gevins AS, Schaffer RE, Doyle JC (1983) Shadows of thought: Shifting lateralization of human brain electrical patterns during brief visuomotor task. Science 220: 97-99

Gevins AS, Morgan NH, Bressler SL (1987) Human neuroelectric patterns predict performance accuracy. Science 235: 580-585

Gevins AS, Cutillo BA, Bressler SL (1989) Event-related covariances during a bimanual visuomotor task. II. Preparation and feedback. Electroencephalogr Clin Neurophysiol 74: 147-160

Glonek T, Kopp SJ, Kot E, Pettegrew JW (1982) P-31 nuclear magnetic resonance analysis of brain: The perchloric acid extract spectrum. J Neurochem 39: 1210-19

Goldman-Rakic PS (1987) Development of cortical circuitry and cognitive function. Child Dev 58: 601-622.

Gruetter R, Rothman DL, Novotny EJ, Shulman RG (1992) Localized ^{13}C NMR spectroscopy of myo-inositol in the human brain *in vivo*. Magn Reson Med 25: 204-210

Haier RJ, Siegel BV, MacLachlan (1992) Regional glucose metabolic changes after learning a complex visuospatial/motor task: A positron emission tomographic study. Brain Res 570: 134-143

Horwitz B, Rumsey JM, Grady CL, Rapoport SI (1988) The cerebral metabolic landscape in autism: Intercorrelations of regional glucose utilization. Arch Neurol 45: 749-755

Huttenlocher PR (1975) Synaptic and dendritic development and mental defect. In: Buchwald NA, Brazier MAB (eds). Brain Mechanisms in Mental Retardation. Academic Press, New York, p 129

Kilby PM, Bolas NM, Radda GK. (1991) 31P-NMR study of brain phospholipid structures in vivo. Biochem Biophys Acta 1085: 257-264

Klausner JD, Sweeney JP, Deck MD (1992) Clinical correlates of cerebral ventricular enlargement in schizophrenia. J Nerv Ment Dis 180:407

Klunk WE, Xu CJ, Panchalingam K (1994) Analysis of magnetic resonance spectra by mole percent: Comparison to absolute units. Neurobiol Aging 15: 133-140

Lim KO, Pauly J, Webb P (1994) Short TE phosphorus spectroscopy using a spin-echo pulse. Magn Reson Med 32: 98-103

McClure RJ, Panchalingam K, Klunk WE, Pettegrew JW (1996) Magnetic resonance spectroscopy of neural tissue. Meth Neurosci 30: 178-208
McIlwain H, Bachelard HS (1985) Biochemistry and the central nervous system, (5th ed.) Churchill Livingstone-,New York, p.41-43
Minshew NJ, Pettegrew JW (1996) Nuclear magnetic resonance spectroscopic studies of cortical development. In: Thatcher RW, Lyon GR, Rumsey J, Krasnegor N (eds) Developmental Neuroimaging: Mapping the Development of Brain and Behavior. Academic Press,San Diego, p 107-125
Minshew NJ, Goldstein G, Siegel DJ (in press) Neuropsychologic functioning in autism: Profile of a complex information processing disorder. J Int Neuropsychol Soc
Minshew NJ, Sweeney JA, Furman JM (1995) Evidence for a primary neocortical system abnormality in autism. Soc Neurosci Abs 21: 735
Minshew NJ, Goldstein G, Dombrowski SM (1993) A preliminary ^{31}P MRS study of autism: Evidence for undersynthesis and increased degradation of brain membranes. Biol Psychiat 33: 762-773
Murphy DGM, Bottomley PA, Salerno J (1992) In vivo brain glucose and phosphorus metabolism in Alzheimer's disease (abstract). Soc Neurosci 18: 567
Novick B, Kurtzberg D, Vaughn HG Jr (1979) An electrophysiologic indication of defective information storage in childhood autism. Psychiat Res 1: 101-108
Novick B, Kurtzberg D, Vaughn HG Jr (1980) An electrophysiologic indication of auditory processing defects in autism. Psychiat Res 3: 107-114
Oppenheim RW (1985) Naturally occurring cell death during neural development. Trends Neurosci 8: 487-493
Petroff OAC, Prichard JW, Behar KL (1985) Cerebral intracellular pH by ^{31}P nuclear magnetic resonance spectroscopy. Neurology 35: 781-788
Pettegrew JW, Minshew NJ, Cohen MM (1984) P-31 NMR changes in Alzheimer's and Huntington's disease brain (abstract). Neurology 34(Suppl 1): 281
Pettegrew JW, Withers G, Panchalingam K (1988) Considerations for Brain pH assessment by ^{31}P NMR. Magn Res Imag 6: 135-142
Pettegrew JW, Panchalingam K, Wither G (1990) Changes in brain energy and phospholipid metabolism during development and aging in the Fischer 344 rat. J Neuropath Exp Neurol 49: 237-249
Pettegrew JW, Keshavan MS, Panchalingam K (1991a) Alterations in brain high-energy phosphate and membrane phospholipid metabolism in first-episode, drug-naive schizophrenics. Arch Gen Psychiat 48: 563-568
Pettegrew JW, Klunk WE, McClure K (1991b) Phosphomonoesters, phospholipids and high-energy phosphates in Alzheimer's disease: Alterations and physiological significance. In: Khachaturian ZS, Blass JP (eds) Alzheimer's Disease: New Treatment Strategies. Marcel Dekker Inc,New York, p 193-212
Pettegrew JW, Panchalingam K, Klunk WE (1994) Alterations of cerebral metabolism in probable Alzheimer's disease; A preliminary study. Neurobiol Aging 15: 117-132
Pittman R, Oppenheim RW (1979) Cell death of motoneurons in the chick embryo spinal cord. IV. Evidence that a functional neuromuscular interaction is involved in the regulation of naturally occurring cell death and the stabilization of synapses. J Comp Neurol 187: 425-446
Piven J, Arndt S, Bailey J, Andreasen N (1996) Regional brain enlargement in autism: A magnetic resonance imaging study. J Am Acad Child Psychiat 35: 1-7
Piven J, Arndt S, Bailey J, Havercamp S, Andreasen NC, Palmer P (1995) An MRI study of brain size in autism. Am J Psychiat 152: 1145-1149
Purpura DP (1979) Pathobiology of cortical neurons in metabolic and unclassified amentias. In: Katzman R (ed) Congneital and Acquired Cognitive Disorders. Raven Press, New York, p 43-68
Sappy-Marinier D, Calabrese G, Hetherington HP, Fisher SN, Deicken R, Van Dyke C, Fein G, Weiner MW (1992) Proton magnetic resonance spectroscopy of human brain: Applications to normal white matter, chronic infarction, and MRI white matter signal hyperintensities. Magn Reson Med 26: 313-327
Siesjo B (1978) Brain energy metabolism. In: Siesjo B (ed) Brain energy metabolism (Chapter 1 and 2). John Wiley and Sons,New York
Silverstein RM, Bassler GC, Morrill TC (1991) Spectrometric Identification of Organic Compounds. Wiley, New York
Squire LR, Ojemann JG, Miezin FM (1992) Activation of the hippocampus in normal humans: A functional anatomical study of memory. Proc Natl Acad Sci 89: 1837-1841
Vance DE (1991) Phospholipid metabolism and cell signalling in eucaryotes. In: Vance DE, Vance J (eds) Biochemistry of lipids, lipoproteins and membranes, Volume 20. Elsevier, New York, p 205-240
Venter A, Lord C, Schopler E (1992) A follow-up study of high-functioning autistic children. J Child Psychol Psychiat 3: 489-507
Volpe JJ (1995) Neuronal proliferation, migration, organization, and myelination. In: Neurology of the Newborn, 3rd ed, Saunders WB:Philadelphia, p 43-92.
Zilbovicius M, Garreau B, Samson Y, Remy P, Barthelemy C, Syrota A, Lelord G (1995) Delayed maturation of frontal cortex in childhood autism. Am J Psychiat 152: 248-252

8. EEG investigations in autistic children

S. COCHIN, J. MARTINEAU

For the past three decades, the search for the locus of brain dysfunction in autism has been the focus of great attention and effort. But the neurobiological substrate of infantile autism is still unknown, as is its a etiology. In the 20 years following Kanner's original description (1943), research focussed on psychogenic explanations of autism, even though Kanner initially concluded that autism was probably due to a biological disorder. It was not until Rimland (1964) presented the first neurobiological explanation of autism, and a review of evidence from twins studies, that research began to focus on the biology of autism. It is now clear that autism is a condition with many varied manifestations and that change with age. In recent years, new methods for studying human brain-behaviour relationships have been developed. Extraction of anatomical and functional brain indices from the intact human head can be performed via CT, MRI, PET and SPECT images. These technical innovations constitute unique, valuable windows on brain development. Each of these brain-imaging techniques has its own research applications involving children and infants. Parallel technological advances in electroencephalography have led to the new field of quantitative EEG (qEEG) which can provide a readily available, reasonably inexpensive, and completely noninvasive probe of brain function. The goal of this chapter is to describe qEEG technology, the main research findings in autism and one of the first applications of qEEG technology in autistic children exploring the function of imitation.

From EEG to quantitative EEG (qEEG)

More than 60 years ago, Hans Berger (1929) reported the first recordings of electrical activity from the human brain, and interest this organ and its electrical activity continues to grow. We persist in our attempts to decipher the code of electrical activity produced by the brain and continue to use this information to guide our understanding of behavioural characteristics and aspects of cognitive function. The limitations of this understanding have remained much the same as they were in Berger's time; advances mainly parallel the development of instrumentation, the accumulated knowledge base, and current conceptual orientation. The EEG changes during various mental activities in man have been the subject of many investigations since the beginning of EEG research. During visual examination of the EEG, most attention has been directed to changes in the alpha and beta ranges. "Blocking" (Adrian and Matthews, 1934) and "attenuation" (Knott, 1938) of alpha activity, and topographical (Jung, 1939) and interindividual (Ruf and Vattuone, 1943) differences in these changes have been reported during cognitive tasks. These changes have often been found in combination with increased fast activity.

Interpretations of classic EEG data have traditionally relied on visual estimates of spectral content. Amounts of activity in the delta (0-3 Hz), theta (4-7 Hz), alpha (8-12 Hz) and beta (above 12 Hz) spectral bands are typically used to generate clinical opinions.

Although all frequencies can be seen in all subjects or patients, delta and theta "slow activity" predominates in regions overlying pathology. Similarly, alpha and especially beta "fast activity" may be deficient in regions overlying pathology. Research applications of EEG include description and localisation of electrophysiological abnormality in patients and localisation of patterns of regional activation in normal subjects in response to specific tasks.

Over the past decade, parallel technological advances in electroencephalography have led to the new field of "quantitative EEG". The quantitative EEG can be traced retrospectively through the entire history of EEG research and development. Three years after Berger's discovery of the human EEG, Dietsch (1932) applied Fourier analysis to it. Later, Gibbs (1937) and Grass and Gibbs (1938) applied the Fourier transform to the analysis of the EEG. From 1961 to 1963, Adey, Walter and their associates (Adey et al., 1961; Walter, 1963; Walter and Adey, 1963) applied Fourier analysis based on fast Fourier transform (FFT) and phase analysis to EEG signals. This was the starting point of computerised spectral analysis.

The field of quantitative EEG is also known as "quantified neurophysiology" or "neurometrics". The method consists of calculating spectral power in each frequency band of the standard EEG recording. In qEEG, the "EEG" refers to classic electroencephalography. Indeed, the same types of scalp electrodes are used for both qEEG and EEG. The "q" refers to quantification; quantification of the EEG is realised by spectral analysis thanks to a computational algorithm such as the FFT (Cooley and Tukey, 1965). Although the mechanism is complex, the results are easy to appreciate. Indeed, EEG spectral analysis by FFT results in a histogram of spectral content, and values across chosen spectral frequencies can be summed to provide estimates of classic delta, theta, alpha and beta bands.

In qEEG many investigators use energy spectra, since the classic EEG is traditionally analysed in the microvolt domain. Once spectra are formed, many workers recalculate spectral values. Outputs from the FFT calculation are referred to as "absolute" or "relative spectra". Relative power is the amount in all bands, while absolute power is the amount of EEG in one band without reference to other bands.

Different features of the spontaneous EEG can then be displayed topographically in the form of a map. Bechtereva et al. (1963) localised focal brain lesions by EEG studies, anticipating EEG cartographic representation. This pioneering research was followed by a growing number of findings and new analyses (Etevenon, 1985). EEG cartography started with the article by Lehmann (1971) on multichannel topography of human alpha EEG fields. This described a common technique of displaying results of quantified analyses as black and white or colour topographical maps. "Mapping" can demonstrate the distribution of absolute or relative spectral values over the scalp, in each spectral band (delta, theta, alpha and beta). After spectral analysis is performed, background EEG magnitude is determined by summation across the different frequency bands, resulting in a single number at each electrode site. Data are interpolated, contour lines drawn, and regions filled in with colour. Unusual regions of changes in frequency band can then readily be recognised. Classic EEG analysis by unassisted visual inspection typically involves estimation of background frequency content over a desired time span and across the scalp. The interpolation process which precedes mapping does not create new information; it simply displays data so as to make their information content more visible in the spatial domain. Several methods are used for interpolation. Buchsbaum et al. (1982) and Duffy et al. (1981) applied quadrilateral and triangular interpolation. However, such interpolation seems unlikely to represent the true scalp field. Etevenon et al. (1985) chose to use a nonlinear interpolation algorithm (using a quadrilateral polygon). This subtle computational process may be important when computed EEG maps are used as aids to diagnosis in neurosurgery or neurology.

The study of the quantitative EEG during task performance is based on the hypothesis that specific engagement of cortical areas should be reflected by localised changes in background EEG and thus be detected by significant changes in qEEG data. It is to be expected that group studies could show common patterns of EEG activation, although qEEG data and task performance involve many sources of intra and interindividual variability. It is also to be anticipated that the resulting patterns would be closely related to the classical models of neuropsychology, especially for lateralised cortical functions. Various reports were published as techniques became more sophisticated. On the one hand, special care was taken to carrying out and controling very selective tasks (Autret et al., 1985; Gevins et al., 1979), and on the other hand, data analysis was extended to large numbers of leads and spectral parameters, resulting in more precise topographical and spectral display of the patterns (Duffy et al., 1981; Pfurtscheller, 1986, 1988).

EEG research findings in autism

The frequency of EEG abnormalities reported in autistic children ranges from 10 % (White et al., 1964) to 31 % (Guillemet et al., 1997), 47 % (DeLong, 1978), 60 % (DeMyer et al., 1973) and even 83 % (Creak and Pampiglione, 1969), with an average of 52 % (DeMyer et al., 1981). Such variability is due to both clinical and technical factors. From the clinical point of view, studies of autistic children group together various conditions, including autism, schizophrenia and psychosis. The outstanding study of Small in 1975, which refers to the nosological criteria of DeMyer et al. (1973), offered a classification including different clinical groups such as infantile autism. Furthermore, peri- and postnatal antecedents or neurological signs are not detailed. Technical factors include the difficulties in obtaining EEG data from these children; this can at least in part explain the varied results. Workers who obtained two or more EEGs in autistic children found EEG abnormalities in 60 % - 80 % (Hutt et al., 1965; Small et al., 1969) while those who recorded only one EEG have found a lower frequency. Despite this variability, significantly more EEG abnormalities were found in autistic children than in normals. However, there are no EEG abnormalities unique to this disorder and there is minimal evidence concerning localisation of any abnormalities, most commonly they are diffusely distributed. We can divide the abnormalities into two main groups: abnormal EEG recordings when the subject is at rest (standard EEG) and those obtained when the subject is stimulated.

Abnormalities in the EEG at rest

White et al. (1964) reported prominent spike and/or spike and wave abnormalities in autistic individuals. Small (1975) found that regional and/or generalised spike and/or spike and wave paroxysms represented 64 % of EEG abnormalities in autistics; thus was confirmed by Barthelemy et al. (1983). Since 1943, an association between autism and epileptic seizures has been observed by many groups (Gillberg, 1991; Gillberg et al., 1983, 1987; Kanner, 1943; Rutter, 1970; Tuchman et al., 1991). In the literature the prevalence of epilepsy in autism has ranged from 4 to 32 %, levels generally higher than in children as a whole (0.5 %). In a recent study, Rossi et al. (1995) examined 106 autistic patients divided into three groups on the basis of the presence or absence of paroxysmal EEG abnormalities and/or epilepsy. The prevalence of epilepsy and paroxysmal EEG abnormalities was 23.6 %. One significant difference between the three groups was in EEG fast activity; other abnormalities involved rhythms. In traditional EEG studies, Hermelin and O'Connor (1970) reported high mean alpha frequencies; apart from Stevens and Milstein (1970) who described autistic children as "hypermature", with unusually persistent alpha rhythms, most workers noted a predominance of either rapid or slow rhythms. For example, Hutt et al. (1965) and Fish and Shapiro (1965) observed numerous slow rhythms, delta or theta of great magnitude, with fast, low voltage activity, but no alpha rhythm. Kolvin et al. (1971) found that 27 % of their autistic subjects showed a low voltage EEG, they thought this suggestive of hyperactivity or over-arousal. Hutt et al. (1965) observed a relationship between the frequency of low voltage, fast rhythms and frequency of stereotyped actions. Gibbs and Gibbs (1973) compared some EEG abnormalities and the developmental level of language.

Applying a computerised EEG technique to low-functioning children with autism, Cantor et al. (1986) demonstrated that they resembled 2 year old toddlers in their EEG measures. Like the toddlers, autistic children have significantly higher percent delta and less alpha activity in all regions than age-matched normals or age-matched mentally handicapped children. Autistic children also look like toddlers in having greater coherence and less asymmetry of amplitude.

Two recent studies reported that the EEG of autistic children, recorded in the rest condition, shows a decrease in spectral power in alpha 1 (7.5-9 Hz) and alpha 2 (9.5-11 Hz) rhythms all over the cortex, although a spectral power increase is observed in delta (1.5-3.5 Hz), alpha 3 (11.5-13 Hz) and beta (13.5-20 Hz) frequency bands in frontal, central and temporal regions (Bashina et al., 1994; Gorvachevskaia et al., 1992).

In recent work, Garreau (1994) recorded from 17 autistic children (mean age 7 years, mean DQ 44) and 17 normal children (mean age 7 years 1 month) and studied the resting qEEG. He showed smaller spectral power in the alpha band in the autistic children than in the normals (Fig 1), statistically significant on frontal (F3, F4, F7, F8, Fz), temporal (T3, T4, T5, T6), central (C3, C4), parietal (Pz) and occipital leads (O1, o2). Lower spectral power was also found in autistic children in the beta1 band for Fz, C3, Pz, O1, O2 and in the beta2 band for C3, C4 and Pz. These results have been interpreted as showing a deficit in synchronisation of alpha generators, provoking functional cortical dissociation in autism.

Other studies dealing with EEG findings and autism showed no particular EEG pattern. In 1969, Creak and Pampiglione reported that 29 of their 35 subjects showed EEG abnormalities without uniformity, distribution or severity of type. Gubbay et al. (1970) found 65 % EEG abnormalities with no particular pattern. Furthermore, Ritvo et al. (1970) reported that 35 % of abnormal EEG findings have no relationship with the clinical diagnosis. In 1982, Tsai et al. studied the correlation between handedness and EEG findings in 40 autistic patients aged from 4 to 12 years. They found that of 43 % of right-handed subjects, 35 % had an abnormal EEG with a pattern of diffuse or focal spikes, slow waves, or paroxysms of spike and wave; 43 % of the non-right-handed children had an abnormal EEG. Thus, they found no EEG pattern unique to autism. The findings of bilateral abnormalities in all autistic children who had an abnormal EEG adds weight to the idea that the autistic syndrome results from dysfunction in both sides of the brain (Cohen et al., 1976; Damasio and Maurer, 1978; DeLong et al., 1981). Furthermore, this study showed no relationship between handedness and the EEG patterns.

Another study (Dawson et al., 1995) showed that, compared to normally developing children, autistic subjects had reduced EEG power in the frontal and

Fig. 1
Grand averages of topographical mapping of spectral power of EEG bands for 17 normal (left) and 17 autistic children (right). Significant differences between the two groups in spectral power in the alpha band are observed for all leads (from Garreau, 1994). *See colour illustrations appendix.*

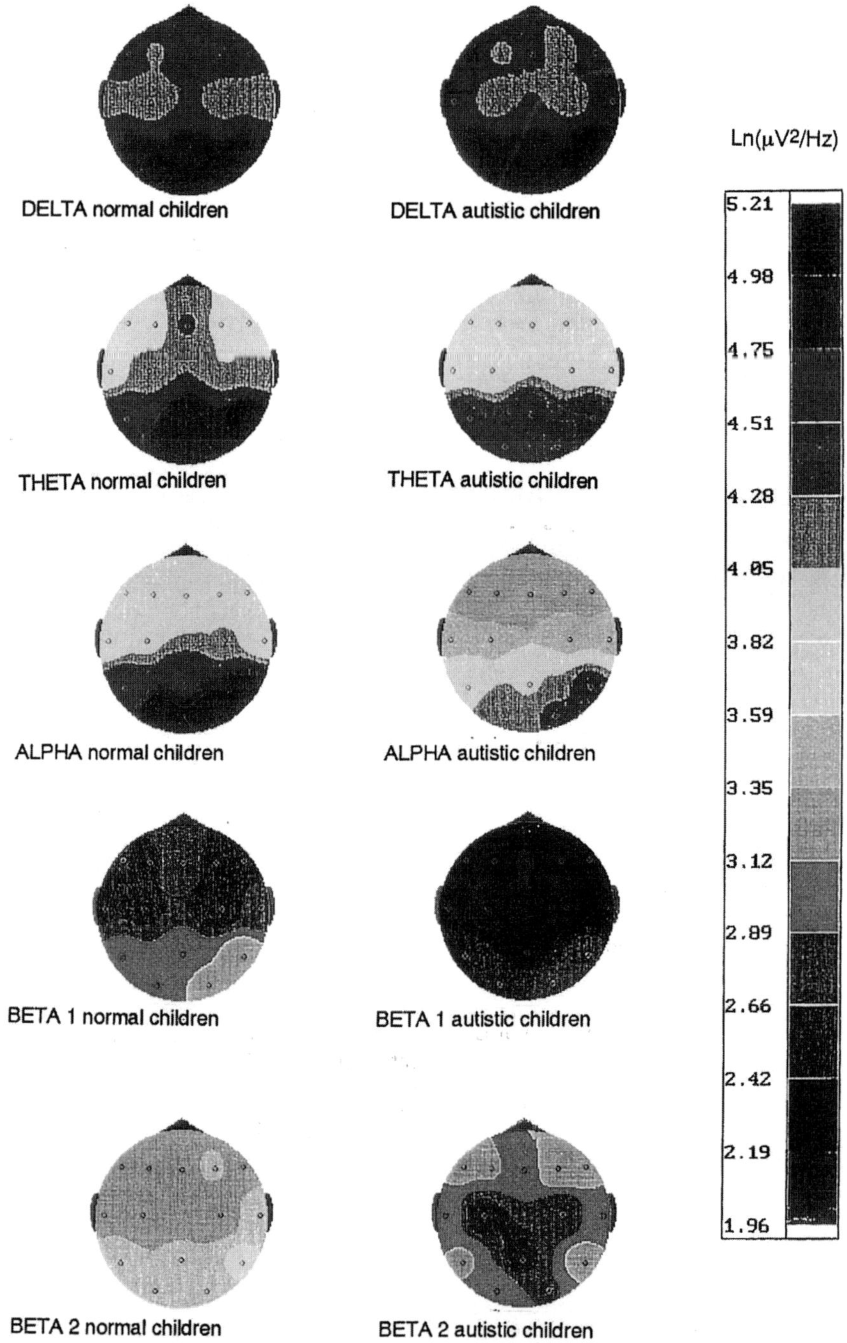

temporal regions, but not in the parietal region. Differences were more prominent in the left hemisphere than the right. Furthermore, subgroups of autistic children based on Wing and Gould's system displayed distinct patterns of brain activity. Compared to autistic children classified as "active-but-odd", "passive" autistic children displayed reduced alpha EEG power in the frontal region.

EEG and asymmetrical hemisphere impairment during stimulation tasks

The most consistent finding to emerge from previous EEG studies is a pattern of reduced or reversed hemisphere asymmetry (Dawson et al., 1982; 1995; Small, 1975). In all cases in which hemisphere differences were found, autistic children showed significantly reduced EEG power in the left hemisphere but not in the right.

A variety of data indicates that in normal development of brain specialisation, the two hemispheres are functionally and anatomically asymmetrical at birth (Best et al., 1982; Glanville et al., 1977; Molfese and Molfese, 1979). Current views on the development of brain lateralisation hold that, although increasing specialisation of the hemispheres occurs as an individual acquires functional capabilities, the propensity for certain functions to be lateralised to the right or left hemisphere is probably present at birth and does not change with age (Witelson, 1977). Thus, the failure of autistic children to exhibit normal patterns of functional brain lateralisation cannot easily be attributed to a simple delay in the development of hemisphere specialisation. Rather, autistic individuals appear to be exhibiting a deviant pattern of brain activity and development. Autism could result from a disorder of hemisphere lateralisation, the neural substrates in the left hemisphere necessary for sequential forms of information processing failing to develop (Prior and Bradshaw, 1979; Tanguay, 1977).

Quantitative EEG studies indicate an abnormal pattern of hemisphere lateralisation, during both wakefulness, without and with tasks, and sleep. Small (1975) suggested that a failure of cerebral lateralisation might underlie the autistic syndrome. She found that normal children have higher EEG voltages over the left hemisphere than over the right during a standard EEG, whereas children with autism do not show this hemispheric difference. Ogawa et al. (1982) studied the EEG during stage 2 sleep in right handed autistic children and in normal children in the same age range. There was significant hemisphere lateralisation in the EEG of normal children but not in the autistics, supporting Small's thesis. They found that during click stimulation, 42 % of normal children but no autistic children showed significant hemisphere asymmetry. During flash stimulation, 64 % of normal subjects showed hemisphere asymmetry, only 28 % of autistic children did so. In normal children, Garreau (1994) showed that auditory stimulations (tone-bursts 750 Hz, 80dB) increased spectral power in the delta band and decreased it in the theta, alpha and beta bands in both hemispheres. These auditory stimulations did not modify the qEEG in autistic children (Fig. 2).

An electrophysiological technique commonly used to study hemisphere lateralisation is the alpha blocking method. This involves the measurement of EEG activity during various cognitive tasks. Differential

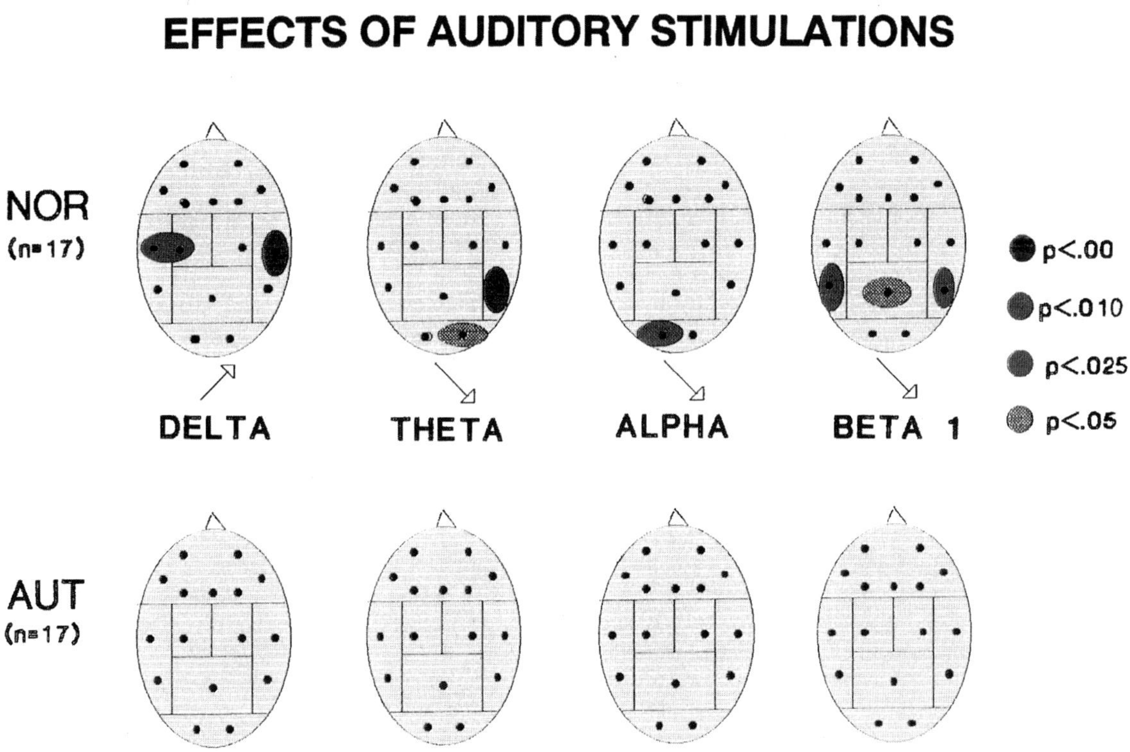

Fig. 2. Effects of auditory stimulation on the qEEG. In normal children, auditory stimulation increased spectral power in the delta band and decreased it in the theta, alpha and beta bands in both hemispheres. No such change was observed in autistic children (from Garreau, 1994). *See colour illustrations appendix.*

attenuation of EEG in the 8 to 12 Hz frequency band (alpha) is used to infer localised brain activity (Butler and Glass, 1974; Doyle et al., 1974). The alpha-blocking method, used in two main studies (Dawson et al., 1982, 1983), showed that a higher than normal percentage of autistic subjects had a reversed pattern of lateralisation of brain activity during tasks involving language or other left hemisphere mediated functions, such as motor imitation. In the study by Dawson et al. (1982), right and left parietal alpha were recorded during four cognitive tasks, two verbal and two spatial. Autistic and normal subjects did not differ during spatial tasks, but 7 of the 10 autistic subjects showed greater than normal right hemisphere activation during verbal tasks. This greater asymmetry was related to increases in IQ and age. The same method was used by Dawson et al. (1983) during four motor imitation tasks; two manual and two oral. Since a major characteristic of autism is impaired use of gesture, it was predicted that autistic persons would also show atypical hemisphere specialisation for motor imitation. Then it was found that autistic subjects showed significantly greater right hemisphere activation during the imitation tasks (particularly evident during oral rather than manual tasks) than normal subjects. These findings are relevant to autistic language and motor imitation impairment. Thus, it is clear that autism is associated with atypical patterns of hemisphere activity namely, right dominant or symmetrical activity during language and other left hemisphere related tasks.

Three hypotheses can be adduced to explain the high frequency of abnormal brain lateralisation in autism. The first postulates subgroups, that is, that variations in patterns of speech lateralisation may reflect distinct subgroups of autistic individuals who differ in the degree of specific left hemisphere pathology (Soper and Satz, 1984). The second involves abnormal cortical neural organisation. This hypothesis is supported in two ways. First, Dawson (1983) suggested that atypical patterns of cerebral lateralisation in autism may reflect inherent differences in underlying brain organisation caused by an early left hemisphere insult, genetic influences or other prenatal influences on cortical development. Second, abnormal cerebral dominance for language caused by intrauterine hormonal influences, occurs in several developmental disabilities such as dyslexia, dysphasia and autism (Geschwind and Galaburda, 1985a, b, c). A third hypothesis involves with abnormal hemisphere activation (Dawson, 1988). It consists of reversed asymmetries which reflect abnormal activation of the hemispheres. These findings suggest that patterns of speech lateralisation are strongly related to levels of language acquisition and raise the possibility that patterns of hemisphere asymmetry for speech processing may actually shift towards normal left hemisphere dominance as the autistic individual acquires language abilities. This suggest that the autistic individual's pattern of hemisphere activation may change during development.

Arousal and novelty detection hypotheses can be proposed to explain these irregularities. In 1980, James and Barry concluded that "characteristic spontaneous EEG irregularities, indicating some CNS disability may exist in autism" but the question of interpretation of abnormalities as indicating under or overarousal remained unresolved. Sokolov's (1963, 1975) attention arousal model involves both cortical analysis of the stimulus for specific properties, novelty and significance, and reticular thalamic mediation of cortical arousal. Based on research on both brain-damaged and normal persons, Heilman and Van Den Abell (1979, 1980) and others (Kinsbourne and Bemporad, 1984) suggested that each hemisphere has its own cortical limbic reticular loop, the right hemisphere exhibiting dominance for novelty detection, involuntary and voluntary attention and arousal. Specifically, there is evidence that the temporoparietal area has a large number of "fixation" cells which activate mechanisms to direct attention (Bushnell et al., 1981; Goldberg and Robinson, 1977). The temporoparietal area receives polymodal sensory, limbic and frontal input related to stimulus properties and significance. Temporoparietal damage results in failure to report, respond to or orientate towards novel or meaningful stimuli (Heilman et al., 1986). However, this neglect is more frequent and more severe after right than left hemisphere lesions (Brain, 1941; Critchley, 1966).

In autism, enhanced right hemisphere activity may reflect overactivation of the right hemisphere mediated cortical limbic reticular system, which is involved in novelty detection, involuntary and voluntary attention and arousal. Admittedly, the evidence for right hemisphere overactivation in autism rests on only three studies (Dawson et al., 1982, 1983, 1986), and must be considered tentative.

Theoretically, such right hemisphere overactivation may lead to increased sensitivity to novelty and arousal; this increased sensitivity would account for the autistic child's tendency to respond to novel stimuli of normal intensity with aversive reactions (Kinsbourne, 1987). Since aversive responses are associated with reduced stimulus intake and processing (Lacey, 1967), higher levels of right hemisphere activation would be expected to be correlated with more severe functional impairment, as found in a study of the relationship between hemisphere activity and language abilities (Dawson et al., 1986). Right hemisphere overactivation may be caused by dysfunctional subcortical mechanisms which influence cortical arousal. Because the cortical, limbic and reticular subsystems which regulate arousal and attention are interdependent, dysfunction of any part of the larger system would be manifest at all levels of brain function.

An orientating response, typically elicited by novel, unpredictable stimuli, is accompanied by several physiological changes, including EEG desynchronisation.

The act of attending to novel, unpredictable stimuli is based on a complex interaction of cortical and subcortical systems (Thatcher and John, 1977). According to the model of Sokolov (1975), analysis of the stimulus properties is mediated by the primary sensory cortex and hippocampus. Furthermore, the novelty detectors of the hippocampus, excited by the novel stimulus, influence the activity of the reticular system, which in turn enhances the activity of the cortex. This enhancement includes EEG desynchronisation and is part of several physiological changes which comprise the orientating response.

It has been suggested (Sokolov, 1975) that, in relaxed states, the neurons of the hippocampus maintain the activity of a tonic synchronising system of the thalamus. When a novel stimulus is presented, there is a decrease in the spontaneous activity of these neurons, which disrupts the thalamic synchronising system and its influence on the cortical EEG. The novel stimulus enhances the functional state of the cerebral cortex by both increasing the activity of the reticular activating systems and disrupting the synchronising mechanisms of the thalamus, so that desynchronisation of neural generators occurs.

Enhanced attention is associated with desynchronisation of the EEG, since, presumably, desynchronisation allows more generators to be available to respond to the stimulus. An arousal state is characterised by relatively independent but co-operative neural groupings, which are available to process different aspects of information.

Thus attention to a novel stimulus involves changes in neural coherence. There is tonic desynchronisation of neural generators, as evidenced by EEG desynchronisation. With development, social and language representational systems exert increasing influence on attentional control. These representational systems allow the young child to go beyond a basic reflex type attentional response to novelty, described above, to acquire voluntary attentional control. Stored representations interact with stimulus properties to influence stimulus value for the child. These higher-order cortical processes influence the direction of voluntary attention (Thatcher, 1976).

Some workers have argued that, in normal populations, high levels of arousal may be associated with specific information processing impairments. Easterbrook (1959) argued that overarousal leads to a restriction of cue utilisation — an idea consistent with studies of overselectivity in autism (Lovaas et al., 1971). Experimental studies with normal infants, children and adults have demonstrated that stimulus recognition and recall are correlated with physiological indices (such as heart rate) which reflect optimal states of arousal (Clarkson and Berg, 1983; Linnemeyer and Porges, 1986). Thus, if autistic children are in a chronic state of high arousal, this may be associated with specific information processing deficits.

Hutt et al. (1965) demonstrated that autistic children showed high levels of desynchronised EEG indicative of increased arousal, which attenuated after bouts of stereotyped motor activities. Like Zentall and Zentall (1983), Hutt and his coworkers interpreted these findings according to a feedback model in which behavioural responses (in this case, stereotyped motor activities) function to regulate the level of stimulus input and arousal.

The study of physiological indices of arousal is further complicated by two factors. First, since physiological measures of arousal, such as EEG desynchronisation and heart rate, correlate poorly with one another in normal individuals (Lacey, 1967), we should not expect different measures to yield consistent results across studies for autistic children. A more reasonable approach may be to look for patterns of physiological response among such measures. Second, if the homoeostatic model is correct in positing that organisms will work to optimise levels of arousal by modulating the level of stimulation (Zentall and Zentall, 1983), then measures of physiological arousal may deviate from normal levels only prior to behavioural compensation. As Kinsbourne (1987) has argued, an organism biased toward overarousal may also be unstable, permitting arousal levels to swing to both maladaptive extremes as compensatory mechanisms come into play. Thus, it may be necessary to study an individual over time in a variety of situations to detect patterns of physiological arousal in response to changes in the environment.

Autistic individuals often fail to exhibit normal, adaptive orientating responses to a variety of stimuli. Experimental studies of the electrodermal, respiratory and heart rate orienting responses in autistic children have shown absent or reduced habituation (James and Barry, 1984; van Engeland, 1984), consistent with an aversive response to novelty and reduced stimulus intake. Adequate studies of physiological correlates of attention in more complex sustained attention tasks are lacking. In studies of spontaneous autonomic and cortical activity, indices of arousal have often been found to be high in autistic children (Palkovitz and Wiesenfeld, 1980; Stevens and Gruzelier, 1984). Although some studies report negative findings, lower than normal values on measures of autonomic and cortical arousal have not been reported. Although the research is by no means conclusive, it suggests that many autistic individuals have chronically high levels of arousal.

Attempts to find predictable relationships between environmental complexity, physiological measures of arousal and autistic behaviour (e.g., stereotyped motor activities) have not always succeeded. Since the level of arousal is likely to be influenced by the stage of development, environmental conditions and the severity of the disorder, both intra- and interindividual variability in physiological and behavioural indices of arousal in autistic persons are to be expected. Future studies which control carefully for subject variables, such as developmental level and degree of autistic impairment, and assess individuals in a variety of conditions differing in complexity and familiarity, may yield a better understanding of the complex relationship between levels of physiological arousal and behaviour in autism. The orientating response which usually occurs upon detection of novelty appears to be abnormal in autistic individuals; physiological responses to novel stimuli are more consistent with an aversive response. Since aversive responses in normal individuals occur when stimuli are perceived as intense, noxious, or painful, the occurrence of these responses to novel stimuli of moderate intensity in autistic persons suggests that they may be overstimulating for them. The behavioural responses of autistic individuals to novel situations suggest that they too may be aversive to them.

qEEG and imitation in autism

Patients with autism are strikingly deficient in social imitation, social turn taking, shared social attention, social sharing of experiences and emotions, and representational play. Our hypothesis is that imitative disturbances are present very early in child development and interact with a good development of social interaction between the child and his environment.

Although the original description of the syndrome by Kanner (1943) did not refer specifically to imitative skills, deficiencies in this area are frequently observed clinically and have been suggested in many studies (DeMyer et al., 1972; Hammes and Langdell, 1981; Lovaas et al., 1967; Ohta, 1987; Ritvo and Provence, 1953). A lack of imitative capacity has been included by some investigators as one of the early signs of autism (Krug et al., 1980; LeCouteur et al., 1989; Rogers and Pennington, 1991; Sauvage et al., 1987). In one of the earliest reports on imitation in young children with autism, Ritvo and Provence (1953) noted poor responses on tasks requiring motor responses as well as tasks focussing on manipulation of objects, sound and drawing. They concluded that imitation is part of the identification process and that the low levels of imitation noted among the autistic indicated an insufficient differentiation between self and nonself. Later, Lovaas et al. (1967) also noted an imitation deficit among autistic children and started training of imitation skills. Today support exits for the positive effect of imitative play on the child's behaviour (Dawson and Galpert, 1987; Nadel, 1988). Mutual imitation is a prominent component of early care-giver/infant social interactions essential to the development of self-awareness and awareness of others (Meltzoff, 1990). Rogers and Pennington (1991) have developed a theoretical framework for understanding the early signs of autism in which abnormalities in early interpersonal abilities affect subsequent stages in a cascading fashion. They suggest that early imitation should be viewed as a social skill and such lower level deficits in autistic children may be quite handicapping for development of higher level social understanding. In a earlier article, Dawson and Lewy (1989) suggested that the complex processing demands of the information inherent in social situations exceed the capabilities of autistic infants, leading to an impaired capacity to engage in social exchanges. More recently, Malvy (1992, 1994) found that children with autism exhibit in early infancy abnormalities not only in communication function but also in intentional and imitative functions. Thus, this deficit in imitation seems to appear very early in the development of the autistic child.

Several studies of neonatal imitation (Meltzoff, 1988; Meltzoff and Moore, 1977) have resulted in increasing acceptance of the idea that very young infants are capable of "real" imitation (Mandler, 1988) based on representational capacities. Thus, imitation of some body movements appears to be present essentially from birth.

Lhermitte et al. (1986) found that excessive imitation is observed with cortical brain damage. Studies of electrical brain activity can be used to detect imitative processing. Kimura (1977) demonstrated that patients with left hemisphere damage are impaired in performing meaningless motor movements. She suggested that the "left hemisphere is adapted for the execution of some categories of motor activity which happened to lend themselves readily to communication" (Kimura, 1973). Later, Dawson et al. (1985) found that the left hemisphere is specialised for production of manual and facial motor imitation. The measure of hemisphere specialisation was EEG recordings of alpha rhythm asymmetries from homologous parietal sites during spatial, verbal and motor imitation tasks.

Lastly, as the theoretical discussion in autism focusses more and more on the presence or absence of empathy in these patients, neurophysiology can bring an important, long neglected contribution to the understanding of deficits (Cohen-Seat et al., 1956, Heuyer et al., 1957; Lelord, 1957, 1966). When normal adults, attached to EEG equipment, are watching a film of motor activity by human actors, an electrocortical modification in the motor area (centroparietal changes in the alpha band) of the spectator occurs, synchronised with the actor's movements. Lelord et al. (1991) have shown that this phenomenon requires physiological curiosity. This EEG "motor or free imitation" (so called by Lelord et al.) of another human being's action indicates a focus on, and possibly identification with, the person on the screen.

While studying "free imitation" by electrophysiological methods, we observed in a very preliminary study that the evidence of such imitation is disturbed in autistic children. The children were presented with the same television sequences showing first a city and then an actor performing large movements. In normal children, changes in the centroparietal area seem to accompany the movement of the actor. In autistic children, this phenomenon appears as soon as the sequence of the city begins. These children with autism pay attention to everything on the screen but do not focus on the people in the film and do not exhibit EEG "motor imitation", as physiological curiosity is scattered. These children seem very sensitive to minimal movement in television sequences. They possibly tend to imitate everything which prevents them from focussing imitation towards others.

Imitation can be defined as sensori-motor processing. Sensory processing refers to the perception of objects, and space but also motion. Motion perception is thus crucial to social communication. Our assumption is that impairments affecting development of motion perception might therefore result in perceptual and social deficits. Gepner et al. (1995) found that autistic children have movement perception impairment. They suggested that the disturbed motor output of autistic subjects may be due to this impairment. Being impaired in visual motion processing might result in impairment in perception and production of gestures, social or otherwise. It seems obvious that spontaneous use of conventional gestures follows learning of gestures through imitation and therefore through adequate perception of motion.

Current research involves identifying motion perception impairment in autistic children. It carries on Lelord's work, using electrophysiological methods, and tries to demonstrate changes in cortical rhythms, showing the general characteristics of this

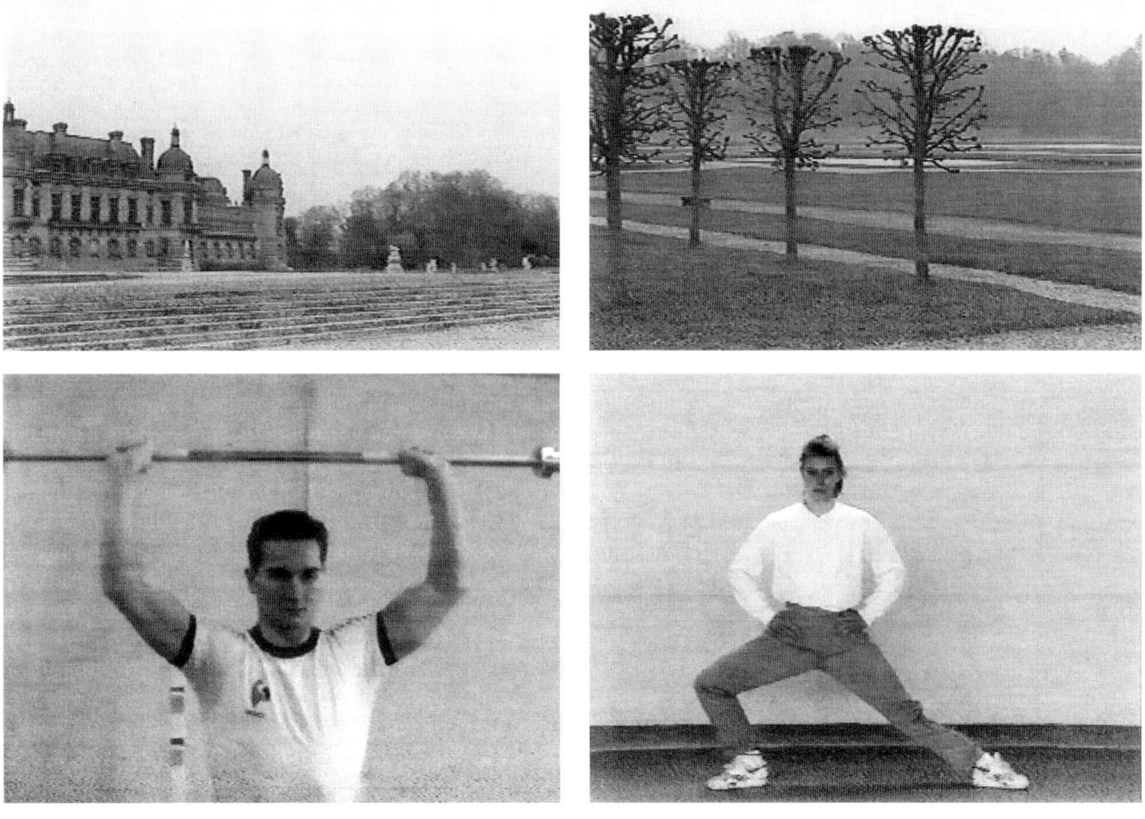

Fig. 3. Four examples of the video film sequences used to study motion perception.

motion perception. Recordings of electrical cerebral activity are performed at rest in standard conditions, and when the subject is looking at a video film alternating neutral fixed grounds, fixed grounds with persons, animated grounds with human movements, and with animal and object movements (Fig 3). Spectral analysis and topographical mapping are then performed during the different sequences of the film.

In children with autism this method can be used to show the individual child's disability, not only with clinical observations but also with quantified data. Bringing specific difficulties of autistic subjects to the fore would allow us to specify in each case suitable therapeutic procedures to alleviate, or even to detect social handicap.

References

Adey WR, Walter DO, Hendrix CE (1961) Computer techniques in correlation and spectral analysis of cerebral slow waves during discriminative behavior. Exp Neurol 3: 501-524

Adrian ED, Matthews BHC (1934) The Berger rhythm: potential changes from the occipital lobes in man. Brain 57: 355-385

Autret A, Auvert L, Laffont F, Larmande P (1985) Electroencephalographic spectral power and lateralized motor activities. Electroencephalogr Clin Neurophysiol 60: 228-236

Bashina VM, Gorbachevskaia NL, Simashkova NV, Iznak AF, Kozhushko LF, Iakupova LP (1994) Klinicheskie, neirofiziologicheskie differentsial'no-diagnostiches kie aspekty izucheniia tiazhelykh form rannego detskogo autizma. Z Nevropatol Psikhiat 94 (4): 68-71

Barthélémy C, Garreau B, Leddet I, Sauvage D, Lelord G, Callaway E (1983) Intérêt des échelles de comportement et des dosages de l'acide homovanilique urinaire pour le contrôle des effets d'un traitement associant vitamine B6 et magnésium chez des enfants ayant un comportement autistique. Neuropsychiat Enfance 31: 289-301

Bechtereva NP, Vvedenskaia IV, Dubikaitis YV, Stepanova TS, Ovnatanov BS, Usov VV (1963) Localisation of focal brain lesions by electroencephalography. Electroencephalogr Clin Neurophysiol 15: 177-196

Berger H (1929) Über das Elektroenkephalogram des menschen. Arch Psychiat Nervenkrank 87: 527-570

Best CT, Hoffman H, Glanville BB (1982) Development of right ear asymmetries for speech and music. Percept Psychophys 31: 75-85

Brain WR (1941) Visual disorientation with special reference to lesions of the right cerebral hemisphere. Brain 64: 244-271

Buchsbaum MS, Rigal F, Coppola R, Cappelletti J, King C, Johnson J (1982) A new system for gray-level surface distribution maps of electrical activity. Electroencephalogr Clin Neurophysiol 53: 237-242

Bushnell MC, Goldberg ME, Robinson DL (1981) Behavioral enhancement of visual responses in monkey cerebral cortex: modulation on posterior parietal cortex related to selected visual attention. J Neurophysiol 46: 755-772

Butler SR, Glass A (1974) Asymmetries in the electroencephalogram associated with cerebral dominance. Electroencephalogr Clin Neurophysiol 36: 481-491

Cantor DS, Thatcher RW, Hrybyk M (1986) Computerized EEG analyses of autistic children. J Autism Dev Disord 16: 169-187

Clarkson MG, Berg WK (1983) Cardiac orienting and vowel discrimination in new-borns: crucial stimulus parameters. Child Dev 54: 162-171

Cohen DJ, Caparulo BS, Schaywitz B (1976) Primary childhood aphasia and childhood autism. J Am Acad Child Psychiat 15: 604-645

Cohen-Seat G, Lelord G, Rebeillard M (1956) Conditions actuelles d'utilisation de l'EEG dans la recherche filmologique. Rev Int Filmol 7: 157-176

Cooley JW, Tukey JW (1965) An algorithm for the machine calculation of complex Fourier series. Math Comput 19: 297-301

Creak M, Pampiglione G (1969) Clinical and EEG studies on a group of 35 psychotic children. Dev Med Child Neurol 11: 218-227

Critchley M (1966) The parietal lobes. New York: Hafner

Damasio AR, Maurer RG (1978) A neurological model for childhood autism. Arch Neurol 35: 777-786

Dawson G (1983) Lateralized brain dysfunction in autism: evidence from the Halstead-Beitan neuropsychological battery. J Autism Dev Disord 13: 269-286

Dawson G (1987) The role of abnormal hemispheric specialization in autism. In: Schopler E, Mesibov G (eds) Neurobiological issues in autism. Plenum, New York p 234-256

Dawson G (1988) Cerebral lateralisation in autism: clues to its role in language and affective development. In: Segalowitz SJ and Molfese DL (eds) Developmental implications of brain lateralisation. New York, Guilford Press p 437-461

Dawson G, Finley C, Phillips S, Galpert L (1986) Hemisphere specialization and the language abilities of autistic children. Child Dev 57: 1440-1453

Dawson G, Galpert L (1987) A developmental model for facilitating the social behavior of autistic children. In: Schopler E and Mesibov G (eds) Social behavior in autism. Plenum, New York p 237-261

Dawson G, Klinger LG, Panagiotides H, Lewy A, Castelloe P (1995) Subgroups of autistic children based on social behavior display distinct patterns of brain activity. J Abn Child Psychol 23 (5): 569-583

Dawson G, Lewy A (1989) Reciprocal subcortical-cortical influences in autism: the role of attentional mechanisms. In: Dawson G (ed) Autism: nature, diagnosis, and treatment. Guilford Press, New York, p 144-173

Dawson G, Warrenburg S, Fuller P (1982) Cerebral lateralisation in individuals diagnosed as autistic in early childhood. Brain Lang 15: 353-368

Dawson G, Warrenburg S, Fuller P (1983) Hemisphere functioning and motor imitation in autistic persons. Brain Cogn 2: 346-354

Dawson G, Warrenburg S, Fuller P (1985) Left hemisphere specialization for facial and manual imitation. Psychophysiology 22 (2): 237-243

DeLong GR (1978) A neurophysiologic interpretation of infantile autism. In: Rutter M and Schopler E (eds) Autism: a reappraisal of concepts and treatment. Plenum Press, New York, p 207-217
DeLong GR, Bean SC, Brown FR (1981) Acquired reversible autistic syndrome in acute encephalopathic illness in children. Arch Neurol 38: 191-194
DeMyer MK, Alpern GD, Barton S, DeMyer WE, Churchill DW, Hingten JN, Bryson CQ, Pontius W, Kimberlin C (1972) Imitation in autistic, early schizophrenic, and non-psychotic subnormal children. J Autism Child Schizophr 2: 264-287
DeMyer MK, Barton S, DeMyer WE, Norton JA, Allen J, Steele R (1973) Prognosis in autism: a follow-up study. J Autism Child Schizophr 3: 199-246
DeMyer MK, Hingigen JN, Jackson RK (1981) Infantile autism reviewed: a decade of research. Schizophrenia Bull 7: 388-451
Dietsch G (1932) Fourier analyse von elektrenkephalogramment des menschen. Arch Gen Physiol 230: 106-112
Doyle J, Galin D, Ornstein RE (1974) Lateral specialization of cognitive mode: EEG frequency analysis. Psychophysiology 11: 567-578
Duffy FH, Bartels PH, Burchfield JL (1981) Significance probability mapping: an aid in the topographic analysis of brain electrical activity. Electroencephalogr Clin Neurophysiol 51: 455-462
Easterbrook JA (1959) The effect of emotion on cue utilization and the organization of behavior. Psychol Rev 66: 183-201
Etevenon P (1985) Applications and perspectives of EEG cartography. In: Duffy FH (ed) Topography mapping of brain electrical activity. Butterworths, Boston p 113-141
Etevenon P, Gaches J, Debouzy C, Gueguen B, Peron-Magnan P (1985) EEG cartography. I. By means of mini or micro-computers. Reliability and interest of this electrical non-invasive brain imagery. Neuropsychobiol 13: 141-146
Fish B, Shapiro T (1965) A typology of children's psychiatric disorders. J Am Acad Child Psychiat 4: 32-39
Garreau B (1994) Etude physiologique d'activités perceptives dans les troubles du développement. Doctoral dissertation. Tours
Gepner B, Mestre D, Masson G, de Schonen S (1995) Postural effects of motion vision in young autistic children. Neuroreport 6: 1211-1214
Geschwind N, Galaburda AM (1985a) Cerebral lateralisation: biological mechanisms, association, and pathology. I.: A hypothesis and a program for research. Arch Neurol 42: 428-459
Geschwind N, Galaburda AM (1985b) Cerebral lateralisation: biological mechanisms, association, and pathology. II.: A hypothesis and a program for research. Arch Neurol 42: 521-552
Geschwind N, Galaburda AM (1985c) Cerebral lateralisation: biological mechanisms, association, and pathology. III.: A hypothesis and a program for research. Arch Neurol 42: 634-654
Gevins AS, Zeitlin GM, Doyle JC, Schaffer RE, Callaway E (1979) EEG patterns during "cognitive" tasks. II. Analysis of controlled tasks. Electroencephalogr Clin Neurophysiol 47: 704-710
Gibbs FA (1937) Regulation of frequency in cerebral cortex. Am J Physiol 119: 317-318
Gibbs EL, Gibbs FA (1973) Clinical correlates of various types of extreme spindles. Clin Electroencephalogr 4: 89-97
Gillberg C, Schaumann H (1983) Epilepsy presenting as infantile autism? two case studies. Neuropediatrics 14: 206-212
Gillberg C, Steffenburg S (1987) Outcome and prognosis factors in infantile autism and similar conditions: a population based study of 46 cases followed through puberty. J Autism Dev Disord 17: 273-287
Gillberg C (1991) The treatment of epilepsy in autism. J Autism Dev Disord 21: 61-77
Glanville BB, Best CT, Levinson R (1977) A cardiac measure of cerebral asymmetries in infant auditory perception. Dev Psychol 13: 54-59
Goldberg ME, Robinson DL (1977) Visual responses of neurons in monkey inferior parietal lobule: the physiologic substrate of attention and neglect. Neurology 27: 350
Gorvachevskaia NL, Iakupova LP, Kozhushko LF, Bashina VM, Simashkova NV, Amelin SN (1992) Topograficheskoe EEG-kartirovanie v detska psikhiatrii. Fiziol Cheloveka 18: 40-48
Grass AM, Gibbs FA (1938) A Fourier transform of the electroencephalogram. J Neurophysiol 1: 521-526
Gubbay SS, Lobascher M, Kingerlee P (1970) A neurological appraisal of autistic children: results of a Western Australian survey. Dev Med Child Neurol 12: 422-429
Guillemet I, Briche I, Roux S, Rossetto S, Garreau B (1997) Autism and epilepsy. Submitted to Am J Psychiatr
Hammes JG, Langdell T (1981) Precursors of symbol formation and childhood autism. J Autism Dev Disord 11: 331-344
Heilman KM, Van Den Abell T (1979) Right hemispheric dominance for mediating cerebral activation. Neuropsychologia 17: 315-321
Heilman KM, Van Den Abell T (1980) Right hemisphere dominance for attention: the mechanism underlying hemispheric asymmetries of inattention. Neurology 30: 327-330
Heilman KM, Bowers D, Valenstien E, Watson RT (1986) The right hemisphere: neurophysiological functions. J Neurosurg 64: 693-704
Hermelin B, O'Connor N (1970) Psychological experiments with autistic children. Pergamon, Oxford
Heuyer G, Cohen-Seat G, Lelord G, Rebeillard M (1957) Etudes EEG d'enfants inadaptés soumis à la stimulation filmique. Neuropsy Inf Hygièn Ment Enfance 9-10: 494-511
Hutt SJ, Hutt C, Lee D, Ounsted C (1965) A behavioral and electroencephalographic study of autistic children. J Psychiat Res 3: 181-197
James AL, Barry RJ (1980) A review of psychophysiology in early onset psychosis. Schizophrenia Bull 6: 506-525
James AL, Barry RJ (1984) Cardiovascular and electrodermal responses to simple stimuli in autistic retarded and normal children. Int J Psychophysiol 1: 179-193
Jung R (1939) Ein Apparat zur mehrfachen Registrierung von Tätigkeit und Funktionen des animalen und vegetativen Nervensystems. Z Neurol 165: 374-397
Kanner L (1943) Autistic disturbances of affective contact. Nerv Child 2: 217-250
Kimura D (1973) The asymmetry of the human brain. Sci Am 228: 70-78
Kimura D (1977) Acquisition of a motor skill after left hemisphere damage. Brain 100: 527-542
Kinsbourne M, Bemporad B (1984) Lateralisation of emotion: a model and the evidence. In: Fox NA, Davidson RJ (eds) The psychobiology of affective development. Erlbaum Hillsdale, NJ, p 234-256

Kinsbourne M (1987) Cerebral brainstem relations in infantile autism. In: Schopler E, Mesibov G (eds) Neurobiological issues in autism. Plenum, NewYork, 107-126

Knott JR (1938) Brain potentials during silent and oral reading. J Gen Psychol 18: 57-62

Kolvin I, Ounsted C, Humphrey M, McNay A (1971) Studies in childhood psychoses: the phenomenology in childhood psychoses. British J Psychiat 118: 385-395

Krug DA, Arick J, Almond P (1980) Behavior checklist for identifying severely handicapped individuals with high levels of autistic behavior. J Child Psychol Psychiat 21: 221-229

Lacey JI (1967) Somatic response in patterning and stress: some revisions of activation theory. In: Appley MH, Trumbull R (eds) Psychological stress: Issues in research. Appleton-Century-Crofts, New York, p 107-124

LeCouteur A, Rutter M, Lord C, Rios P, Robertson S, Holdgrafer M, McLennan J (1989) Autism diagnostic interview: a standardized investigator based instrument. J Autism Dev Disord 19: 363-387

Lehmann D (1971) Multichannel topography of human alpha EEG fields. Electroencephalogr Clin Neurophysiol 31: 439-449

Lelord G (1957) Modalités réactionnelles différentes de rythmes moyens et antérieurs autour de 10 c/s. Rev Neurol 96: 524-526

Lelord G (1966) Intérêt des méthodes électrophysiologiques dans l'étude de l'action du film cinématographique chez l'enfant et l'adolescent. Pédopsychiatrie 1: 159-166

Lelord G, Barthélémy C, Martineau J, Bruneau N, Garreau B, Hameury L (1991) Free acquisition, free imitation, physiological curiosity and exchange and development therapies in autistic children. Brain Dysfunct 4: 335-347

Lhermitte F, Pillon B, Serdaru M (1986) Human autonomy and the frontal lobes. Part I: Imitation and utilization behavior: a neuropsychological study of 75 patients. Ann Neurol 19: 326-334

Linnemeyer SA, Porges SW (1986) Recognition memory and cardiac vagal tone in 6 month old infants. Inf Behav Dev 9: 43-56

Lovaas OI, Freitas L, Nelson K, Whalen C (1967) The establishment of imitation and its use for the development of complex behavior in schizophrenic children. Behav Res Ther 5: 171-181

Lovaas OI, Schreibman L, Koegel RL, Rehm R (1971) Selective responding by autistic children to multiple sensory input. J Abn Psychol 77: 211-222

Malvy J (1992) Analyse fonctionnelle des déficiences observées précocément chez les enfants autistes à l'aide de films familiaux. Mémoire de DEA, Université de Tours, France

Malvy J (1994) Autisme infantile et films familiaux. Evaluation fonctionnelle des premiers signes. ANAE 26: 33-37

Mandler JM (1988) How to build a baby: on the development of an accessible representational system. Cogn Dev 3: 113-136

Meltzoff AN, Moore MK(1977) Imitation of facial and manual gestures by human neonates. Science 198: 5-78

Meltzoff AN (1988) Infant imitation and memory: nine month olds in immediate and deferred tests. Child Dev 59: 217-225

Meltzoff AN (1990) Foundations for developing a concept of self: the role of imitation in relating self to other and the value of social modeling and self practice in infancy. In: Cicchetti D, Beeghly M (eds) The self in transition: infancy to childhood. The University of Chicago Press, Chicago, p 139

Molfese DL, Molfese VJ (1979) Hemisphere and stimulus differences as reflect in the cortical responses of newborn infants to speech stimulus. Dev Psychol 15: 505-511

Nadel J (1988) L'imitation immédiate: bilan et perspectives ou: pourquoi Platon nous a-t-il fait ça? Psychol Fran

Ogawa T, Sugiyama A, Ishiwa S, Suzuki M, Ishihara T, Sato K (1982) Ontogenic development of EEG-asymmetry in early infantile autism. Brain Dev 4: 439-449

Ohta M (1987) Cognitive disorders of infantile autism: a study employing the WISC, spatial relationship conceptualization, and gesture imitation. J Autism Dev Disord 17: 45-62

Palkovitz RJ, Wiesenfeld AR (1980) Differential autonomic responses of autistic and normal children. J Autistic Dev Disord 10: 347-360

Prior MR, Bradshaw JL (1979) Hemisphere functioning in autistic children. Cortex 15: 73-81

Pfurtscheller G (1986) Event related desynchronisation mapping: visualisation of cortical activation patterns. In: Duffy FH (ed) Topographic mapping of brain electrical activity, Butterworths, Boston, p 99-110

Pfurtscheller G (1988) Mapping of event-related desynchronization: temporal and spatial aspects. In: Samson-Dollfus D (ed) Statistics and topography in quantitative EEG. Elsevier, Amsterdam, p 184-195

Rimland B (1964) Infantile autism: the syndrome and its implications. Appleton-Century-Crofts, New York

Ritvo S, Provence S (1953) Form perception and imitation in some autistic children: diagnostic findings and their contextual interpretation. Psychoanal Study Child 8: 155-161

Ritvo ER, Ornitz EM, Walter RD, Hanley J (1970) Correlation of psychiatric diagnoses and EEG findings: a double-blind study of 184 hospitalized children. Am J Psychiat 126: 988-996

Rogers SJ, Pennington BF (1991) A theoretical approach to the deficits in infantile autism. Dev Psychopathol 3: 137-162

Rossi PG, Parmeggiani A, Bach V, Santucci M, Visconti P (1995) EEG features and epilepsy in patients with autism. Brain Dev 17: 169-174

Ruf H, Vattuone G (1943) Die Hirnpotentiale beim Lesen. Arch Psychiat Nervenkr 116: 329-338

Rutter M (1970) Autistic children. Infancy of adulthood. Sem Psychiat 2: 435-450

Small JG, DeMyer MK, Kendall JK (1969) Experiences with response averaging in autistic children. Electroencephalogr Clin Neurophysiol 26: 110

Small JG (1975) EEG and neurophysiological studies of early infantile autism. Biol Psychiat 10: 385-397

Sauvage D, Hameury L, Adrien J L, Larmande C, Perrot-Beaugerie A, Barthélémy C, Peyraud A (1987) Signes d'autisme avant deux ans: évaluation et signification. Ann Psychiat 2: 338-350

Sokolov EN (1963) Perception and the conditioned reflex. Macmillan, New York

Sokolov EN (1975) The neuronal mechanisms of the orienting reflex. In: Sokolov EN Vinogradova OS(eds) Neuronal mechanisms of the orienting reflex. Erlbaum, Hillsdale, NJ, p 145-156

Soper HV, Satz P (1984) Pathological left-handedness and ambiguous handedness: a new explanatory model. Neuropsychologia 22: 511-515

Stevens JR, Milstein V (1970) Severe psychiatric disorders of childhood. Am J Dis Child 120: 182-192

Stevens S, Gruzelier J (1984) Electrodermal activity to auditory stimuli in autistic, retarded, and normal children. J Autism Dev Disord 14: 245-260

Tanguay PE (1977) Clinical and electrophysiological research. In: Ritvo E (ed) Autism: diagnosis, current research and management. Spectrum, New York p 75-84

Thatcher RW (1976) Electrophysiological correlates of animal and human memory. In: Terry R, Gershon S (eds) The neurobiology of aging. Raven Press, New York, p 345-367

Thatcher RW, John ER (1977) Foundations of cognitive processes: functional neuroscience. Wiley, New York

Tsai L, Jacoby CG, Stewart MA, Beisler JM (1982) Unfavorable left-right asymmetries of the brain and autism. British J Psychiat 140: 312-319

Tuchman RF, Rapin I, Shinnar S (1991) Autistic and dysphasic children II. Epilepsy. Pediatrics 88: 1219-1225

van Engeland H (1984) The electrodermal orienting response to auditive stimuli in autistic children, normal children, mentally retarded children, and child psychiatric patients. J Autism Dev Disord 14: 261-279

Walter DO (1963) Spectral analysis for electroencephalogram: mathematical determination of neurophysiological relationships from records of limited duration. Exp Neurol 8:155-181

Walter DO, Adey WR (1963) Spectral analysis of EEGs recorded during learning in the cat, before and after subthalamic lesions. Exp Neurol 7: 481-501

White PT, DeMyer WE, DeMyer MK (1964) EEG abnormalities in early childhood schizophrenia: a double-blind study of psychiatrically disturbed and normal children during promazine sedation. Am J Psychiat 120: 950-958

Witelson SF (1977) Early hemisphere specialization and inter-hemispheric plasticity: an empirical and theoretical review. In: Segalowitz SJ, Gruber FA (eds) Language development and neurological theory. Academic Press, New York, p 243-269

Zentall SS, Zentall TR (1983) Optimal stimulation: a model of disordered activity and performance in normal and deviant children. Psychol Bull 94: 446-471

9. Neuroimaging in eating disorders in youth

V. DELVENNE

Eating disorders classically begin in adolescence. Anorexia nervosa most often occurs near the time of puberty while bulimia has a later age of onset, at about 18 years. They are often considered as two different aspects of the same illness. Indeed, almost half of the patients with anorexia nervosa experience episodes of bulimia and follow-up studies have demonstrated that 44 % of them later develop bulimia. Similarly, most bulimic patients have vomiting and fasting periods several times a week (Casper et al., 1980; Hsu et al., 1979).

Anorexia nervosa is a complex syndrome whose most prominent feature is weight loss. However, different clinical characteristics such as disturbances in perception of body shape, high levels of motor restlessness and hyperactivity are associated with strategies to induce weight loss such as restricting food, vomiting, purging or abuse of diuretics or appetite suppressants.

As first described by Russell (1979), bulimia nervosa is characterised by recurrent episodes of binge-eating and compensatory behaviours, such as purging or fasting, to prevent weight gain. Although anorectic and bulimic patients differ in eating behaviour and its consequences (fasting, weight loss, menstrual pattern), they show similar mental symptoms such as preoccupation with food and appearance and disturbed body image (Van der Ham et al., 1990).

A number of metabolic and endocrine abnormalities, mainly at the hypothalamic level, are seen in bulimia in a milder form than in anorexia nervosa. For example, patients with eating disorder have amenorrhoea or oligomenorrhoea, and disturbed cortisol suppression or blunted thyrotropin-releasing hormone (TRH) tests (Fichter et al., 1990). Much evidence suggests that most of these changes are secondary to low weight or reduced caloric intake, as they revert to normal with weight restoration and eating a normal diet.

Concerning central nervous system neurotransmitters, a significant reduction of cerebrospinal fluid (CSF) metabolites of serotonine and dopamine (Kaye et al., 1984) or opiate-related peptides (Kaye et al., 1987) has been observed in anorexia nervosa. These levels do become normal with restoration of weight. However, long-term weight-restored anorectics have elevated concentrations of CSF 5-HIAA (Kaye et al., 1991) and a reduction of CSF noradrenaline levels (Kaye et al., 1984). Changes in monoaminergic systems have also been observed in normal-weight bulimic patients (Pirke et al. 1992; Brewerton et al., 1992). These findings might correlate with some of the clinical characteristics such as altered mood, anxiety or obsessional thinking, observed in eating disorders. It has also been postulated that these neurochemical changes precede the onset of abnormal eating behaviour and are the consequence of a primary stress reaction (Donohoe, 1984).

A possible genetic vulnerability to environmental stress has also been suggested, following family and twin studies (Holland et al., 1988). What is not known is the nature and the importance of this vulnerability in the etiology and development of eating disorders.

The hypothesis of some central nervous system dysfunction in patients with eating disorders has been proposed following neuropsychological investigations. Attention and vigilance disabilities and impaired levels of performance in arithmetic have been described in anorectic patients (Fox, 1981; Small et al, 1983). These impaired cognitive performances appeared to be a sign of poor prognosis at follow-up. Lower vigilance performance and lower speed of drawing geometric figures are also impaired in bulimic patients (Mc Kay et al., 1986; Williamson et al., 1989). Moreover, alteration of body image perception was first suggested by Bruch (1977) as an important pathognomonic and pronostic sign of anorexia nervosa. Of the various experimental procedures to assess body image disturbances, the authors using "size estimation" and "image making" techniques (Slade, 1985; Horne et al., 1991), have identified a tendency to overestimate body width in a variety of female groups, including normals, but the greatest distortion was observed in anorectic patients. This body image distortion has also been demonstrated in bulimic patients (Slade, 1985).

CT studies

Neuro imaging studies in eating disorders are scarce except for CT scan studies.The first morphological study, carried out in 1961 by means of pneumoencephalography in three anorectic patients (Heidrich and Schmidt-Matthias, 1961), showed ventricular and sulcal enlargement.

Since 1977 Enzman and Lane (1971), numerous studies have been done on patients with anorexia nervosa bulimia nervosa, using cranial computed tomography (CT)(Nussbaum et al., 1980; Datlof et al., 1986). All have demonstrated, in varying degree, enlargement of the external cerebrospinal fluid space with diffuse sulcal widening, often associated with increased ventricular size. These abnormalities are partly reversible after weight restoration. The most constant finding is cortical sulcal enlargement. No satisfactory explanation has been proposed for these changes in brain morphology. Different pathogenic mechanisms have been suggested: malnourishment (Artman et al., 1985; Krieg et al., 1988); reduction of total protein or inhibition of brain protein biosynthesis (Artman et al., 1985), hypercortisolemia causing cerebral dehydration or low plasma levels of triiodothyronine (Krieg et al., 1988). Neuronal brain damage has also been suggested in those cases which did not reverse with weight recovery (Artman et al., 1985; Martin, 1958). Another possible explanation is offered by Artmann et al. (1985), who described minimal early acquired brain lesion in 60 % of their anorectic patients. The most frequently proposed hypothesis links the increase of the cerebrospinal fluid to an increase of the extra cellular space following starvation. Indeed, malnourishment provokes a reduction in muscular and adipose tissue which induces an increase of the ratio total water / body weight. However, these morphological changes were also observed in other psychiatric and somatic problems but discrepancies between studies limit our understanding of them (Schlegel and Kretzchmar, 1987).

MRI studies

MRI studies in anorectic patients have shown a smaller pituitary gland (Kornreich et al., 1991; Doraiswany et al., 1990) and a reduction in size of the thalamus and midbrain (Husain et al., 1992). The smaller pituitary size seems to reflect pituitary atrophy secondary to nutritional or endocrine changes. In addition, abnormalities of the neuronal circuits or in monoamine function have been suggested as an explanation.

SPECT studies

Two studies have been performed with single photon emission tomography in eating disorders, yielding different results. Krieg et al. (1989 b), found normal cerebral blood flow in anorectic patients suggesting no reduction in function of brain regions in anorexia nervosa. In other studies (Nozoe et al., 1991; Nozoe et al., 1993), Nozoe et al. described an increase in resting blood flow in the inferior frontal and left temporal cortex in bulimic patients, while anorectic patients showed a reduction in the left parietal cortex. After a meal, no differences appeared between patients with eating disorders and controls. It was concluded that there was possible hypoactivity of the cerebral cortex in anorexia nervosa.

PET studies

A few studies have been done on patients with eating disorders, using positron emission tomography and FDG the results are somewhat different in anorexia nervosa and bulimia nervosa.

PET in anorexia nervosa

Investigation of cerebral function, with positron emission tomography (PET) and ^{18}F-fluorodeoxyglucose (FDG) is limited in anorexia nervosa (Herholz et al., 12987; Delvenne et al., in press). A relative hypermetabolism in the caudate nuclei, which falls to normal after weight improvement was first reported in a group of 5 anorectic patients (Herholz et al., 1987).

Global and regional glucose cerebral hypometabolism was reported in a group of 20 underweight anorectic patients (Delvenne et al., 1995). The hypometabolism was more marked in the frontal and parietal cortex in both absolute and relative values (Fig. 1). In relative values, expressed as the ratio to mean cortical values, comparisons within regions showed hypometabolism in the parietal and superior frontal cortex, associated with relative hypermetabolism in the caudate nuclei and in inferior frontal cortex. After weight gain, following cognitive therapy and admission to hospital, the absolute hypometabolism returned towards normal in all regions, while the relative metabolism of glucose tended to remain abnormal in the parietal and inferior frontal cortex (Delvenne et al., in press).

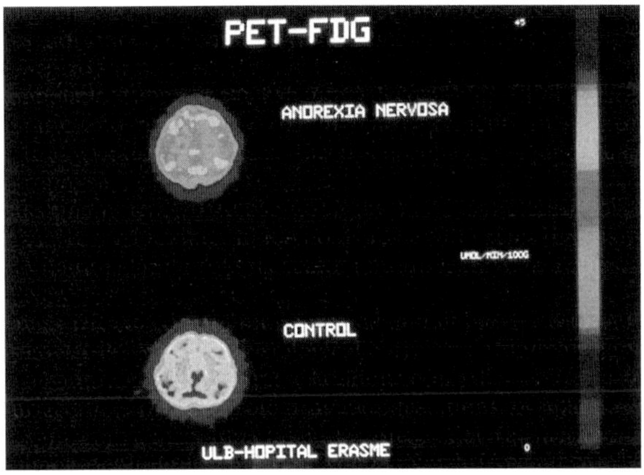

Fig. 1. Superior horizontal tomographic slice passing through the frontal and parietal cortices from an anorectic patient (upper slice) and a control subject (lower slice).
Absolute global and regional glucose cerebral hypometabolism was observed in anorectic patient.
See colour illustrations appendix.

Methodological and technical differences may explain discrepancies between studies. Relative hypermetabolism in the caudate nuclei was not observed in all studies. This seems to be a consequence of the method used for normalisation, and a reflection of differences in glucose hypometabolism, which is lower in cortical than in subcortical regions. Indeed, when relative metabolism of glucose was expressed as a ratio to whole slice glucose metabolic rates, no caudate nucleus hypermetabolism was observed. When relative values were expressed as ratios to the global cortical grey matter values of glucose metabolism, relative caudate nucleus hypermetabolism was apparent. Normalisation to the cortex was chosen as it reduces the impact of white matter and takes account of most of the ROI, which are mainly cortical. Relative caudate nucleus hypermetabolism thus seems to represent a reflection of differences in glucose hypometabolism between cortical and subcortical regions.

PET in bulimia nervosa

PET was first carried out in bulimic patients during cognitive stimulation. Changes in lateralisation of cerebral function with a left greater than right hemisphere activity, have been described in normal-weight bulimic patients performing to a visual vigilance task during uptake of FDG (Wu et al., 1990; Hagman et al., 1990). This particular task causes strong activation of the right hemisphere (Dupont et al., 1993) in normal subjects and lower perceptual sensitivity has been demonstrated in bulimic patients (Laessle et al., 1990). In another study (Andreason et al., 1992), bulimic subjects were submitted to an auditory discrimination task which in normal subjects provokes, increased rCMRGlu in the right prefrontal cortex and a decrease in the parietal and anterior cingulate cortex (Cohen et al., 1988). In addition, a correlation between lower left anterolateral prefrontal glucose metabolism of patients with bulimia and depressive symptoms was observed and a left greater than right hemisphere asymmetry in the temporal lobes of patients with bulimia associated with bilateral inferior temporal relative hypermetabolism.

When the PET examination was conducted at rest, no lateralized differences of activation were found (Delvenne et al., in press). As in anorectic patients, bulimic patients show an absolute global and regional hypometabolism of glucose in most cerebral regions and a relative hypometabolism in the parietal cortex. This supports the hypothesis of a continuum within the eating disorders differentiated on a clinical basis.

Hypothesis concerning PET scan findings in eating disorders

Neuroimaging observations in eating disorders might derive from metabolic, neurophysiological or morphological abnormalities possibly associated with low body weight or nutritional factors. These may also be the consequences of associated symptoms such as anxiety or depression. A primary cerebral dysfunction in anorexia nervosa and bulimia has also been suggested.

The influence of nutritional factors

Low body weight or prolonged starvation states can be put forward as explanations of the absolute glucose hypometabolism observed in the brain in patients with eating disorders as a global return to normal was observed after weight gain. Consequences of low body weight can be excluded in the bulimic patients, whose body weight was normal. Starvation usually induces keto-acidosis, which has been suggested as explaining selective hypometabolism of glucose in the cortex (Hawkins et al., 1979; Herholz et al. 1987). However, anorectic and bulimic patients, at the time of the PET studies were in a stable metabolic state, with no ketone bodies in the urine and constantly normal plasma glucose levels. They received normal feeding. However, chronic effect of ketosis on the brain following chronic periods of starvation, frequently seen not only in anorectic but also in bulimic patients, cannot be totally excluded. When anorectic patients were re-examined after gain, completely normal cerebral glucose metabolism was not observed in the parietal cortex: hypometabolism persisted. At this time, the patients received stable caloric intake but most were still gaining weight. So, we can not exclude the possibility that this might contribute to the persistent abnormalities.

Abnormal hypothalamic function, characterised by neuroendocrine dysfunction such as amenorrhea, was observed in underweight anorectic and bulimic patients. This is partly related to low body weight or nutritional factors. Disturbances in hypothalamic glucose metabolism cannot be assessed because of the limited resolution of the PET camera. However, as some hypothalamic areas project to both subcortical and cortical regions (Saper, 1990), this may also be suggested as an explanation of brain glucose hypometabolism. However, neuroendocrine dysfunction shows frequently delayed recovery after weight gain and our anorectic patients who had gained weight and who had a normal rCMRglu, were still amenorrheic.

Disturbances in function related to glucose utilisation are the result of changes occurring predominantly in nerve terminals rather than cell bodies (Roland, 1992). Some central neurotransmitter systems have been shown to be disturbed in patients with eating disorder with significant reduction in cerebrospinal fluid (CSF) 5-hydroxyindole-acetic acid, noradrenaline and MHPG or homovanillic acid levels in the underweight anorectics (Fava et al., 1989). These levels became normal with weight restoration in anorectic patients. Elevated concentrations of CSF 5-HIAA have also been described in long-term weight-restored anorectics (Kaye et al., 1991). Abnormalities of these modulatory amine transmitter systems could contribute to the absolute global hypometabolism but not to the relative regional glucose hypometabolism. Indeed, serotoninergic and noradrenergic fibres distributed diffusely in all cortical regions, while dopaminergic fibres are found only in certain cortical regions, such as the prefrontal, cingulate and archicortex. Apart from this cerebral glucose hypometabolism, anorectic patients were also hyperactive and showed no global cerebral dysfunction on cognitive testing.

The impact of morphology

It has been suggested that partial volume effects secondary to morphological modifications influence brain glucose metabolism (Mazziotta et al., 1991; Herholz et al., 1987). In low-weight anorectic patients and in bulimic patients, CT studies have shown enlargement of the cortical sulci and sometimes of the ventricles, partially corrected after normalisation of weight (Enzman and Lane, 1971; Datlof et al., 1986). However, potential errors from partial volume effect cannot be considered when regions of interest were drawn to delineate precisely the structure and were larger than the spatial resolution of the imaging device.

The impact of the clinical features.

Clinical characteristics of the anorectic patients, such as restrictive or binge-eating or purging, might be thought to explain metabolic changes. These subtypes did not seem to account for statistical differences:differences in regional cerebral glucose metabolism among subgroups of anorectic patients were not significant (Delvenne et al., 1995).

Psychopathological disturbances such as depression or anxiety have been demonstrated to influence cerebral glucose metabolism in different ways.

The relationship between eating disorders and depression is still the subject of controversy. Anorectic patients often display depressive symptoms during the course of their illness, prior to the eating disorder, or more frequently within the time of chronic progression (Cantwell et al., 1977; Hudson et al., 1983). Studies which demonstrate familial associations between eating disorders and affective illness also support a link between the two (Cantwell et al., 1977; Gershon et al., 1984). In addition, neuroendocrine abnormalities such as abnormal cortisol suppression or thyrotropin-releasing hormone (TRH) tests, classically described in affective disorders, have frequently been observed in anorectic patients (Gwirtsman and Gerner, 1981). However, the influence of starvation on these biological disturbances and on the development and persistence of depressive symptoms must also be considered (Laessle et al., 1988). As depression is not associated with preoccupation with food and appearance or disturbed body image, loss of appetite and weight reduction is frequently observed. The nature of the relationship between the two illnesses appears complex and cannot be described in terms of simple models. PET studies conducted in affective disorders have shown, among other things, a hypometabolism of glucose which may be global (Phelps et al., 1984; Martinot et al., 1990), frontal (Martinot et al., 1990; Biver et al., 1994) and parietal (Cohen et al.,? ; Biver et al., 1994). Brain glucose metabolism has been compared in depressed patients with normal and low weight and low weight anorectic patients (Delvenne et al., in press; Delvenne et al., in press). Low weight patients, both anorectics and depressives, showed global hypometabolism in comparison with controls and depressed of normal weight patients, the lowest values being seen in anorectic patients. In addition, absolute metabolism of glucose throughout the cortex, as in various brain regions, correlated significantly with the body mass index. Thus, low weight and its consequences seem to influence cerebral glucose metabolism much more than depressive symptoms.

In PET studies, anorectics or bulimics are more anxious than control subjects (Delvenne et al., in press; Delvenne et al., 1995). Changes in cerebral glucose metabolism related to anxiety are complex, showing differences according to the intensity and type of anxiety. Studies with PET and FDG in normal volunteers have demonstrated a decrease of the cerebral glucose metabolism with increased anxiety (Gur et al., 1987). Lower metabolic rates of glucose were found in the basal ganglia in patients with a generalised anxiety disorder performing a passive viewing task, (Wu et al., 1991) while decreased metabolism in the left inferior parietal region has been described in panic disorder (Nordahl, 1990). Anxiety might therefore be a potential factor for modifications of cerebral glucose metabolism in eating disorders but the relationship is was not clear. Anxiety scores have not been found to correlate with rCMRGlu within anorectic or bulimic groups.

Relative hypometabolism in the parietal cortex, with relative hypermetabolism in the caudate nuclei and inferior frontal cortex was observed in anorectic patients (Herholz et al., 1987; Delvenne et al., in press). This relative hypermetabolism raises questions about the relationship between anorexia nervosa and obsessive compulsive disorder. Indeed, obsessional features focussed on eating patterns are common in anorexia nervosa (Rothenberg, 1990; Holden, 1990) and a relative hypermetabolism of the orbitofrontal gyri, corresponding to our inferior frontal cortex, and of the head of the caudate nuclei, has also been described in obsessive compulsive patients (Baxter et al., 1987; Nordahl et al., 1989). Persistence of these abnormalities after weight gain might be related to persistence of obsessions concerning food, weight and body shape in weight-restored anorectic patients.

Interestingly, significant hypometabolism has also been found in parietal structures (Nordahl et al., 1989) in obsessive compulsive patients although it was less marked than in anorectic patients.

Hypothesis of primary cerebral dysfunction in eating disorders

Relative parietal hypometabolism remains constant in anorectic patients, with a trend to persistence after weight gain (Delvenne et al., 1995; Delvenne et al., in press). This observation might support the suggestion of a possible primary cerebral dysfunction or a particular regional sensitivity to consequences of nutritional deficiency with different rates of restoration according to the region. Indeed, a significant correlation appeared between parietal hypometabolism and BMI in different groups of patients with eating disorder and depressed patients with normal and low weight (Fig. 2).

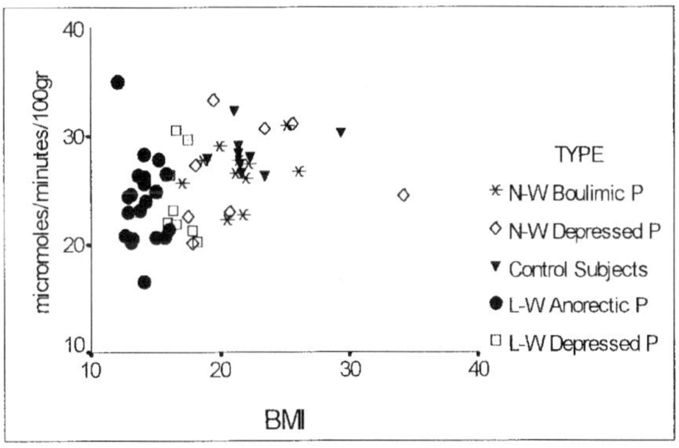

Fig. 2. Correlation between global cortical glucose metabolim and body mass index in 5 groups of patients and controls: normal weight bulimic patients, normal weight depressed patients, control subjects, low weight anorectic patients and low weight depressed patients.
Spearman rank correlation coefficient: $p = 0.001$.

Cognitive studies in anorectic patients showed distortions of body image (Bowden et al., 1989; Horne et al., 1991), associated with impairment of awareness of emaciation and low performance in arithmetic (Fox, 1981; Hamsher et al., 1981; Bowden et al., 1989). These disabilities are specifically marked in operations such as correct placing of a decimal point, division and fractions, and associated with impaired ability to copy complex geometrical figures, supporting possible parietal lobe dysfunction (Botez, 1987). Similarly, implication of parietal cortex has been recognised (Horne et al., 1991)in perception of the body image (Botez, 1987), which is altered in eating disorders. In addition, an elevated pain threshold has been observed in eating disorder patients (Lautenbacher et al., 1990) which was not the consequence of a peripheral polyneuropathy (Pauls, 1991). All these observations might relate to the observed parietal hypometabolism. However, establishing a cause and effect relationship is particularly difficult.

Conclusions

Despite clinical evidence of normal intellectual function, neuroimaging studies in eating disorders reveal abnormal cerebral function. The correlation between brain glucose hypometabolism and morphological abnormalities on CT remains questionable but no correlations were observed between cerebral hypometabolism of glucose and cortical sulcal enlargement.

Absolute cerebral hypometabolism of glucose was observed in patients with eating disorders and in low weight depressed patients; it seems to be influenced by weight loss or bad nutrition. However, relative hypometabolism in the parietal cortex seems to be more specific to anorexia nervosa.

PET FDG studies in cohort of psychiatric patients often produce conflicting results. As not only absolute glucose metabolism, but perhaps also some particular differences in relative values seems to be influenced by nutritional factors, this might be suggested as explaining the variability in results. Depressed patients and schizophrenics often have irregular eating patterns and fluctuations in weight. It would therefore appear important to evaluate alimentary parameters at the time of PET studies with fluorodeoxyglucose but also in the period preceding them.

References

Andreasson PJ, Semple WE, Gross M, Holcomb HH, Dowling MS, Nordahl TE (1988) Functional localization of sustained attention: comparison to sensory stimulation in the absence of instruction. Neuropsychiat Neuropsychol Behav Neurol 1: 3-20

Artman H, Grau H, Adelmann M, Schleiffer R (1985) Reversible and non-reversible enlargement of cerebrospinal fluid in anorexia nervosa. Neuroradiology 27: 304-312

Baxter LR, Schwartz JM, Phelps ME, Mazziotta JC, Guze BH, Selin CE, Gerner RH, Sumida RM. Reduction of prefrontal cortex glucose metabolism common to three types of depression. Arch Gen Psychiat 46: 243-250

Baxter LR, Phelps ME, Mazziotta JC, Schwartz JM, Gerner RH, Selin CE, Sumida RM (1985) Cerebral metabolic rates for glucose in mood disorders. Arch Gen Psychiat 42: 441-447

Baxter LR, Phelps ME, Mazziotta JC, Guze BH, Swartz JM, Selin CE (1987) Local cerebral glucose metabolic rates in obsessive compulsive disorder. Arch Gen Psychiat 44: 211-218

Biver F, Goldman S, Delvenne V, Luxen A, De Maertelaer V, Hubain P, Mendlewicz J, Lotstra F (1994) Frontal and parietal metabolic disturbances in unipolar depression. Biol Psychiat 36: 381-388

Botez MI (1987) Le syndrome parietal. In: Botez MI (ed) Neuropsychologie clinique et neurologie du comportement. Masson, Montreal p135-154

Bowden PK, Touyz SW, Rodriguez PJ, Hensley R, Beumont PJV (1989) Distorting patient or distorting instrument? British J Psychiat 155: 196-201

Brewerton TD, Lydiard RB, Laraia MT, Shook JE, Ballenger JC (1992) CSF β-endorphin and dynorphin in bulimia nervosa. Am J Psychiat 149: 1086-1090

Bruch H (1977) Les yeux et le ventre. Payot, Paris

Buchsbaum MS, De Lisi LE, Holcomb H, Cappelletti J, King AC, Johnson J, Hazlett E, Dowling-Zimmerman S, Post RM, Morihisa J, Carpenter W, Cohen R, Pickar D, Weinberger DR, Margolin R Kessler RM (1984) Anteroposterior gradients in cerebral glucose use in schizophrenia and affective disorder. Arch Gen Psychiat 41: 1159-1166

Cantwell DP, Sturzenberger S, Burroughs J, Salkin B, Green JK (1977) Anorexia nervosa. An affective disorder? Arch Gen Psychiat 34: 1087-1093

Casper RC, Eckert ED, Halmi KA, Goldberg SC, Davis JM (1980) Bulimia. Its incidence and clinical importance in patients with anorexia nervosa. Arch Gen Psychiat 37: 1030-1035

Cohen RM, Semple WE, Gross M, Nordhal TE, King AC, Pickar D, Post RM. Evidence for common alterations in cerebral glucose metabolism in major affective disorders and schizophrenia. Neuropsychopharmacology 2: 241-254

Cohen RM, Semple WE, Gross M Holcomb HH, Dowling MS, Nordhal TE (1988) Functional localization of sustained attention: comparison to sensory stimulation in the absence of instruction. Neuropsychiat Neuropsychol Behav Neurol 1: 3-20

Datlof S, Coleman PD, Forbes GB, Kreipe RE (1986) Ventricular dilatation on CAT scans of patients with anorexia nervosa. Am J Psychiat 143: 96-98

Delvenne V, Lotstra F, Goldman S, Biver F, De Maertelaer V, Appelboom-Fondu J, Schoutens A, Bidaut LM, Luxen A, Mendlewicz J (1995). Brain hypometabolism of glucose in anorexia nervosa: a Pet-Scan study. Biol Psychiat 37: 161-169

Delvenne V, Goldman S, Simon Y, De Maertelaer V, Luxen A, Lotstra F. Brain hypometabolism of glucose in anorexia nervosa: normalization after weight gain. Biol Psychiat (sous presse)

Delvenne V, Goldman S, Simon Y, De Maertelaer V, Lotstra F. Brain hypometabolism of glucose in bulimia. Int J Eating Dis (sous presse)

Delvenne V, Goldman S, Biver F, De Maertelaer V, Wikler D, Damhaut P, Lotstra F. Brain hypometabolism of glucose in low weight depressed patients and in anorectic patients: a consequence of starvation. Submitted in J Affect Dis

Delvenne V, Goldman S, De Maertelaer V, Wikler D, Damhaut P, Lotstra F. Brain metabolism in anorectic pa-

tients and in affective disorder patients: influence of weight loss and depressive symptomatology. Submitted in Psychiat Res Neuroimag
Donohoe TP (1984) Stress-induced anorexia nervosa: implications for anorexia nervosa. Life sci 34: 203-218
Doraiswamy PM, Krichnan KRR, Figiel GS, Husain MM, Boyko OB, Rockwell WJK, Ellinwood EH (1990) A brain magnetic resonance imaging study of pituitary gland morphology in anorexia nervosa and bulimia. Biol Psychiat 28: 110-116
Dupont P, Orban GA, Vogels R, Bormans G, Nuyts J, Schiepers C, De Roo M, Mortelmans L (1993) Different perceptual tasks performed with the same visual stimulus attribute activate different regions of the human brain: a positron emission tomography study. Proc Nat Acad Sci 90: 10927-10931
Enzman DR, Lane B (1971) Cranial computed tomography findings in anorexia nervosa. J Comput Assist Tomogr 1: 410-414
Fava M, Copeland PM, Schweiger U, Herzog DB (1989) Neurochemical abnormalities of anorexia nervosa and bulimia nervosa. Am J Psychiat 146: 963-971
Fichter MM, Pirke KM, Pöllinger J, Wolfram G, Brunner E (1990) Disturbances in the hypothalamo pituitary adrenal and other neuroendocrine axes in bulimia. Biol Psychiat 27: 1021-1031
Fichter MM, Meister I, Koch HJ (1986) The measurement of body image disturbances in anorexia nervosa. British J Psychiat 148: 453-461
Fox CF (1981) Neuropsychological correlates of anorexia nervosa. Int J Psychiat Med 11: 285-290
Gershon, E.S., Schreiber, J.L., Hamovit, J.R., Dibble, E.D., Kaye, W., Nurnberger, J.I., Andersen, A.E., Ebert, M. (1984) Clinical findings in patients with anorexia nervosa and affective illness in their relatives. Am. J. Psychiat 141: 1419-1422
Gur RC, Gur RE, Resnick SM, Skolnick BE, Alavi A, Reivich M (1987) The effect of anxiety and cortical cerebral blood flow and metabolism. J Cereb Blood Flow Metab 7: 173-177
Gwirtsman HE, Gerner RH (1981) Neurochemical abnormalities in anorexia nervosa: similarities to affective disorders. Biol Psychiat 16: 991-995
Hagman JO, Buchsbaum MS, Wu JC, Rao SJ, Reynolds CA, Blinder BJ (1990) Comparison of regional brain metabolism in bulimia nervosa and affective disorder assessed with positron emission tomography. J Affect Dis 19: 153-162
Hamsher KS, Halmi KA, Benton AL (1981) Prediction of outcome of anorexia nervosa from neuropsychological status. Psychiat Res 4: 79-88
Hawkins RA, Biebuyck JF. Ketone bodies are selectively used by individual brain regions (1979) Science 205: 325-327
Heidrich R, Schmidt-Matthias H (1961) Encephalographische befunde bei anorexia nervosa. Arch Psychiat Nervenkr 202: 183-201
Herholz K, Krieg JC, Emrich HM, Pawlik G, Beil C, Pirke KM, Pahl JJ,Wagner R, Wienhard K, Ploog D, Heiss WD (1987) Regional cerebral glucose metabolism in anorexia nervosa measured by Positron Emission Tomography. Biol Psychiat 22: 43-51
Holden NL (1990) Is anorexia nervosa an obsessive-compulsive disorder? British J Psychiat 157, 1-5
Holland AJ, Sicotte N, Treasure J (1988) Anorexia nervoas: evidence for a genetic basis. J psychosom Res 32: 561-571
Horne RL, Van Vactor JC, Emerson S (1991) Disturbed body image in patients with eating disorders. Am J Psychiat 148: 211-215
Hsu LK, Crisp AH, Harding B. Outcome of anorexia nervosa (1979) Lancet 1: 61-65
Hudson JI, Pope HG, Jonas JM, Yurgelun-Todd D (1983) Family history study of anorexia nervosa and bulimia. British J Psychiat 142: 133-138
Husain MM, Black KJ, Doraiswamy PM, Shah SA, Rockwell WJK, Ellinwood EH, Krichnan KRR (1992) Subcortical brain anatomy in anorexia and bulimia. Biol Psychiat 31: 735-738
Jimerson DC, Lesem MD, Kaye WH, Brewerton TD (1992) Low serotonin and dopamine metabolite concentrations in cerebrospinal fluid from bulimic patients with frequent binge episodes. Arch Gen Psychiat 49: 132-138
Kaye WH, Ebert MH, Raleigh M, Lake RC (1984) Abnormalities in CNS monoamine metabolism in anorexia nervosa. Arch Gen Psychiat 41: 350-355
Kaye WH, Berrettini W, Gwirstsman H, Chretien M, Gold PW,George DT, Jimerson DC Ebert MH (1987) Reduced cerebrospinal fluid levels of immunoreactive pro-opiomelanocortin related peptides (including beta-endorphin) in anorexia nervosa. Life Sci. 41: 2147-2155
Kaye WH, Gwirtsman HE, George DT, Ebert MH (1991) Altered serotonin activity in anorexia nervosa after long-term weight restoration. Arch Gen Psychiat 48: 556-562
Kornreich L, Shapira A, Horev G, Danziger Y, Tyano S, Mimouni M (1991) CT et MR evaluation of the brain in patients with anorexia nervosa. Am J Neurol Radiol 12: 1213-1216
Krieg JC, Pirke KM, Lauer C, Backmund H (1988) Endocrine, metabolic, and cranial computed tomographic findings in anorexia nervosa. Biol Psychiat 23: 377-387
Krieg JC, Lauer C, Pirke KM (1989a) Structural Brain Abnormalities in Patients With Bulimia Nervosa. Psychiat Res 27: 39-48
Krieg JC, Lauer C, Leinsinger G, Pahl J, Schreiber W, Pirke KM, Moser EA (1989b) Brain morphology and regional cerebral blood flow in anorexia nervosa. Biol Psychiat 25: 1041-1048
Krieg JC, Holthoff V, Schreiber W, Pirke KM, Herholz K (1991). Glucose metabolism in the caudate nuclei of patients with eating disorders, measured by PET. Eur Arch Psychiat Clin Neurosci 240: 331-333
Laessle RG, Scheiger U, Pirke KM (1988). Depression as a correlate of starvation in patients with eating disorders. Biol Psychiat 23, 719-725
Laessle RG, Bossert S, Hank G, Hahlweg K and Pirke KM (1990) Cognitive performance in patients with bulimia nervosa: relationship to intermittent starvation. Biol Psychiat 27: 549-551
Lankenau H, Swigar ME, Bhimani S, Luchins D, Quinlan DM (1985) Cranial CT-scans in eating disorders and controls. Compreh Psychiat 26: 136-147
Lautenbacher S, Pauls AM, Strian F, Pirke KM, Krieg JC (1990) Pain perception in patients with eating disorders. Psychosom Med 52: 673-682
Martin F (1958) Pathologie des aspects neurologiques et psychiatriques de quelques manifestations carentielles avec troubles digestifs et neuro-endocriniens. Etude des altérations du système nerveux central dans deux cas d'anorexia survenue chez la jeune fille (dite anorexie mentale). Acta Neurol Belg 58: 816-830
Martinot J-L, Hardy P, Feline A, Huret J-D, Mazoyer B, Attar-Levy D, Pappata S, Syrota A (1990) Left prefrontal glucose hypometabolism in the depressed state: a confirmation. Am J Psychiat 147: 1313-1317

Maxwell JK, Tucker DM, Townes BD (1984) Asymmetric cognitive function in anorexia nervosa. Int J Neurosci 24: 37-44

Mazziotta JC, Phelps ME, Plummer D, Kuhl DE (1981) Quantification in positron emission tomography: 5. Physical-anatomical effects. J Comp Assist Tomogr 5: 734-743

McKay SE, Humphries LL, Allen ME, Clawson DR (1986) Neuropsychological test performance of bulimic patients. Int J Neurosci 30: 73-80

Nordahl TE, Benkelfat C, Semple WE, Gross M, King AC, Cohen RM (1989) Cerebral glucose metabolic rates in obsessive compulsive disorder. Neuropsychopharmacology 2: 23-28

Nordahl TE, Semple WE, Gross M, Mellman TA, Stein MB, Goyer P, King AC, Uhde TW, Cohen RM (1990) Cerebral glucose metabolic differences in patients with panic disorder. Neuropsychopharmacology 3: 261-272

Nozoe S, Naruo T, Yonekura R, Nakabeppu Y, Soejima Y, Nagai N, Nakajo M, Tanaka H (1991) Comparison of regional cerebral blood flow in patients with eating disorders. Brain Res Bull 36: 251-255

Nozoe S, Naruo T, Nakabeppu Y, Soejima Y, Nakajo M, Tanaka H (1993) Changes in regional cerebral blood flow in patients with anorexia nervosa detected through single photon emission tomography imaging. Biol Psychiat 34: 578-580

Nussbaum M, Shenker IR, Marc J, Klein M (1980) Cerebral atrophy in anorexia nervosa. J Pediat 96: 867-869

Pauls AM, Lautenbacher S, Strian F, Pirke KM, Krieg JC (1991) Assessment of somatosensory indicators of polyneuropathy in patients with eating disorders. Eur Arch Psychiat Clin Neurosci 241: 8-12

Phelps ME, Mazziotta JC, Baxter L, Gerner R (1984) Positron emission tomographic study of affective disorders: problems and strategies. Ann Neurol 15 (suppl) 149-156

Pirke KM, Platte P, Laessle R, Seidl M, Fichter MM (1992) The effect of a mental challenge test of plasma norepinephrine and cortisol in bulimia nervosa and in controls. Biol Psychiat 32: 202-206

Rivinus TM, Biederman J, Herzog DB, Kemper K, Harper GP, Harmatz JS Houseworth S (1988) Anorexia nervosa and affective disorders: a controlled family history study. Am. J. Psychiat 141: 1414-1418

Roland P (1992) Cortical representation of pain. Trans Int Neurosci 15: 3-5

Rothenberger A (1990) Adolescence and eating disorder: the obsessive compulsive syndrome. Psychiat Clin North Am 13: 469-488

Russell GFM (1979) Bulimia nervosa: an ominous variant of anorexia nervosa. Psychol Med 9: 429-448

Saper CB (1990) Hypothalamus. In: Paxinos G The human nervous system. Edit. Academic Press, San Diego: 389-413

Schlegel S, Kretzschmar K (1987) Computarize tomography in affective disorders. Part. I. Ventricular and sulcal measurements. Biol Psychiat 22: 4-14

Slade P (1985) A review of body-image studies in anorexia nervosa and bulimia nervosa. J Psychiat Res 19: 255-265

Small A, Madero J, Teagno L and Ebert M (1983) Intellect, perceptual characteristics and weight gain in anorexia nervosa. J Clin Psychol 39: 780-782

Van der Ham T, Van Strien DC, Van Engeland H (1994) Acta Psychiat Scand 90: 229-235.

Whitehouse AM, Freeman CPL, Annandale A (1988) Body size estimation in anorexia nervosa. British J Psychiat 153 (suppl. 2): 23-26

Williamson DA, Davis CJ, Goreczny AJ, Blouin DC (1989) Body image disturbances in bulimia nervosa: influences of actual body size. J Abn psychol 98: 97-99

Winokur, A., March, V., Mendels, J. (1980) Primary affective disorder in relatives of patients with anorexia nervosa. Am. J. Psychiat 137: 695-698

Wu JC, Hagman J, Buchsbaum MS, Blinder B, Derrfler M, Ye Tai W, Hazlett E, Sicotte N (1990) Greater left cerebral hemispheric metabolism in bulimia assessed by positron emission tomography. Am J Psychiat 147: 309-312

Wu JC, Buchsbaum MS, Hershey TG, Hazlett E, Sicotte N, Johnson JC (1991) PET in generalized anxiety disorder. Biol Psychiat 29: 1181-1199

Part three

Neurophysiological investigations and treatment

1. The influence of neuropeptides and methylphenidate on evoked potentials in autistic and hyperkinetic children

H. VAN ENGELAND, M.N. VERBATEN, L. JONKMAN, C. KEMNER

Neuropsychological studies suggest evidence that autistic and attention deficit disordered (ADHD) children suffer from attention and information processing deficits (Kootz et al., 1981; Prior, 1987; Corkum and Siegel, 1995). Autistic and ADHD children show deficits in particular on dichotic listening tasks, continuous performance tasks and so-called "frontal tasks" (Pennington and Ozonoff, 1996).

Neuropsychological tests offer information about the performance of children in a specific task situation (percentages of correct detections, false alarms, reaction times, perseveration). However, before a response is given, both stimulus and response related brain processes are completed and the performance measures show only the outcome of these processes. Psychophysiological studies have shown that by measuring event related brain potentials (ERPs) in addition to performance, one can say more about the cause of the different attention and information processes which precede the response. Besides that, ERP studies are able to give us information about the part of the brain involved in processing these stimuli.

In the past decade our research group has carried out a series of ERP studies in childhood psychiatric patients, in particular children suffering from autism or ADHD. Our primary interest was to find syndrome specific ERP deviances and to find out in what way drugs with a beneficial effect on the behaviour of autistic children and ADHD are able to normalise these ERP abnormalities. In this chapter we give an overview of our work and compare the results with studies reported in the literature.

Event related brain potentials (ERP)

The electrical activity of the brain can be measured from electrodes that are placed on the scalp; this is called an electroencephalogram (EEG). Event related brain potentials are short lasting changes in the electrical activity of the brain are time locked to an external event, for example a stimulus. ERP can be evoked by different stimuli, e.g., visual, auditory or somatosensory, and are considered as the cortical representations of perceptual and cognitive processes involved in the processing of a stimulus. Compared to the spontaneous electrical activity of the brain, ERP have a very small amplitude and are most often extracted from the EEG by averaging stretches of the EEG which follow of a presentation stimulus. By using this averaging method, electrical changes in brain activity which are time locked to the stimulus are amplified with respect to other electrical changes in the EEG which have no relation to the stimulus. The resulting ERP consists of a sequence of waves which are defined mainly by their polarity (positive or negative), latency (the time after presentation of the stimulus at which the wave occurs) and scalp distribution. A distinction can be made between very early waves, with a latency of less than 50-100 ms and later waves with a latency in excess of 100 ms.

The early waves are thought to reflect automatic processing of physical perceptual characteristics of stimuli and are called exogenous since they are less sensitive to psychological manipulation. The later waves are thought to reflect the processing of the cognitive semantic properties of a stimulus and are called endogenous, since they are more sensitive to psychological manipulation.

The ERP wave used to study selective attention processes is an early negative wave called processing negativity (PN). This is best measured in the dichotic listening task as used by e.g. Hillyard et al. (1973). In this task a different series of frequent and infrequent tones is presented to each ear; the subject's task is to direct attention to the tones in only one ear and to respond whenever a deviant tone (a target) appears in it. The attended ear is called the relevant channel, while the nonattended ear is the irrelevant channel. Two different types of selection process are involved in this task, namely, inter- and intra channel selection. Inter channel selection is needed for distinguishing between the relevant and irrelevant channels; these selection processes are referred to as the selective attention processes. There is a larger negativity to attended than to nonattended stimuli, so by subtracting ERP to unattended stimuli from ERP to attended stimuli, a negative wave, the PN, is obtained which reflects attentional processing of relevant information. Intra channel selection processes, i.e., selection between standard and deviant stimuli in the attended channel, are measured by the P3. This wave, which is of primary importance in studying stimulus evaluation processes is, a positive wave which occurs between 300 and 800 ms after stimulus presentation. Although the P3 has been described as being sensitive to a host of variables (Polich and Kok, 1995), for the purposes of the this chapter we will focus on the P3 in a particular task paradigm, the so-called oddball tasks. In such tasks, infrequently occurring stimuli (deviants) are presented in a series of frequently occurring stimuli (standards), and in 'active' oddball paradigms the task of the subject is to detect the deviant stimuli (targets) by responding to them. The P3 amplitude has been found to be larger to target than to standard stimuli and thus manifests target selection processes. Although it was formerly thought that the P3 only occurs to target stimuli to which subjects have to respond, P3 waves have also been found in response to deviant stimuli in "passive" task situations in which no response was required (Kemner et al., 1996). However, in most of these passive task paradigms P3 amplitudes were smaller than in active task situations. Dual task studies have further shown that the processes manifest in the P3 amplitude are dependent on the availability of capacity from specific resources. In such studies, a primary and a secondary task have to be performed at the same time, the subject being instructed to keep performance of the primary task at an optimal level. It is assumed that when the primary task is made more difficult, more processing capacity has to be invested in this task, and therefore less capacity will be available for processing of secondary task. The reduction of processing resources available for the processing of the secondary task stimuli is reflected by smaller P3 amplitudes to these stimuli. In contrast, the investment of more capacity in the primary task assumed to occur with increasing task difficulty is reflected by a P3 increment (Wickens et al., 1983).

In the oddball paradigm novelty and stimulus relevance are manipulated, inducing so-called orientating responses (OR). The OR can be observed in humans and animals as the result of the presentation of a novel stimulus. It involves a shift in attention to the newly presented stimulus and very often is called the "what is it?" reflex. Sokolov (1963) has intensively investigated the OR. In his view the physical and temporal features of a stimulus are encoded, after several stimulus presentations, in a neural model and each incoming stimulus is compared with this model. When a novel, stimulus is presented, an OR occurs, due to the mismatch between the stimulus and the neural model. The N1 is the ERP wave associated with the initial OR (Verbaten et al., 1986). The ERP wave associated with the change OR is the so-called "mismatch negativity (MMN)". The mismatch between the neural model and the properties of the novel stimulus produces a negative wave, i.e., the MMN, with a frontal or central maximum. The MMN is measured as a difference wave, obtained by subtracting the ERP to a standard stimulus from the ERP to a deviant stimulus. The amplitude of the MMN is larger, the larger the difference between the stimuli (Näätänen, 1990).

Differences in ERP waves between children and adults

Although the PN and P3 do occur in adults as well as in children there are some developmental differences in their latency, amplitude and topography. Berman and Friedman (1995) studied the development of (auditory) selective attention as reflected by the PN, by comparing normal children with adolescents and adults, mean ages 8, 14, and 23 years respectively. They reported that at the Fz electrode, both early (150-300 ms) and late (450-700 ms) portions of the PN were smaller in amplitude and longer in latency in children than in adolescents and adults. The smaller PN amplitude in children appeared to be caused by the fact that they had larger amplitudes to nonattended stimuli than adolescents and adults. It was concluded that "with age there is an improvement in the narrowing of attentional focus, with the major change taking form of greater facility in rejecting stimuli in the unattended channel". Furthermore, a difference in scalp topography was found: the early PN, was more frontally orientated in both children and adolescents than in adults, in whom there was a greater spread of negative activity to posterior and temporal scalp sites. The same pattern was found for the late component of the PN, except that children differed from both adolescents and adults. P3 amplitudes are consistently higher and latencies longer in children than in adults (Courchesne, 1978; Taylor, 1988). Recently, Fuchigami et al. (1995) reported that the developmental changes in P3 latency are different for attended and ignored stimuli; the latency of the task relevant P3 gradually shortened from 4 to 17 years of age, while the P3 latency in the ignore condition also shortened with age but stabilised at 12 years. Furthermore, the scalp distribution of the P3 is more posterior in younger children than in older children and adults.

Autism, brain event-related potentials and the effects of ORG-2766

Some ERP waves have been reported to be abnormal in autistic patients. In a number of studies, the auditory P3b component (parietal P3 with a latency of 300-600 ms to target stimuli) has been reported to be abnormally small in autistic patients (Courchesne et al., 1984, 1985, 1989; Dawson et al., 1988; Oades et al., 1988; Lincoln et al., 1993). A recent study (Kemner et al., 1995), however, failed to confirm this effect. Courchesne et al. (1984,1985) reported another abnormality in autistic patients pertaining to the Auditory PCz300 (auditory P3 at Cz in reaction to so-called novel auditory stimuli, i.e., infrequent, bizarre and unexpected sounds, presented in an auditory oddball task). The Auditory PCz300 was smaller in autistic patients than in normal subjects. Kemner et al. (1995) replicated and extended this finding by showing that autistic children differed not only from normal subjects, but also from children with attention deficit disorder with hyperactivity (ADDH) and or dyslexia. With respect to visual parietal P3b (target P3) responses, Pritchard et al. (1987) and Courchesne et al. (1985, 1989) found no differences between autistic and normal subjects.

Verbaten et al. (1991) found smaller visual occipital P3 components to (non task relevant) habituation stimuli, and a smaller P3 target standard difference in a task condition in autistic subjects than in normal and psychiatric control groups. The P3 amplitude had an occipital maximum in these groups of children (mean age of the autistic group 9.8 years).The smaller P3 components at Oz in response to standard stimuli in a passive condition were replicated by Kemner et al. (1994) in autistic children (mean age 9.8 years). They did not, however replicate the finding of smaller visual target P3 components in the autistic group, although the trend was in the same direction. In the study of Verbaten et al. (1991) where autistic children performed worse than normal children in a counting task), only high performing autistic children and normal children were taken into account; the high performing autistic children also showed the target standard difference at the Oz lead. These results suggest that relative task difficulty might have played a role; i.e., smaller P3 differences between autistic and control subjects in easy tasks. The absence of a significant OzP3 difference between autistic and control subjects with regard to visual targets in the study of Kemner et al. (1994) might also be understood thus; in that study, there was no significant between group difference in performance.

The ERP waves which precede the P3 component have not shown clear differences between autistic and control subjects. With visual stimuli, no differences between autistic and normal children were found for the amplitude of the N1 or the N2 component, and only one study (Kemner et al., 1994) found a larger P2 N2 wave to visual target stimuli in autistic subjects. More differences in early ERP waves between normal and autistic children were found with auditory stimuli, but findings have been inconsistent. Courchesne et al. (1984) found no differences in N1 amplitude between autistic and normal subjects, but in a replication study, (Courchesne et al., 1985) reported smaller N1 amplitudes (Fz) to infrequent stimuli, whereas Oades et al. (1988) found larger N1 (Fz) amplitudes to infrequent stimuli in autistic children. Kemner et al. (1995) did not find differences between autistic and control subjects for N1, N2, or mismatch negativity measures.

There is thus firm evidence that so called cognitive P3 waves are abnormal in autistic children.

Although infantile autism has come to be regarded as a neurologically based disorder (Prior, 1987), pharmacotherapy has not yet produced clear beneficial clinical effects on the core symptoms of autism.

Our group reported positive effects on the social behaviour of autistic children after a 4 week trial of the adrenocorticotropin (ACTH) analog ORG-2766 (20 mg/day). ORG-2766 is resistant to enzymatic degradation and thus can be administered orally. Its mode of action is unclear, but there is general agreement that it has an effect on the central nervous system and thereby on behaviour, possibly through actions on endogenous opioid systems (Wolterink and Van Ree, 1989). Buitelaar et al. (1990) found that children treated with ORG-2766 manifested more goal directed looking behaviour and less stereotyped behaviour in semi standardised playroom observation. A second study, in which autistic children were given ORG-2766 (40 mg/day) for 8 weeks (Buitelaar et al., 1992), confirmed the earlier results. The positive effects of ORG-2766 were attributed to improved visual attention.

We recently examined the effects of 6 weeks of treatment with ORG-2766 (40 mg/day) on brain event related potentials of autistic children in a double blind placebo controlled study (Verbaten et al., 1996) of 36 autistic children (10 girls, 26 boys, age range 6.9-14.0 years, mean 10.5 years). Mean performance, verbal, and total IQ on the Wechsler intelligence scale for children (revised) were 84.2 ± 20.2, 81.5 ± 20.6, and 81.2 ± 20.2 respectively. Subjects fulfilled DSM III-R criteria for autistic disorder. Mean CARS score is 39.0 (s.d. 4.1). The children performed oddball tests in visual and auditory modalities. Half the children (18) received ORG-2766 (40 mg/day) for 6 weeks and the other 18 received a placebo during the same period. All children were tested twice; once before either ORG-2766 or placebo was administered, and once during 6 weeks of medication (randomised parallel design). The occipital P3 waves in reaction to visible target stimuli, but not to visual standard stimuli, increased in amplitude after 6 weeks of treatment with ORG-2766. This effect of ORG-2766 on the occipital P3 to visual targets might mean, given the fact that the P3 is generally associated with controlled evaluative processes (Donchin, 1981), that these processes improve with ORG-2766 treatment.

Another abnormality in autistic children involving the occipital P3, described by Kemner et al. (1995), was a larger occipital P3 to auditory deviant stimuli in the task condition in autistic children than in normal and psychiatric controls. Our study revealed that this auditory occipital target P3 decreased in autistic children under the influence of ORG-2766. This decrease was not restricted to the occipital lead. The P3 component also decreased significantly at Cz, to both standard and deviant stimuli. Although such decreases were not significant at Fz and Pz, there was a trend at Pz in the same direction. Administration of ORG-2766 did not affect the so-called Auditory PCz300 in response to novel auditory stimuli.

Pertaining to the auditory modality and also to novel stimuli, an effect of ORG-2766 was found on early processing. The N1 wave at the frontal lead in response to novel stimuli increased under the influence of ORG-2766, but only in the non-task condition; in the task-condition, no increase was found. Born et al. (1989) had a similar finding in normal subjects, reporting that ORG-2766 increased the auditory N1 wave to task irrelevant stimuli in a dichotic listening task, whereas it decreased the P3 wave to auditory targets.

We thus found an effect of ORG-2766 on task relevant visual information processing as reflected by the occipital P3 wave to target stimuli in autistic children, while the early automatic components of such processing (N1) were not influenced by the drug. Controlled auditory processing, manifest in the auditory P3 wave, decreased under the influence of ORG-2766, probably as a result of a disinhibiting effect of the drug on an earlier phase of processing, as indicated by an increased frontal N1 wave to task irrelevant novel stimuli. A remarkable finding was that, despite beneficial effects of ORG-2766 on visual information processing, no effects were found at the behavioural level; ORG-2766 did not affect task performance in the oddball tasks in this study.

ADHD, ERP and methylphenidate

Of the ERP measures the P3 is the one most studied in children with ADHD. In most of the P3 studies in these children, oddball tasks, or so called continuous performance tasks (CPT), were used; in the literature one also often encounters the term "vigilance tasks" for these types of task. In a CPT, ordered displays of letters, numbers, or colours, etc., are presented to the subjects and the task is to press a reaction time button to an infrequently presented subset of these characters (targets), and to withold responding to all other, more frequently presented, stimuli. Targets can be e.g. the letter X (CPT-X), or the letter X preceded by the letter A (CPT-AX version) or any letter preceded by the same letter (CPT-Double). In the CPT and oddball studies in which the performance and P3 of children with ADHD was compared to that of controls, children with ADHD generally performed worse and had smaller P3 amplitudes (Klorman et al., 1979; Michael et al., 1981; Holcomb et al., 1985, 1986; Robaey et al., 1992; Taylor et al., 1993; Winsberg et al., 1993; Kemner et al., 1996). From these studies it can be concluded that the finding of smaller P3 amplitudes in children with ADHD is fairly consistent across paradigms, although in some studies P3 amplitudes appear to be smaller to only *target* stimuli and in other studies it is a more general phenomenon across stimulus types. Regarding target P3 amplitudes, it has to be noted that it is not always clear whether in the different studies the target P3 was computed on the basis of stimulus or response categories (to all targets irrespective of the response or only to correctly detected targets). However, in almost all of these studies differences from P3 in normals were found, whereas Corkum and Siegel (1993) reported that differences in performance occurred in only half of the studies.

Dual task studies have produced evidence that the P3 amplitude can be considered a measure of processing capacity. In these studies, a primary and a secondary task have to be performed at the same time, with the subject instructed to keep performance of the primary task at an optimal level. It is assumed that when the primary task is made more difficult, more processing capacity has to be invested in this task, and therefore less capacity will be available for processing of the secondary task. Since the processes that underly the P3 are capacity limited, the reduction of processing resources available for the processing of secondary task stimuli is usually reflected by smaller P3 amplitudes to these stimuli (Wickens et al., 1983). In contrast, the investment of more capacity in the primary task that is assumed to occur with increasing task difficulty, is reflected by a P3 increment (Wickens et al., 1983).

Another technique which can be used for studying capacity trade-off is the so-called irrelevant probe technique. In probe studies, task irrelevant stimuli (probes) are presented against the background of an ongoing task. The advantage of the probe method over the dual task procedure is that there are minimal interference effects of the task irrelevant probe stimuli with the processing of task stimuli, which is especially important when working with children.

In a study by Kenemans et al. (1992) the effects of task difficulty manipulations on the N1, P2, P2 N2 and P3 in response to irrelevant visual probes were studied by presenting adult subjects an active decision task (also visual) that varied in difficulty. During hard and easy versions of the active decision task the same visual probes were presented and probe amplitudes were compared across conditions to study load effects. The P2 N2 complex showed a standard deviant effect (higher deviant amplitudes) independent of the load manipulation; a similar standard deviant effect was noted for the P3 but seemed to occur in only the easy task. It was concluded that the P2 N2 and P3 reflect different stages of the attention orientating reaction to deviant irrelevant probes in which only the latter (P3) process is capacity limited.

We recently studied attention capacity in 14 children with ADHD and 14 normal children by measuring performance and ERP with an irrelevant probe technique (as used by Kenemans et al., 1992), adjusted for children (Jonkman et al., in press). Three types of task irrelevant visual probes (standard, deviant and novel) were presented against the background of one of two visual tasks which varied in difficulty. The parietal P3 wave was measured in response to task stimuli and probes. The children with ADHD made significantly fewer correct detections than the normal children in both easy and hard task, but compared to normals they showed only a trend towards a larger performance deterioration with increasing task difficulty. P3 analysis suggested that the children with ADHD subjects invested the same amount of capacity as the normal subjects in the easy task but less in the hard task. Both groups showed a similar reduction of novel-probe P3 amplitude with increasing task load. It was concluded that children with ADHD do not suffer from a shortage in attention capacity; the evidence is in favour of a capacity allocation defect rather than a capacity availability deficit. The probe P3 showed that the children with ADHD had spare capacity, but were unable to invest it in the hard task.

Smaller P3 in children with ADHD might be caused by abnormal early ERP waves (N1, N2 and PN) reflecting selective attention processes. Verbaten et al. (1994), using a CPT, found that these children showed significantly smaller frontal N2 waves and PN waves than normal children.

Two dichotic listening studies in which both performance and ERP waves of hyperactive boys were compared with those of normal controls (Zambelli et al., 1977; Loiselle et al., 1980) showed that hyperactive boys performed worse (lower hit percentages and more false alarms, i.e., errors of commission) than the controls. They also failed to show enhanced N1 amplitudes in response to attended stimuli when compared to nonattended stimuli, while controls did show such a selective attention effect. Later, Satterfield et al. (1988,1990) performed two selective attention experiments in which the visual and auditory modalities were the relevant and irrelevant input channels, respectively, and vice versa. Only data from the condition in which auditory stimuli had to be attended were reported, however. In the first study (Satterfield et al., 1988) the performance and ERP of 6 year old children with ADHD were compared with those of normal controls of the same age. It was found that these boys performed worse (lower percentage of hits and more false alarms) than their normal peers. Also, pointing to a deficit in selective attention, they did not show a significant frontal PN (to standard stimuli) while the normal controls did. In the second study, 6 and 8 year olds were compared (Satterfield et al., 1990). Both 6 and 8 year old controls showed frontal PN, while children with ADHD showed this frontal PN only at age eight, but they did not show a PN with a central maximum, which was present in the 8 year old controls.

Thus, ERP studies have shown that children with ADHD have deficits in selective attention (N1, N2 and PN) as well as in cognitive evaluative processes (P3). The latter deficit seems to be a capacity allocation rather than a capacity availability deficit.

Most methylphenidate (MPH) studies have focused on the P3 in CPT or oddball tasks. The most common finding from these studies is that, besides improving behavioural performance, MPH enhances P3 amplitudes to targets only, or to both targets and non targets (Klorman et al., 1979, 1983, 1988, 1991; Michael et al., 1981; Halliday et al., 1983; Coons et al., 1987; Syrigou-Papavasiiiou et al., 1988; Fitzpatrick et al., 1992; Bailey et al., 1993; Frank, 1993; Taylor et al., 1993; Winsberg et al., 1993; Verbaten et al., 1994; Klorman et al., 1994).

The number of studies focussing on the effect of methylphenidate on selective attention processes in ADHD is only small. Klorman et al. (1990) found MPH effects on only early ERP waves to auditory stimuli. Novak et al. (1995), using a visuo spatial selective attention task found that although correct detections were enhanced by MPH, the stimulant does not alter the attention effects on the N1. Verbaten et al. (1994), using a CPT task, found that MPH increased frontal N2 waves. These inconclusive results stimulated our group to study the effects of methylphenidates on the ERP of children with ADHD in more detail, with special attention for the effects of MPH on selective attention processes and on possible capacity related deficits in ADHD. In a first study 18 children participated in a double blind placebo controlled study in which the effect of 15 mg MPH on auditory and visual selective attention tasks was determined by presenting frequent (90 %) and infrequent (10 %) stimuli in both relevant and irrelevant input channels (Jonkman et al., 1997). The subjects' task was to respond to the infrequent tones in the relevant input channel. Processing activity (negative and positive) was assessed for both tasks. N1, P2, N2 and P3 peaks were scored in the auditory tasks and N1, P1, N2, P2 and P3 peaks were scored in the visual tasks. The effects of MPH appeared to be more prevalent in the visual than in the auditory condition. In the visual condition MPH enhanced the percentage of hits, caused higher central parietal and occipital P3 amplitudes to attended stimuli (both standards and deviants), and also enhanced the frontal processing negativity (PN). In the auditory task MPH did not influence performance, but it enhanced the frontal PN as well as the parietal and occipital P3 amplitudes to all stimulus types. It was therefore concluded that some visual and auditory "deficits" detected in ADHD in an earlier study (Jonkman et al., 1997) were "normalised" by MPH, but others were not. Abnormalities in later stimulus processing, as evidenced by abnormally small P3 amplitudes at different leads in both visual and auditory modalities, were "normalised" by MPH. In the visual condition this effect was more specific (only to attended stimuli) than in the auditory condition (to all stimulus types). Furthermore MPH had a beneficial effect on the frontal PN in visual as well as in auditory modalities. So MPH does affect selective attention (PN) as well as cognitive evaluative processing (P3) in children with ADHD. However, these effects do not necessarily lead to a higher level of performance, as can be seen in the auditory condition. Further, MPH changed some correlations between performance (hits, reaction times) and P3 in the direction of "normality" but only in the auditory modality.

In a second study we investigated whether MPH had beneficial effects on attention capacity allocation deficits that earlier were found in a group of 14 children with ADHD (Jonkman et al., in press). A so-called irrelevant probe technique was used to measure MPH effects on ERP and performance. Three types of irrelevant visual probe (standard, deviant and novel) were presented against the background of visual tasks which varied in difficulty. The parietal P3 wave was measured in response to task stimuli and probes. MPH was expected to enhance the task P3 and percentage of hits, particularly in the hard task since in this task allocation defects were established in the earlier study (Jonkman et al., 1997). However MPH enhanced the percentage of correct responses and task P3 amplitudes in both easy and hard tasks. Probe P3 amplitudes, indicating spare capacity, were not influenced by MPH. It was concluded that MPH does not improve the capacity-allocation deficit that was found earlier in these children, but that MPH has some less specific enhancing effects on performance and ERP.

To summarise, the most important conclusions from our recent selective attention (dichotic listening) studies are that, when compared to normal children, children with ADHD showed deficits in early auditory selective attention processes; and later cognitive evaluation processes to target stimuli in demanding task situations (probably due to deficient allocation strategies), as well as to non-target stimuli in all situations. Thus, there is little evidence for specific attention deficits in ADHD, since deficits occur at all processing levels. In our studies methylphenidate has found to improve the performance of children of ADHD by enhancing the overall level of performance (accuracy) rather than alleviating specific deficits; and to enhance PN and P3 amplitudes in a non specific way. In interpreting these results one has to keep in mind that only small groups of ADHD children have been investigated and it is not clear to what extent the results are applicable to the total ADHD population. Furthermore, no "pure" ADHD groups were used, and this leaves the possibility that some of the results are caused by the comorbidity of other disorders such as conduct disorder and learning disabilities. In future research this has to be investigated by comparing the results of pure and comorbid ADHD groups.

References

Bailey K, Perros P, Price G (1993) ERP changes after a single dose of methylphenidate on a visual continuous performance task. Biol Psychol 37: 45

Berman S, Friedman D (1995) The development of selective attention as reflected by event-related brain potentials. J Exp Child Psychol 59: 1-31

Born J, Kern W, Pietrowsky R, Sittig W, Fehm HL (1989) Fragments of ACTH affect electrophysiological signs of controlled processing in humans. Psychopharmacology 99: 439-444

Buitelaar JK, Van Engeland H, De Kogel FH, De Vries H, Van Hooff J, Van Ree JM (1992) The adrenocorticotropic hormone (4-9) analog ORG-2766 benefits autistic children: report on a second controlled clinical trial. J Am Acad Child Adolesc Psychiat 31: 1149-1156

Buitelaar JK, Van Engeland H, Van Ree JM, De Wied D (1990) Behavioral effects of ORG-2766, a synthetic analog of the adrenocorticotropic hormone (4-9) analog, in 14 outpatient autistic children. J Autism Dev Disord 20: 467-478

Coons HW, Klorman R, Borgstedt AD (1987) Effects of methylphenidate on adolescents with a childhood history of attention deficit disorder. II. Information processing. J Am Acad Child Adolesc Psychiat 26: 368-374

Corkum PV, Siegel LS (1993) Is the continuous performance task a valuable research tool for use with children with Attention Deficit Hyperactivity Disorder? J Child Psychol Psychiat 34: 1217-1239

Courchesne E, Lincoln AJ, Kilman BA, Galambos R (1985) Event-related brain correlates of the processing of novel visual and auditory information processing in autism. J Autism Dev Disord 15: 55-76

Courchesne E, Kilman BA, Galambos R, Lincoln AJ (1984) Autism: processing of novel auditory information assessed by event-related potentials. Electroencephalogr Clin Neurophysiol 59: 238-248

Courchesne E, Lincoln AJ, Yeung-Courchesne R, Elmasian R, Grillon C (1989) Pathophysiologic findings in nonretarded autism and receptive developmental disorder. J Autism Dev Disord 19: 1-17

Courchesne E (1978) Neurophysiological correlates of cognitive development: changes in long-latency event-related potentials from childhood to adulthood. Electroencephalogr Clin Neurophysiol 45: 468-482

Dawson G, Finley C, Phillips S, Galpert L, Lewy A (1988) Reduced P3 amplitude of the event-related brain potential: its relationship to language ability in autism. J Autism Dev Disord 18: 493-504

Donchin E (1981) Psychophysiology 18: 493-513

Fitzpatrick PA, Klorman R, Brumaghim JT, Borgstedt AD (1992) Effects of sustained release and standard preparations of methylphenidate on attention deficit disorder. J Am Acad Child Adolesc Psychiat 31: 226-234

Frank Y (1993) Visual event related potentials after methylphenidate and sodium valproate in children with attention deficit hyperactivity disorder. Clin Electroencephalogr 24: 19-23

Halliday R, Rosenthal JH, Naylor H, Callaway E (1976) Averaged evoked potential predictors of clinical improvement in hyperactive children treated with methylphenidate: An initial study and replication. Psychophysiology 13: 429-440

Hillyard SA, Hink RF, Schwent VL, Picton TW (1973) Electrical signs of selective attention in the human brain. Science 182: 177-180

Holcomb PJ, Ackerman PT, Dykman RA (1986) Auditory event-related potentials in attention and reading disabled boys. Int J Psychophysiol 3: 263-273

Holcomb PJ, Ackerman PT, Dykman RA (1985) Cognitive event-related brain potentials in children with attention and reading deficits. Psychophysiology 22: 656-667

Jonkman LM, Kemner C, Verbaten MN, Koelega HS, Camfferman G, Van der Gaag R, Buitelaar JK, Van Engeland H (1997) Effects of methylphenidate on event-related potentials and performance of attention deficit hyperactivity disorder children in auditory and visual selective attention tasks. Biol Psychiat 41: 690-702

Kemner C, Verbaten MN, Cuperus J, Camfferman G, Slangen JL, Van Engeland H (1994) Visual and somatosensory event-related brain potentials in autistic children and three different control groups. Electroencephalogr Clin Neurophysiol 92: 225-237

Kemner C, Verbaten MN, Cuperus JM, Camfferman G, Van Engeland H (1995) Auditory event-related brain potentials in autistic children and three different control groups. Biol Psychiat 38: 150-165

Kemner C, Verbaten MN, Koelega HS, Buitelaar JK, van der Gaag RJ, Camfferman G, van Engeland H (1996) Event-related brain potentials in children with attention deficit and hyperactivity disorder (ADDH): effects of stimulus deviancy and task relevance in the visual and auditory modality. Biol Psychiat

Kenemans JL, Verbaten MN, Melis CJ, Slangen JL (1992) Visual stimulus change and the orienting reaction: event-related potential evidence for a two stage process. Biol Psychol 33: 97-114

Klorman R, Salzman LF, Pass HL, Borgstedt AD, Dainer KB (1979): Effect of methylphenidate on hyperactive children's evoked responses during passive and active attention. Psychophysiology 16: 23-29

Klorman R, Salzman LF, Bauer LO, Coons HW, Borgstedt AD, Halpern WI (1983) Effects of two doses of methylphenidate on cross situational and borderline hyperactive children's evoked potential. Electroencephalogr Clin Neurophysiol 56: 169-185

Klorman R, Brumaghim JT, Salzman LF, Strauss J, Borgstedt AD, McBride MC, Loeb S (1990) Effects of methylphenidate on processing negatives in patients with attention deficit hyperactivity disorder. Psycholphysiology 27: 328-337

Klorman R, Brumaghim JT, Fitzpatrick PA, Borgstedt AD, Strauss J (1994) Clinical and cognitive effects of methylphenidate on children with attention deficit disorder as a function of aggresion oppositionality and age. J Abn Psychol 103: 206-221

Lincoln AJ, Courchesne E, Harms L, Allen M (1993) Contextual probability evaluation in autistic, receptive developmental disorder and control children: event-related potential evidence. J Autism Dev Disord 23: 37-58

Loiselle D, Stamm JS, Maitinsky S, Whipple SC (1980) Evoked potential and behavioral signs of attentive dysfunctions in hyperactive boys. Psychophysiology 17: 193-201

Michael RL, Klorman R, Salzman F, Borgstedt AD, Dainer KB (1981) Normalizing effects of methylphenidate on hyperactive children's vigilance performance and evoked potentials. Psychophysiology 18: 665-677

Michael RL, Klorman R, Salzman F, Borgstedt AD, Dainer KB (1981) Normalizing effects of methylphenidate on hyperactive children's vigilance performance and evoked potentials. Psychophysiology 18: 665-677

Näätänen R (1990) The role of attention in auditory information processing as revealed by event-related potentials and other brain measures of cognitive functioning. Behav Brain Sci 13: 201-288

Novak GP, Solanto M, Abikoff H (1995) Spatial orienting and focused attention in attention deficit hyperactivity disorder. Psychophysiology 32: 546-559

Oades RD, Walker MK, Geffe LB, Stern LM (1988) Event-related potentials in autistic and healthy children on an auditory choice reaction time test. Int J Psychophysiol 6: 25-37

Pennington BF, Ozonoff S (1996) Executive functions and developmental psychopathology. J Child Psychol Psychiat 1: 51-87

Polich J, Kok A (1995) Cognitive and biological determinants of P300: an integrative review. Biol Psychol 41: 103-146

Prior MR (1987) Biological and neuropsychological approaches to childhood autism. British J Psychiat 150: 8-17

Pritchard WS, Raz N, August GJ (1987) Visual augmenting/reducing and P_{300} in autistic children. J Autism Dev Disord 17: 231-242

Robaey P, Breton F, Dugas M, Renault B (1992) An event-related potential study of controlled and automatic processes in 6-8 year old boys with attention deficit hyperactivity disorder. Electroencephalogr Clin Neurophysiol 82: 330-340

Satterfield JH, Schell AM, Nicholas TW, Satterfield BT, Freese TH (1990) Ontogeny of selective attention effects on event-related potentials in attention deficit hyperactivity disorder and normal boys. Biol Psychiat 28: 879-903

Satterfield JH, Schell AM, Nicholas T, Backs RW (1988) Topographic study of auditory event-related potentials in normal boys and boys with attention deficit disorder with hyperactivity. Psychophysiology 25: 591-606

Syrigou-Papavasiiiou A, Lycaki H, LeWitt PA, Verma NP, Spivak D, Chayasirisobhon S (1988) Dose response effects of chronic methylphenidate administration on late event-related potentials in attention deficit disorder. Clin Electroencephalogr 19: 129-133

Taylor MJ (1988) Developmental changes in ERPs to visual language stimuli. Biol Psychol 26: 321-338

Taylor MJ, Voros JG, Logan WJ, Malone MA (1993) Changes in event-related potentials with stimulant medication in children with attention deficit hyperactivity disorder. Biol Psychol 36: 139-156

Verbaten MN, Roelofs JW, Sjouw W, Slangen JL (1986) Different effects of uncertainty and complexity on single trial visual ERPs and the SCR-OR in non signal conditions. Psychophysiology 23: 254-262

Verbaten MN, Roelofs JW, Van Engeland H, Kenemans JL, Slangen JL (1991) Abnormal visual event-related potentials of autistic children. J Autism Dev Disord 21: 449-470

Verbaten MN, Kemner C, Buitelaar JK, Van Ree JM, Van Beijsterveld CEM, Van Engeland H (1996) Effects of ORG-2766 on brain event-related potentials of autistic children. Psychiat Res 63: 33-45

Verbaten MN, Overtoom CCE, Koelega HS, Swaab-Barneveld H, Van der Gaag RJ, Buitelaar JK, Van Engeland H (1994) Methylphenidate influences both early and late ERP waves of ADHD children in a continuous performance test. J Abn Child Psychol 22: 1-18

Wickens C, Kramer A, Vanasse L, Donchin E (1983) Performance of concurrent tasks: A psychophysiological analysis of the reciprocity of information processing resources. Science 221: 1080-1082

Winsberg BG, Javitt DC, Shanahan Silipo G, Doneshka MD (1993) Mismatch negativity in hyperactive children: effects of methylphenidate. Psychopharmacol Bull 29: 229-233

Wolterink G, Van Ree JM (1989) Opioid systems in the amygdala can serve as substrate for the behavioral effects of the ACTH 4-9 analog ORG-2766. Neuropeptides 14: 129-136

Zambelli AJ, Stamm JS, Maitinsky S, Loiselle DL (1977) Auditory evoked potentials and selective attention in formerly hyperactive adolescent boys. Am J Psychiat 134: 742-747

2. Electrophysiological correlates of vitamin B6 and magnesium treatment in autism

J. MARTINEAU

Autism, one of the most intractable of disorders, has been challenged over the years by numerous alternatives to conventional therapeutic methods. Progress has been made in methodology and design in recent years (Klein et al., 1994). There are a number of theories, with some supportive evidence, that a variety of biochemical abnormalities may exist in autism (Campbell and Shay, 1995). Antidopaminergic and antiserotoninergic agents, serotonin reuptake blockers, opiate antagonists and dopamine agonists have been explored (Campbell and Cueva, 1995). Only haloperidol has been studied systematically. Although its effectiveness has been demonstrated, some investigators felt that the drug does not alter the core of autism (Rapoport and Kruesi, 1985) and it is associated with tardive dyskinesia (Campbell et al, 1988a); furthermore, not all patients respond to it (Locascio et al., 1991). The psychoactive agents studied in autism differ in their mechanisms of action, but all reduce hyperactivity: L-Dopa (Campbell et al., 1972, 1976), methylphenidate (Strayhorn et al., 1988), haloperidol (Anderson et al., 1989; Perry et al., 1989), pimozide (Ernst et al., 1992), fenfluramine (Campbell et al., 1988b), naltrexone (Campbell et al., 1993; Herman et al., 1989), clomipramine (Gordon et al., 1993) and desipramine (Gordon et al., 1993).

Other treatments used in children with autism include vitamins. Among them, vitamin B6 has been reported to give promising results in some autistic patients.

In 1965, Heeley and Roberts investigated tryptophan metabolism in a group of 16 psychotic children and reported a defect in 9 cases which may represent impaired function of pyridoxal 5' phosphate dependent systems. Of the 9 children with abnormal tryptophan metabolism, four were treated with an oral pyridoxine supplement of 30 mg/day and when retested with a tryptophan load, showed normal tryptophan metabolism.

At about the same time, Rimland was corresponding with parents of autistic children and tabulating their observations on the effects of various drugs, vitamins, minerals, etc.. He was "struck by the extent to which the trial and error efforts had so often converged to the same four vitamins: ascorbic acid, niacin, pyridoxine and to a lesser extent, pantothenic acid" (Rimland, 1973). He then conducted an experiment with 190 autistic children of parents who had agreed to participate in a high dosage vitamin study. Children were given multiple vitamins B and C for two weeks; then vitamin B6 and niacin amide were introduced. Two weeks after that, pantothenic acid was added. It was a 24 week-study, and 6 weeks before the end of the study, a 4 week no treatment period was introduced, so that the effects of discontinuing the vitamins could be noted. Rimland (1974) wrote that "the most obvious and dramatic changes attributable to a single vitamin were brought about by vitamin B6".

Then, Callaway (1977) and Rimland et al (1979) carried out a double blind vitamin B6 withdrawal study using 16 autistic children who had already participated in megavitamin treatment regimens. Children were selected only if their parents stated that: B6 improved their children, its withdrawal resulted in a return of symptoms, and a reinstitution of B6 had resulted again in improvement. The children received B6 and magnesium, which was added to prevent possible side-effects due to the vitamin therapy, such as increased activity level, sleeplessness, enuresis, sound sensitivity and irritability (Callaway, 1977). This study provided evidence that the double blind withdrawal of B6 produced an increase in disturbed behaviour of these autistic children.

There are six biologically active forms of vitamin B6: pyridoxine, pyridoxal, pyridoxamine and their respective phosphates. In the form of pyridoxal phosphate, vitamin B6 serves as a coenzyme for a wide variety of enzymes of amino acid metabolism. Human beings are unable to synthesise vitamin B6, but it six biologically active forms can be converted into each other. Vitamin B6 is involved in crucial steps in the synthesis of several neurotransmitters (Gualtieri et al., 1983), for instance decarboxylation of glutamic acid into GABA, but also in the formation of serotonin (5-HT), dopamine (DA), noradrenaline (NA) and adrenaline (A). Individuals with autism may have abnormalities in the processes forming these neurotransmitters (Martineau et al., 1994), making vitamin B6 a viable form of treatment. The catecholamine system, including the neurotransmitter dopamine, may play an important role in several notable functions such as motor control, cognition, and regulation of hormone release (Moore and Bloom, 1978). Measures of averaged evoked potentials (AEP), a measure of the brain's ability to process external sensory stimuli, are thought to reflect catecholamine metabolism (Barthélémy et al., 1988; Schafer and MacKean, 1975). Although the relationship between AEP and clinical responses in behaviour has not been firmly established (Martineau et al., 1981), investigators have found lower amplitudes, shorter latency periods, and greater variability in the AEP of autistic children than in control subjects (Barthélémy et al., 1988; Martineau et al., 1988; Small et al., 1969). Barthélémy et al. (1988) suggested that these differences in AEP may be a reflection of abnormal function of the dopamine system and furthermore, may be linked to autistic behaviour such as selective attention.

The purpose of the present study is, firstly, to review studies we conducted with vitamin B6 and magnesium and the electrophysiological correlates of this treatment in autistic subjects and secondly, to present new data concerning the relationships between behavioural and electrophysiological changes during treatment with vitamin B6 and magnesium.

Review of prior studies

Methods

Three types of paradigm were used to investigate electrophysiological effects of vitamin B6 and magnesium in autistic children. For each paradigm, evoked potentials were recorded at a time when the child was able to remain relatively quiet and immobile for half an hour and each child was familiarised with the laboratory. The nurse who usually took care of the child was present. The child was in a dark, soundproof room, seated in a confortable armchair. Silver chloride electrodes were placed on the scalp at central (Cz) and occipital (Oz) locations according to the 10-20 system and were referred to linked electrodes placed on the earlobes. The ground electrode was placed on the middle of the forehead. Electrodes positioned 1cm above and 1cm below the external canthus of each eye recorded eye movements (EOG). All electrode impedances were less than 5 KOhms.

Paradigm 1

The EEG amplifiers were set at a bandpass for the low frequencies of 2500 Hz (3 dB down). Auditory and visual evoked responses (AER and VER) were recorded. The session consisted of 100 tone bursts (100 ms, 1000 Hz, 90 dB) and 100 flashes of light (0.1 ms, 1200 lux). The stimuli were given regularly every 2 s. A PDP 11/10 was used for averaging and measuring AER and VER amplitudes and latencies. EOG artefacts were rejected automatically.

Paradigm 2

The signals were amplified by an Alvar Electronic AC amplifier set for a bandpass down 3 dB at 0.1 Hz and 100 Hz and providing a gain of 10^5. The conditioned stimulus was a brief (4 ms) sound at 1 KHz, 25 dB above threshold, presented through two speakers placed 35 cm directly lateral to each ear. AEP recordings and auditory threshold detection were routinely carried out on children admitted in the unit. The unconditioned stimulus was a 0.1 ms, 1200 lux flash of light from a lamp 40 cm in front of the subject's eyes. No specific instruction was given. The experimente checked the EEG recording throughout the experiment. As long as the tracing showed mecanogram, electromyogram or large eye movement, no stimulus was given. There were three types of trial: sound (S), light (L), sound and light (S-L). During each session, there were 12 series of 20 trials. Trials were given after random intervals which ranged from 4 to 30 s. In the first four series of trials, S was used alone (habituation), in the next four series, L was presented 840 ms after S to produce conditioning (S-L) and in the last four series, L was used alone (L). Stimulation was given 100 ms after a synchronisation signal. Baselines were taken as the mean over the 100 ms prior to stimulation. Data were digitised at 200 samples/s. Each epoch was 2 s, and 20 epochs were averaged before being printed out on an X-Y plotter for measurement. In normal children, the auditory stimulus induced a stable AER at the vertex. When the sound was coupled with light, the sound induced a large, stable response recorded at the occipital lead (association) and a decrease in AER amplitude was observed at the vertex (Martineau et al., 1984). In autistic children, regardless of the stimulus used, AER appeared very variable, not well differentiated from the baseline, with short latencies and weak amplitudes. Measurements were made on both auditory and visual evoked potentials, of the latencies of the first positive peak (P1), the first negative peak (N1) and the second positive peak (P2) and the peak to peak amplitude of P1N1 and N1P2.

Paradigm 3

On each trial, the EEG and EOG were amplified by a minihuit Alvar polygraph (3 dB bandwidth, 0.5-2000 Hz). The EEG was digitised every 4 ms for a 2.3 s period which began 500 ms before the stimulus. Presentation of stimuli was stopped whenever the child moved or spoke. All trials contaminated by ocular movements or movement artefacts were rejected online (criterion 100μV).

Auditory stimuli were presented through two speakers 35 cm directly lateral to each ear, and a flash was positioned 30 cm from the subject's face. AER were recorded during two sessions on consecutive days, at the same time of day; each session included 180 nonrejected trials. The first day, a weak tone burst (S: 50 dB SPL, 750 Hz, 100 ms duration with 20 ms rise time) was presented alone in the first 60 trials (S1, day 1, 1-60). A strong flash of light (L: 1200 lux, 200 μs) was then presented 800 ms after S in trials 61 to 180 (SLI, day 1). On the second day, the strong flash of light was presented after S in trials 1 to 120 (SLII, day 2). The weak tone burst was then presented alone in the last 60 trials (S2, day 2, 121 - 180). Intertrial intervals varied randomly between 4 and 12 s. Only the second session (series 10 to 18) was repeated throughout the treatment. Each averaged AER was obtained by averaging 20 AER, using a PDP 11/10, then a PDP 11/24 computer. The standard deviation (SD), which was more appropriate than the amplitude for determining the presence or absence of a response and to characterise it, was computed across time (Callaway 1975) during 400 ms averaged presound and 400 ms averaged postsound EEG (Martineau et al., 1987). The ratio of the standard deviation from the averaged postsound to the averaged presound EEG was chosen as the criterion for determining the presence of the averaged evoked response if ratio > 1.4 (Roux, 1981). The mean of the standard deviations of the averaged AER considered as present was calculated for each condition: S1, SLI, SLII and S2. In one study (Martineau et al., 1989), a measure of variability (SNR: signal to noise ratio) was calculated, in which characteristics of single potentials were considered: the SNR was estimated for each AER (Coppola et al., 1978). Each analysis began at stimulus onset and covered the following 400 ms (with one digitisation each 4 ms). First the averaged AER across 60 single potentials was calculated, then the correlation coefficient between this averaged AER and each of the single potentials was computed. The estimate of SNR used in this study was the average of the Z transforms of the 60 correlation coefficients. A high mean then corresponds to high SNR, i.e. little AER variability. SNR was calculated for S1, SLI, SLII and S2.

Subjects

All children, aged 3-14 years, had a diagnosis of autism made on the basis of the DSM III or DSM III-R criteria (APA, 1980, 1987). Some were inpatients from a day care child psychiatry unit, others were receiving long term institutional care in a rural setting. All had marked autistic symptoms, including social withdrawal, language impairment, stereotypes, tantrums, and hypersensitivity to stimuli. They exhibited aggressive behaviour toward themselves and others and had disordered eating and sleeping behaviours. Patients with gross neurological deficits, severe seizure disorders or endocrine or systemic disease were excluded. The children received oral medication daily at 8 am and 12 am in the following doses: 30 mg/kg/day pyridoxine chlorhydrate (up to 1 g/day), 10-15 mg/kg/day Mg^{++} (magnesium lactate) or a combination of pyridoxine and Mg^{++} (B6+Mg) at these dose levels.

Paradigm 1

A group of 16 autistic children (10 boys, mean age 7.5 years) was used to compare the effects of the association B6+Mg to those of the Mg given alone, in a double-blind therapeutic trial. This trial lasted 8 weeks and was based on 2 week trial periods. After a 2 week drug-free period, children were randomly assigned to two groups. The first group received B6+Mg, the second group received Mg. After two weeks, the medication was switched for 2 weeks. This 4 week treatment period was followed by a 2-week drug free period. Electrophysiological studies were performed at the end of each 2 week period (Martineau et al., 1985).

Paradigm 2

A group of 11 normal children (6 boys, mean age 7.5 years) and 12 autistic children (6 boys, mean age 7 years) took part in an open study of the effects of B6+Mg lasting 15 days. Evoked potentials were recorded prior to and on the 11th day of treatment (Martineau et al., 1981).

Paradigm 3
double-blind trials comparing the effects of either B6+Mg or Mg alone and placebo with two weeks of treatment, two middle-term open studies with eight weeks of treatment and a long term open study with eight months of treatment.

Double blind trials. The therapeutic trials were similar to paradigm 1. After a 2 week drug free period, children were randomly assigned to two groups. The first group received B6+Mg (trial 1) or Mg (trial 2), the second group placebo. After two weeks, the medication and placebo groups were switched for 2 weeks. This 4 week treatment period was followed by a 2 week drug free period. Twelve autistic children (9 boys, mean age 9 years) participated in trial 1 (B6+Mg / placebo) and 20 (15 boys, mean age 8.5 years) in trial 2 (Martineau et al., 1985). Electrophysiological studies were performed at the end of each 2 week period.

Middle-term open studies. Two open trials were performed during 14 weeks, each beginning with a 2 week baseline period. The experimental phase followed, all patients receiving 8 weeks of B6+Mg, followed by a 4 week post treatment period. Eleven autistic children (5 boys, mean age 5.8 years) participated in the first trial (Martineau et al., 1988) and six (6 boys, mean age 6.1 years) in the second which was a part of a study comparing the effects of B6+Mg and fenfluramine (Martineau et al., 1989). Electrophysiological studies were performed before the trial, at two, four and eight weeks during treatment and four weeks after treatment.

Long term open study. tTis study was performed over 10 months, with a 2 week baseline period, 8 months of medication with B6+Mg and a 6 week post treatment period. Only one boy, aged 4.2 years participated in this study (Martineau et al., 1986). Electrophysiological investigations were performed before treatment, at two, four, eight, 16 and 24 weeks during the trial and at two weeks after it.

Clinical testing

The clinical effects of the treatments were assessed by a team composed of doctors, psychologists, teachers and nurses. The families were also included when they were involved in the care of the child. An overall clinical assessment was combined with a daily observation scale (behaviour summarised evaluation BSE, table 1). This scale gave information on the actual behaviour of the child. It consists of about 20 items (according to the studies, from 18 to 25) grouped in 7 categories and rated on a 5 point scale (0: never, 4: always). The first three categories deal particularly with autistic features, the last four with associated abnormalities. Each child was rated every week during the trials by two independent raters who had daily contact with him or her.

Results

Paradigm 1 (double-blind trial with B6+Mg/Mg)
The AER and VER grand average recorded during baseline 1 showed poorly differentiated peaks, particularly AER. During the B6+Mg treatment and the Mg period, the main peaks of AER and VER showed better differentiation. Deterioration was observed during the post treatment period. Clinical data analysis showed decreased global scores during the B6+Mg and Mg treatment, and scores remained low during the post treatment period.

Paradigm 2 (open trial with B6+Mg)
There were several differences between autistic children and the control group. Before treatment, the only significant finding was longer P2 latencies in the occipital lead for the autistic children to sound in SL series. However, P1 latencies in all conditions tended to be shorter in autistic children than in controls; this was true for sound alone and the sound of SL series at the central lead and for light in the occipital lead. During treatment, autistic children showed longer latencies than normals. This was significant for vertex N1 and P2 to sound during the SL series and for occipital N1 and P2 to light alone. However, the B6+Mg treatment also increased P2 latencies to light alone and to sound alone in normals.

Before treatment, P1N1 and N1P2 amplitudes were smaller in the autistic group, particularly at the vertex. Differences were significant only for P1N1 evoked by light alone at the vertex and in the occipital lead. Treatment of normal children with B6+Mg caused a decrease in P1N1 and N1P2, with the exception of waves N1P2 evoked at the vertex by sound alone, and at the occiput by light alone. In autistic children, all amplitudes at the vertex increased with the exception of N1P2 evoked by sound in SL series. At the occiput, the differences were minimal.

Of the 12 autistic children taking part in this study, 6 showed marked clinical improvement during B6+Mg therapy. Improvement consisted principally in decreased withdrawal and improvement of meaningful relationships. Increased alertness and reduced negativism were specifically noted. A slight diminution in emotional outbursts, self-mutilation, and stereotyped behaviour was also noticed. Because of the small number of subjects in the two groups (6 each), comparisons of the improved and unimproved groups can be taken only as indications for future studies. Before treatment, no differences in amplitude nor in AEP latency were found between the two subgroups. Under treatment, the N1P2 wave amplitude was higher at the vertex in B6+Mg responsive children than in non responders, with exception of the response to S of SL series which was decreased in the B6+Mg responders children. At the occipital lead, there was more variability. Whereas the P1 latency and the amplitude of P1N1 and N1P2 were lower during the SL series in the children unresponsive to B6+Mg, the amplitude of P1N1 and N1P2 was higher in the children responsive to the B6+Mg regime.

Paradigm 3: Double blind trials (B6+Mg / Placebo or Mg / Placebo)

The cortical potentials evoked by sound in the SL series were better differentiated during treatment with the B6+Mg combination than during baseline. A lengthening of peak latencies and an increase in amplitude were observed for Cz EP in the sound-alone series and for Oz N1P2 in the SL series. Cz N1P2 amplitude remained stable in the SL series because of two phenomena: an increase in amplitude due to the B6+Mg treatment and a decrease due to the association phenomenon (Martineau et al., 1981). The averaged scores of each item decreased significantly during vitamin B6+Mg treatment for the categories of autistic symptoms I, II, III especially for items 1, 2, 3, 5, 6, 9, 10 and also for item 15 of the associated symptoms.

No change in evoked potentials was observed during the Mg treatment. Neither the averaged scores study, nor the category or item studies showed any significant change. Three children were particularly nervous while receiving this treatment.

Middle-term open studies (B6+Mg)

In the first trial performed on twelve autistic children, a significant increase in AEP frequency was observed at Oz site during the first 2 weeks of treatment, and maintained at 4 weeks. After 8 weeks of B6+Mg and after treatment, a slight decrease in Oz AEP frequency was observed. The Oz AEP amplitude increased during treatment. At the Cz site, the AEP frequency and amplitude did not change with treatment, but there were significant decreases in amplitude variances after 4 and 8 weeks and post treatment, reflecting the decrease in intra- and inter subject variability in AEP amplitude with treatment. A reduction in behavioural disturbance of the autistic children was observed during the first 2 weeks of B6+Mg administration, and was maintained over the 8 weeks of the treatment, in spite of a slight increase of behavioural problems after 4 and 6 weeks of treatment, due to a slight increase of items 5, 11 and 15 in all patients.

In the second trial performed on six autistic children, a significant increase in AEP frequency and amplitude was also observed at Oz, without change at the Cz site. This second study also confirmed the decrease in AEP variability during treatment.

Long-term open study (B6+Mg)

Before treatment, the presence of evoked potentials at the vertex was inconstant and their form atypical. No response was recorded at the occipital lead (no association phenomenon). After 4 weeks of treatment, the amplitude of Cz evoked potentials was increased and their form was less variable. During the six series of sound and light coupling, five evoked potentials were recorded in the occipital lead. Their amplitude was large and their morphology stable, as in a control child of the same age. After 8 weeks of B6+Mg treatment, the presence of Cz evoked potentials was relatively constant, but only two evoked potentials were recorded in the occipital lead. After 16 and 24 weeks and following treatment, a great deterioration in the responses was observed, Cz evoked potentials were inconstant, and no evoked potentials were recorded in the occipital lead. Clinical assessment during treatment showed a decrease in global scores. After 8 weeks of treatment, scores were decreased for autistic features (autistic withdrawal 85%; impairment in communication 50 %; bizarre responses to the environment 75 %) and for an associated sign (inappropriate affective responses 85 %). From the third month, an increase in "movement disturbance" was observed, the child showing an increase in stereotyped motor behaviour, he was more agitated and skipping frequently. After 8 months of B6+Mg, he was stabilised well and medication was stopped. An increase in all scores was then observed, indicating an increase in autistic withdrawal and inappropriate affective responses.

Relationships between behavioural and electrophysiological changes during B6+Mg treatment.

Following these therapeutic trials, the B6+Mg has been given to autistic children during open trials with 4 weeks of observation before treatment, 8 weeks of treatment, and 4 weeks of observation post treatment.

During these 16 weeks, the behavioural changes were assessed every week with the BSE (Table 1) and the electrophysiological changes were recorded before treatment, after 8 weeks of treatment and following treatment (Table 2).

Since 1988, 12 autistic children (7 boys, mean age 5 years 3 months) have taken part. They received oral medication daily at 8 am and 12 noon: 20 mg/kg/daypyridoxine chlorhydrate and 15 mg/kg/day magnesium lactate.

Paradigm 3, which allows study of association function and its deficits, was used for these open trials. Silver chloride electrodes were placed on the scalp, at central (Cz), occipital (Oz), frontal (Fz) and left (T3) and right (T4) temporal leads.

Figure 2 shows (top) the grand averages of AER during the sound and light series for the children before, during and after B6+Mg treatment. AER recorded at Cz, Fz, T3 and T4 were well differentiated with normal amplitude and latency before, during and after treatment. However, this grand average does not highlight either evoked responses in the occipital lead, characteristic of the association function,

Table 1
Behavior summarised evaluation (BSE)

Autistic withdrawal
1 – Is eager aloneness
2 – Ignores people
3 – Poor social interaction
4 – Abnormal eye contact
Impairment in communication
5 – Does not make an effort to communicate using voice and/or words
6 – Lack of appropriate facial expressions and gestures
7 – Stereotyped vocal or voice utterances, echolalia
Bizarre responses ti the environnement
8 – Lack of initiative, poor activity
9 – Inappropriate relating to inanimate objects or to doll
10 – Uses objects in a compulsive and/or ritualistic way
11 – Resistance ti change and to frustration
Motility disorders
12 – Stereotyped sensorimotor activity
13 – Agitation, restlessness
14 – Bizarre posture and gait
Inappropriate affective responses
15 – Autoaggressiveness
16 – Heteroaggressiveness
17 – Soft anxiety signs
18 – Mood difficulties
Impairment in main instinctual functions
19 – Disturbance of feeding behavior
20 – No attempt to control urine and feces
21 – Masturbation
22 – Sleep disturbances
Attention and perception disturbances
23 – Unstable attention, easily distracted
24 – Bizarre responses to audiitory stimuli
25 – Variability

or changes at other sites. Overall clinical assessment showed a decrease in scores during treatment (Figure 1). The children were divided into two subgroups, according to the percentage decrease in their overall assessment. Five children seemed sensitive to the treatment, with a decrease in global scores from 15% to 59 %, and seven seemed insensitive, with no change in scores in three children or an increase in global scores from 2 to 17 %. Figure 1 shows the mean global scores when the group was divided in this way. The decrease of global scores in the sensitive group was statistically significant ($p > .01$). Figure 2 shows the grand averages of evoked responses

Table 2
Study protocol

	Time span: 16 weeks			
	Before	Vitamin B6 + Mg		After
Measure	4 weeks	8 weeks		4 weeks
BSE	* * * *	* * * *	* * * *	* * * *
EP	*	*	*	*

of these two subgroups. For the sensitive children, responses evoked by the sound during the sound and light series were recorded at the occipital lead when the children were under treatment, showing an improvement of their association function. This response was still observed 4 weeks post treatment. On the contrary, no response was recorded in the insensitive children.

Discussion

These experiments yield three main findings:

vitamin B6 with magnesium lead to improvement of a subgroup of autistic children;

the combination of vitamin B6 + magnesium is much more effective than vitamin B6 or magnesium alone;

the therapeutic effects were observed in both short and long term trials.

The electrophysiological changes induced by vitamin B6 + magnesium treatment confirmed the clinical results and raise the question of the mechanism through which the medication is active. The functions of vitamin B6 in humans are multifaceted and interrelated as indicated in Figure 3 (Leklem, 1988). The role of vitamin B6 in the development and function of the nervous system has been reviewed (Dakshinamurti et al., 1985). Pyridoxal 5'-phosphate is the coenzyme of an enzyme in the serotonine pathway: L-aromatic amino acid decarboxylase (L-AAAD), and of two enzymes in the catecholamine pathway: L-AAAD and dopamine beta hydroxylase (DBH) which converts dopamine to noradrenaline. It also affects all nonoxidative enzymatic transformations of the other amino acid pathways, catalysing such reactions as decarboxylation, transamination, racemisation and beta and gamma elimination. Vita-

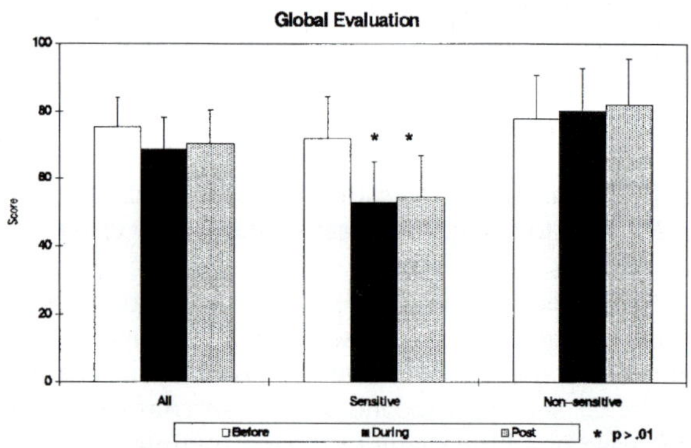

Fig. 1. Global evaluation performed with the Behavior summarized evaluation for the children before, during and after the vitamin B6 + Mg treatment. A significant decrease in scores was observed during treatment for the 5 sensitive children.

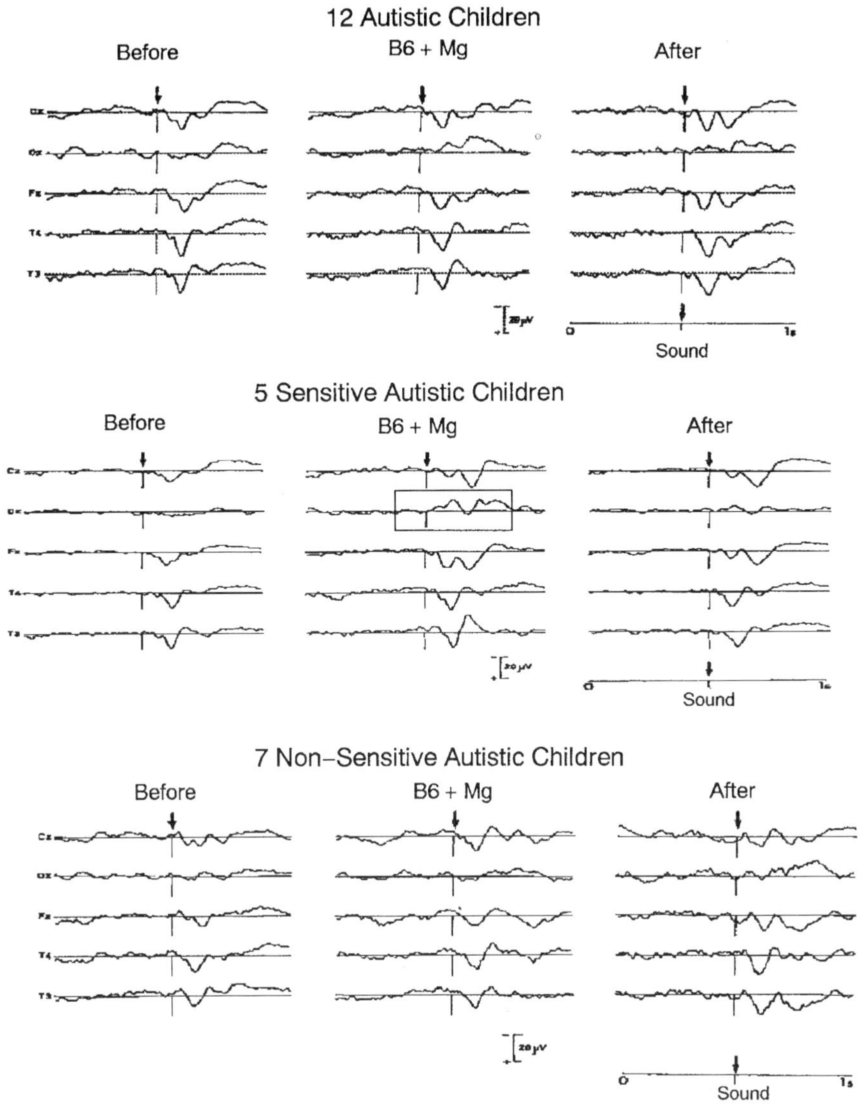

Fig. 2
Grand averages of the auditory evoked responses during the sound and light series before, during and after vitamin B6 + Mg treatment. Top, all children, middle, the five sensitive children, bottom the seven insensitive children. For the sensitive children, responses evoked by the sound during the sound and light series were recorded at Oz when the children were under treatment, showing an improvement of the association function.

min B6 is also involved in the biosynthesis of lipids, protein, carbohydrates, nucleic acids and sphingosine bases; the effects of the vitamin are thus ubiquitous. It has been called the brain vitamin since its affects so many different aspects of CNS metabolism (Gillberg and Coleman, 1992).

The improvement observed during vitamin B6+magnesium treatment could be linked to a beneficial action of these substances on dysfunction of some neurotransmitters in subgroups of autistic children. Several hypotheses have attempted to link the clinical signs of autism to a neurochemical disorder.

Administration of haloperidol, a potent dopamine blocking agent, is associated with reductions in withdrawal, stereotyped movements and abnormal object relations (Campbell et al., 1978, Anderson et al., 1984), while administration of amphetamine, a dopamine agonist, induces increased irritability, hyperactivity and worsening of stereotyped movements (Campbell et al., 1972, 1976). Autistic subjects often show a high level of activity, a variety of involuntary stereotyped movements and ritualistic behaviour problems. These motor disturbances might be modulated by the dopaminergic systems in the brain (Sourkes, 1976, Moore and Bloom, 1978). Simon and Le Moal (1984, 1985) described a dopaminergic mechanism by which neurons in the ventral mesencephalon regulate the function and interaction of prefrontal cortical, limbic and striatal centres. This reticular modulation of higher centres regulates the process of attention in prefrontal and associated medial striatal centres and the process of intention in limbic and associated lateral striatal centres (Simon and Le Moal 1985) . Thus, brain stem reticular structures, which provide the energy for the alerting and sustaining process underlying directed attention

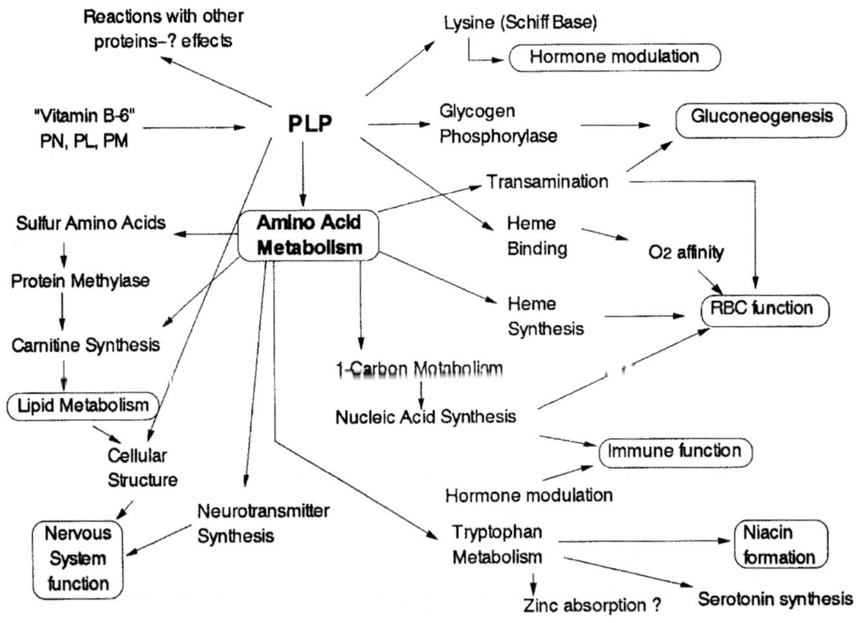

Fig. 3
Cellular processes in which pyridoxal 5'-phosphate (PLP) acts as a coenzyme or binds with proteins and modifies the action of the protein (Leklem, 1988)

(Davies, 1983) influence both the sensory (attention) and motor (intention) contingencies obeyed by inferior parietal lobule neurons as they mediate the process of directed attention (Mesulam, 1983). Simon and Le Moal (1985) attribute the intentional component to the intensive process underlying directed attention. Autistic children suffer from severe distortions of intention, perception and directed attention (Lelord, 1990).

The presence of a dysfunctional serotoninergic system was suggested by Coleman (1973) and Young et al. (1982a) due to the modulatory effects of this neuronal system on a variety of important behavioural and physiological processes (pain and sensory perception, motor function, learning, memory, appetite and sleep) often perturbed in autism.

The involvement of adrenalin and noradrenalin systems in regulating attention and arousal (Moore and Bloom 1979) raises the question of their significance in autism. Moreover, as with dopamine, both animal studies and the activity of pharmacological agents such as desipramine have suggested a role of NA in the expression of various disorders (Young et al., 1982).

There are four possible explanations of the pharmacological action of pyridoxine in autism, which take account of the dopaminergic hypothesis:

1. Enhancement of dopamine turnover with increased dopa decarboxylase activity. This hypothesis is supported by the observation that pyridoxine treatment reduces the L-dopa effects in Parkinsonian patients (Papavasiliou et al., 1972).

2. Increased dopamine receptor sensitivity; this is suggested by the decreased prolactin levels seen during treatment (Gualtieri et al., 1981).

3. Imbalance in GABA production by glutamic acid decarboxylase and degradation by GABA transaminase, as GABA modifies dopaminergic neurons.

4. Functional deficiencies in enzymes requiring pyridoxal 5'-phosphate; these can be corrected by large doses of vitamin B6 (Folkers et al., 1978).

The role of magnesium must not be underestimated. It is the second most prevalent intracellular cation. It has many important functions including key steps in intermediary metabolism, protein synthesis, DNA synthesis and transcription. Since vitamin B6 may restore dopamine balance in the brain (Brooks et al., 1983) and magnesium acts on dopamine storage (Durlach, 1976), one could hypothesise that more dopamine will be synthesised and stored when vitamin B6 and magnesium are given together.

Is there any electrophysiological specificity in vitamin B6+magnesium treatment in autistic children?

In the study analysing relationships between behavioural and electrophysiological changes during vitamin B6+magnesium treatment (Fig 1), it seems that, before treatment, evoked potentials recorded at Cz, Oz, Fz, T3 and T4 are more variable, and less differentiated from baseline in the group of sensitive autistic children. This confirms the observation (Martineau et al., 1989) that the evoked potentials of autistic children responding to vitamin B6+ magnesium or to fenfluramine were different during the baseline period. The frequency of evoked responses recorded at both Cz and Oz sites tended to be highest in the fenfluramine group and the Cz evoked responses amplitude variability tended to be greater in the vitamin B6+magnesium group. We can therefore add to the trends of vitamin B6+magnesium sensitivity previously reported (Barthélémy et al., 1988), i.e., that sensitive children seemed to be younger, with a higher IQ, better language ability and higher urinary homovanillic acid levels than insensitive children, a high variability of evoked responses.

In summary, many complex mechanisms appear to be involved in the pharmacological action of vitamin B6+magnesium, but our results emphasise the value of such anodyne medication for the treatment of some autistic children.

References

American Psychiatric Association (1980) Diagnostic and statistical manual of mental disorders, 3rd edn (DSM III). American Psychiatric Association, Washington DC

American Psychiatric Association (1987) Diagnostic and statistical manual of mental disorders, 3rd revised edn (DSM III-R). American Psychiatric Association, Washington DC

Anderson LT, Campbell M, Grega DM, Perry R, Small AM, Green WH (1984) Haloperidol in the treatment of infantile autism: effects on learning and behavioral symptoms. Am J Psychiat 141: 1195-1202

Anderson LT, Campbell M, Adams P, Small AM, Perry R, Shell J (1989) The effects of haloperidol on discrimination learning and behavioral symptoms in autistic children. J Autism Dev Disord 19: 227-239

Barthélémy C, Martineau J, Bruneau N, Müh JP, Lelord G, Callaway E (1988) Clinical and biological effects of pyridoxine plus magnesium in autistic subjects. In: Leklem JE, Reynolds RD (eds) Clinical and physiological applications of vitamin B6. Alan R Liss, New York, p 329-356

Brooks SC, D'Angelo L, Chalmeta A, Ahern G, Judson JH (1983) An unusual schizophrenic illness responsive to pyridoxine HCl (B-6) subsequent to phenothiazine and butyrophenone toxicities? Biol Psychiat 18: 1321-1328

Callaway E (1975) Brain electrical potentials and individual psychological differences. Grune and Stratton, New York

Callaway E (1977) Response of infantile autism to large doses of B6. Psychopharmacol Bull 13: 57-58

Campbell M, Adams P, Perry R, Spencer EK, Overall JE (1988a) Tardive and withdrawal dyskinesia in autistic children: a prospective study. Psychopharmacol Bull 24: 251-255

Campbell M, Adams P, Small AM, Curren E, Overall JE, Anderson LT, Lynch N, Perry R (1988b) Efficacy and safety of fenfluramine in autistic children. J Am Acad Child Adolesc Psychiat 27: 434-439

Campbell M, Anderson LT, Meier M, Cohen I, Small AM, Samit C, Sachar EJ (1978) A comparison of haloperidol and behaviour therapy and their interaction in autistic children. J Am Acad Child Psychiat 17: 640-655

Campbell M, Anderson LT, Small AM, Adams P, Gonzalez NM, Ernst M (1993) Naltrexone in autistic children: behavioral symptoms and attentional learning. J Am Acad Child Adolesc Psychiat 32: 1283-1291

Campbell M, Cueva JE (1995) Psychopharmacology in child and adolescent psychiatry: a review of the past seven years. Part I. J Am Acad Child Adolesc Psychiat 34: 1124-1132

Campbell M, Fish B, David R, Shapiro T, Collins P, Koh C (1972) Response to triiodothyronine and dextroamphetamine: a study of preschool schizophrenic children. J Autism Child Schizophr 2: 343-358

Campbell M, Shay J (1995) Pervasive developmental disorders. In: Kaplan HI, Sadock BJ (eds) Comprehensive textbook of psychiatry. Vol. IV. Williams and Wilkins, Baltimore, p 2277-2293

Campbell M, Small AM, Collins PJ, Friedman E, David R, Genieser NB (1976) Levodopa and levoamphetamine: a crossover study in schizophrenic children. Curr Ther Res 18: 70-86

Coleman MC (1973) Serotonin and central nervous system syndromes of childhood: a review. J Autism Child Schizophr 3: 27-35

Coppola R, Tabor R, Buchsbaum MS (1978) Signal to noise ratio and response variability measurements in single trial evoked potentials. Electroencephalogr Clin Neurophysiol 44: 214-222

Dakshinamurti K, Paulose CS, Siow YL (1985) Neurobiology of pyridoxine. In: Reynolds RD and Leklem JE (eds) Vitamin B6: its role in health and disease. Alan R Liss, New York, p 99-121

Davies DR (1983) Attention, arousal and effort. In: Gale A, Edwards JA (eds) Physiological correlates of human behaviour. Academic Press, London, p 9-34

Durlach J (1976) Neurological manifestations of magnesium imbalance. In: Vinken PJ, Bruyn GW (eds) Handbook of clinical neurology, vol 28. North Holland, Amsterdam, p 545-579

Ernst M, Magee HJ, Gonzalez NM, Locascio JJ, Rosenberg CR, Campbell M (1992) Pimozide in autistic children. Psychopharmacol Bull 28: 187-191

Folkers K, Ellis J, Watanabe T, Saji S, Kaji M (1978) Biochemical evidence for a deficiency of vitamin B6 in the carpal tunnel syndrome based on a cross-over study. Proc Nat Acad Sci USA 75: 3410-3412

Gillberg C, Coleman M (1992) The biology of autistic syndromes - 2nd Edn. MacKeith Press, London

Gordon CT, State RC, Nelson JE, Hamburger SD, Rapoport JL (1993) A double-blind comparison of clomipramine, desipramine, and placebo in the treatment of autistic disorder. Arch Gen Psychiat 50: 441-447

Gualtieri CT, Golden RN, Fahs JJ (1983) New developments in pediatric psychopharmacology. J Dev Behav Pediatr 4: 202-209

Heeley AF, Roberts GE (1965) Tryptophan metabolism in psychotic children: a preliminary report. Dev Med Child Neurol 7: 46-49

Herman BH, Hammock MK, Arthur-Smith A, Kuehl K, Appelgate K (1989) Effects of acute administration of naltrexone on cardiovascular function, body temperature, body weight and serum concentrations of liver enzymes in autistic children. Dev Pharmacol Ther 12: 118-127

Klein RG, Abikoff H, Barkley RA et al (1994) Clinical trials in children and adolescents. In: Prien RF, Robinson DS (eds) Clinical evaluation of psychotropic drugs: principles and guidelines. Raven Press, New York, p 501-546

Lelord G (1990) Physiopathologie de l'autisme. Les insuffisances modulatrices cérébrales. Neuropsychiat Enfance 38: 43-49

Leklem JE (1988) Vitamin B6 metabolism and functions in humans. In: Leklem JE, Reynolds RD (eds) Clinical and physiological applications of vitamin B-6. Alan R Liss, New York, p 3-28
Locascio JJ, Malone RP, Small AM, Kafantaris V, Ernst M, Lynch NS, Overall JE, Campbell M (1991) Factors related to haloperidol response and dyskinesias in autistic children. Psychopharmacol Bull 27: 119-126
Martineau J, Barthélémy C, Cheliakine C, Lelord G (1988) Brief report: an open middle-term study of combined vitamin B6-magnesium in a subgroup of autistic children selected on their sensitivity to treatment. J Autism Dev Disord 18: 435-447
Martineau J, Barthélémy C, Garreau B, Lelord G (1985) Vitamin B6, magnesium, and combined B6-magnesium: therapeutic effects in childhood autism. Biol Psychiat 20: 467-478
Martineau J, Barthélémy C, Lelord G (1986) Long-term effects of combined vitamin B6-magnesium administration in an autistic child. Biol Psychiat 21: 511-518
Martineau J, Barthélémy C, Roux S, Garreau B, Lelord G (1989) Electrophysiological effects of fenfluramine or combined vitamin B6 and magnesium on children with autistic behavior. Dev Med Child Neurol 31: 721-727
Martineau J, Garreau B, Barthélémy C, Callaway E, Lelord G (1981) Effects of vitamin B6 on averaged evoked potentials in infantile autism. Biol Psychiat 16: 627-640
Martineau J, Garreau B, Roux S, Lelord G (1987) Auditory evoked responses and their modifications during conditioning paradigm in autistic children. J Autism Dev Disord 17: 525-539
Martineau J, Hérault J, Petit E, Guérin P, Perrot A, Mallet J, Sauvage D, Lelord G, Müh JP (1994) Catecholaminergic metabolism and autism. Dev Med Child Neurol 36: 688-697
Martineau J, Tanguay P, Garreau B, Roux S, Lelord G (1984) Are sex differences in averaged evoked responses (AERs) produced by coupling sound and light in children and adults? J Psychophysiol 2: 177-183
Mesulam MM (1983) The functional anatomy and hemispheric specialization for directed attention. The role of the parietal lobe and its connectivity. Trans Int Neurosci 6: 384-387
Moore RY, Bloom FE (1978) Central catecholamine neuron systems: anatomy and physiology of the dopamine systems. Ann Rev Neurosci 1: 129-169
Moore R, Bloom F (1979) Central catecholamine neuron system: anatomy and physiology of the norepinephrine and epinephrine systems. Ann Rev Neuroscience 2: 113-168
Papavasiliou PS, Cotzias GC, Duby SE, Stect JA, Feling C, Bell MA (1972) Levodopa in Parkinsonism: potentialisation of central effects with peripheral inhibitor. N Engl J Med 286: 8-14
Perry R, Campbell M, Adams P, Lynch N, Spencer EK, Curren EL, Overall JE (1989) Long-term efficacy of haloperidol in autistic children: continuous vs discontinuous drug administration. J Am Acad Child Adolesc Psychiat 28: 87-92
Rapoport JL, Kruesi MJP (1985) Organic therapies. In: Kaplan HI, Sadock BJ (eds) Comprehensive textbook of psychiatry. Vol. IV. Williams and Wilkins, Baltimore, p 1793-1798
Rimland B (1973) High dosage levels of certain vitamins in the treatment of children with severe mental disorders. In: Hawkins D, Pauling L (eds) Orthomolecular psychiatry. Freeman, New York, p 531-539
Rimland B (1974) An orthomolecular study of psychotic children. Orthomol Psychiat 3: 146-161
Rimland B, Callaway E, Dreyfus P (1979) The effects of high doses of vitamin B6 on autistic children: a double-blind crossover study. Am J Psychiat 135: 472-475
Roux S (1981) Aspects électrophysiologiques du conditionnement des potentiels corticaux évoqués par des stimulations sensorielles chez l'homme. Doctoral dissertation, third cycle, Poitiers
Schafer E, MacKean C (1975) Evidence that monoamines influence human evoked potentials. Brain Res 99: 49-58
Small J, DeMyer M, Kendall J (1969) Experience with response averaging in autistic children. Electroencephalogr Clin Neurophysiol 26: 112-113
Simon H, Le Moal M (1984) Mesencephalic dopaminergic neurons: functional role. In: Usdin E, Carlsson A, Dahlstrom A, Engel J (eds) Catecholamines: neuropharmacology and central nervous system - theorical aspects. Alan R Liss, New York, p 293-307
Simon H, Le Moal M (1985) Influence des neurones dopaminergiques du mésencéphale sur les processus d'attention et d'intention. Psychol Med 17: 939-945
Sourkes TL (1976) Parkinson's disease and other disorders of the basal ganglia. In: Siegel GJ (ed). Basic neurochemistry. Little, Brown, Boston, p 668-684
Strayhorn JM Jr, Rapp N, Donina W, Strain PS (1988) Randomized trial of methylphenidate for an autistic child. J Am Acad Child Adolesc Psychiat 27: 244-247
Young JG, Kavanagh ME, Anderson GM, Shaywitz BA, Cohen DJ (1982) Clinical neurochemistry of autism and associated disorders. J Autism Dev Disord 12: 147-165

3. Multivariate descriptive statistical methods: an aid to bioclinical studies in populations of developmentally disordered children

S. ROUX

In the field of childhood psychiatric disorders, most bioclinical studies have been carried out on small samples of children selected according to nosological diagnoses. Because the bioclinical data to be analysed are often complex, in this chapter I present and discuss an original, complementary approach to classical bioclinical studies, based on the use of multivariate descriptive statistical methods.

Multivariate descriptive statistical methods have been developed to analyse large quantities of information which are too vast for direct analysis, to extract the most relevant tendencies, and to classify them. These descriptive methods include two main subgroups of analysis: factor analysis — such as the well-known principal component analysis — and cluster analysis. Principal component analysis is essentially a method of data-reduction applied to quantitative variables. The new variables (i.e., factors) may be used in a variety of ways: to provide a convenient summary or an informative visual display of the data or a simplified set of variables for use in later analyses (Everitt, 1989). Cluster analysis is a well-known method for grouping individuals so that those within each group are relatively similar with respect to the initial parameters. Many different clustering algorithms are used, which may vary as to whether they are hierarchical or disjoint, whether distance is calculated by a Euclidian metric or a variance method, and whether the number of clusters obtained is predetermined or selected post hoc. The constraints and limitations of this methodology, such as the characteristics of available clustering methods, have been discussed (Hoffman and Franke, 1986; Rescorla, 1988; Salstone and Fraboni, 1990; Overall et al., 1993). Since principal component analysis provides a possible reduction of the variables, the clustering algorithm is often applied to the principal component factor scores of the variables rather than to the variables themselves. However, there are other techniques for reducing the dimensionality of multivariate data. One of these is correspondence analysis, which is an analogue of principal component analysis but is performed on other types of data. Correspondence analysis, as a geometric approach to multivariate descriptive data analysis, originated in France; Benzécri (1969, 1973) and his colleagues have done much to popularise this technique. The term "correspondence analysis" is a translation of the French "analyse factorielle des correspondances". This method, which will be presented below, has received considerable attention in the statistical and psychometric literature (Hoffman and Franke, 1986).

Multivariate statistical methods have been widely used for many years in the field of psychiatric research. On the one hand, principal component analysis has shown its value for validation of psychometric instruments, to determine their factor structure (Barthélémy and Lelord, 1991). On the other hand, many researchers have advocated the use of cluster analysis as a technique for forming diagnostic categories. As long ago as 1982, however,

Skinner and Blashfield (1982) emphasised the limited impact of cluster analytical studies on clinical practice. They discussed the reasons which underlie this and described directions for upgrading both the scientific quality and clinical acceptance of cluster analytical research. In a most interesting way, these empirical techniques have been used to examine the structure or composition of clinical samples, to approach the heterogeneity of psychiatric pathology, such as attention disorders (Frankel et al., 1992) or schizophrenia (Farmer et al., 1983). This heterogeneity has received considerable attention in publications on autism (Schopler, 1978; Wing and Gould, 1979; Rutter and Schopler, 1987; Waterhouse et al., 1996). Thus, for some time researchers have attempted to define more homogeneous subtypes in large populations of autistic children and more broadly in developmentally-disordered children. These studies, detailed below, essentially used clinical and cognitive data. They participated in the interpretation of clinical data and the increased understanding of the disorders in question.

The value of multidisciplinary approaches has been demonstrated for many years in the field of developmental disorders (Bruneau et al., 1990; Barthélémy et al., 1990; Lelord et al., 1991). These studies have been performed on clinical and biological data mainly gathered from small groups of children during therapeutic studies. For biological research purposes, it is desirable to have a reasonable degree of homogeneity within the populations of children. Thus, the refinement of homogeneous subgroups using multivariate statistical methods can be helpful for these bioclinical studies. Moreover, when large clinical samples can be obtained, the conjoint analysis of clinical and biological data, using multivariate descriptive data analyses, can generate new pathophysiological hypotheses for clinicians and researchers, thus contributing to the understanding of the underlying mechanisms.

In this report, I first review publications which used principal component and cluster analysis in developmental disorders. I then present correspondence analysis as a method and apply it, as an example, to behavioural and electrophysiological data gathered from large populations of developmentally-disordered children in hospital.

Multivariate statistical analyses in developmental disorders

I shall review the principal research concerned with describing homogeneous subgroups within populations of developmentally-disordered children using cluster analysis, sometimes preceded by principal component analysis.

The first study of autistic children which tried to derive categories empirically by the use of multivariate statistical procedures was that of Prior et al (1975). Cluster analysis (a nonhierarchical classification method) was performed on a population of 164 children, ranging in age from 3 to 13 years, and previously diagnosed as autistic, psychotic or psychotic/retarded. Data from the checklist of Rimland (1971) were used for the analysis. The children were grouped into two classes; those with early onset of disease who showed numerous withdrawal and aloneness symptoms and impaired communication, and those with later onset whose symptoms were more heterogeneous and scattered. The second class might be seen as fitting the DSM-III category of childhood onset PDD.

Scherman et al. (1983), using the K-means algorithm, classified 48 developmentally-disordered preschool children. Analysis was applied to data derived from IQ scores and behavioural ratings. The results indicated that diagnostic similarity did not always agree with functional similarity, since a range of diagnoses was found in each of the statistically-derived clusters. The validation of the five subgroups previously obtained by cluster analysis, using cognitive and linguistic data, showed that this classification was more relevant than the clinical diagnosis to clinical practice, research, educational planning and prognosis.

Using only cognitive data, Fein et al. (1985) individualised several profiles in a sample of 54 developmentally-disordered children. Most of them were successfully categorised according to different strengths and weaknesses on verbal, performance, memory and quantitative tests. The authors discussed the limitations of their results, especially the small size of the sample and the factorial complexity of the variables processed. They suggested that future sorting should be attempted with variables chosen on the basis of the factor structure of their neuropsychological battery.

Siegel et al. (1986) performed hierarchical cluster analysis on observational data from 46 autistic and autistic-like children 4-20 years of age. Four clusters were derived from the analysis of profiles of eight factors provided by an initial principal component analysis. The subgroups differed on the basis of several types of behaviour: perseverative thinking and play, motor disturbances, schizoid features, anxiety, negativism, noncommunicative language and bizarre play; they also showed different aetiological profiles. Moreover, mental ability was related to group membership, although the groups were formed on the basis of behavioural characteristics.

The authors stated the need for further cluster analytical research to be applied to larger and more age homogeneous samples.

Dahl et al. (1986) investigated 390 preschool children, including a large number of autistic children. An agglomerative hierarchical algorithm applied to 44 behavioural variables derived from BRIAAC (behaviour rating instrument for autistic and atypical children) and BRS (behaviour rating scale) these scales produced 12 subgroups of children. The cluster analysis revealed a great deal of overlap between groups and produced clusters quite heterogeneous with respect to the DSM-III diagnostic categories. Clusters were ordered roughly on a continuum of severity of impairment. Rescorla (1988), who continued Dahl's study, performed a cluster analysis on a clinical sample of 204 boys aged 3-5 years, spanning a wide spectrum of function, from severely autistic to children with little or no psychiatric impairment. A principal component analysis had previously been applied to 73 symptoms of the CBCL (Achenbach's child behaviour checklist). The eight main factors identified by the factor analysis were entered into a disjoint iterative method of clustering (K-means algorithm). The results were analysed for 2 to 6 cluster solutions. Clustering identified an autistic group when a 3 cluster solution was formed. As more clusters were obtained, this autistic cluster was subdivided according to the presence or absence of anxiety and level of functioning.

Szatmari et al. (1989) applied a K-means partitioning clustering method to a sample of 28 children with Asperger's syndrome and 25 high-functioning autistic children. Cluster analysis was performed on 3 variables concerning restricted range of activities, and social and communication impairment. Three groups of children were identified, separated primarily on the basis of the intensity of the disorders.

Campbell and Overall (1989) performed a principal component analysis on 14 items of the CPRS (children's psychiatric rating scale) in a population of 180 autistic children. The four main factors were then entered in a simultaneous partition method which identified five clusters. These clusters were differentiated by factors 2, 3 and 4 of principal component analysis; i.e. anger/uncooperativeness, hyperactivity and speech deviance. The first main factor, labelled "autism", was present at relatively high levels in all five clusters.

More recently, Eaves et al. (1994) used cluster analysis on a large, relatively homogeneous group of 166 children 3-12 year old in the autistic spectrum. They retained 43 variables, including behavioural and cognitive data and information from medical and family histories. These variables were first factor analysed; four subgroups of children were then identified using a standard clustering algorithm. These four subtypes differed in cognitive (verbal and performance IQ) and behavioural (stereotyped motor activities, abnormal verbal and nonverbal communication, impaired social skills, sensory disturbances, aloofness, hyperactivity, aggressivity) characteristics, but also in family history of learning problems.

Finally, Sevin et al. (1995) conducted a cluster analytic study to derive behaviourally homogeneous subtypes of pervasive developmental disorders. Behavioural variables were measured using several of the standardised psychometric instruments most commonly employed in assessing autistic individuals (CARS, ABC, etc.). Ward's minimum variance method was applied to 34 children and adolescents, aged from 2 to 22 years. The cluster solution indicated the presence of four distinct subgroups according to social, language and stereotyped behaviours.

In our department, Hameury et al. (1995) developed a quantified grouping system based on four developmental assessment parameters: autistic behaviour, intellectual impairment, neurological signs, language and communication disorders. A hierarchical clustering analysis performed on this quantified assessment of 202 developmentally-disordered children, allowed four patterns to be identified, which could be distinguished from the classical DSMIII-R classification; for example, two subgroups of autistic children were identified, one with a pure syndrome, the other with a syndrome associated with severe disorders. We showed the value of this approach by applying it to one of the assays of monoamines routinely performed in our department: dihydroxyphenylacetic acid (DOPAC) and homovanillic acid (HVA), the main urinary dopamine derivatives. Unexpectedly, this method revealed a subgroup of retarded children which had a particular biochemical profile.

These different studies which have been carried out for twenty years can be criticised with regard to the small size of the samples (Fein et al., 1985; Siegel et al., 1986; Szatmari et al., 1989; Sevin et al., 1995), the lack of factor analysis to "filter" the processed variables (Fein et al., 1985) or the use of principal component analysis, which showed a "size effect" on the first main factor (Campbell and Overall, 1989). In the same way, the choice of the clinical populations studied can be criticised in regard to the diagnostic categories, the variables selected or the range of ages and IQs involved. However, these studies provided a real objective contribution to the resolution of the problem of identifying subtypes of autism, and more widely of developmental disorders.

Correspondence analysis

Like principal component analysis, correspondence analysis is a technique for transforming a set of variables into a new set of uncorrelated variables which account for maximal amounts of the variation in the original observations. The use of correspondence analysis instead of principal component analysis enables one to take advantage of one valuable property of this algorithm, which helps in detecting structural relationships among variables; it helps to show how variables are related, not just that a relationship exits (Benzécri, 1969, 1973; Lebart et al., 1979, 1984).

This procedure was initially devised to analyse contingency tables. Although it is a different kind of matrix, the aim of correspondence analysis is similar to the aim of principal component analysis. The difference is determined by the type of transformation applied to the original data matrix and the metrics in which the principal axes are defined. Rows and columns are replaced by their profiles and the similarity between two rows or two columns is defined by the distance between their profiles; this distance is defined as the chi square distance which guarantees invariance according to the property of "distributional equivalence" (i.e. identical profiles imply equal or proportional raw data). Thus, it frees the analysis from the size effect and consequently retains and emphasises relevant secondary characteristics, which would otherwise have been concealed. Because of the inherent symmetry of correspondence analysis, the data matrix for analysis is a contingency table. However, the method can be applied to almost any matrix of categorical data, provided the entries are non-negative. It can also be applied to ordered categories and "discretised" quantitative variables, whose study requires, for example, a classification of the lines (i.e., patients) through their profiles. Consequently, this procedure allows investigation of possible nonlinearity among categories with respect to the principal axes. It can lead to the discovery of relationships between scale value categories which are obscured if methods are used which recognise only the metric properties of the data. Thus, a "loss of information" in ignoring the ordered or interval nature of the data yields a meaningful gain in understanding (Hoffman and Franke, 1986).

Another distinct advantage of correspondence analysis over other methods is that all variables can be plotted in the same space for ease of interpretation. Thus, it produces two dual displays whose row and column geometries have similar interpretations, facilitating the analysis and detection of relationships. In other multivariate approaches, as commonly employed, this duality does not exit.

The first step in interpreting the graphic display produced by correspondence analysis is to determine the "absolute contribution to inertia". This quantifies the importance of each variable in determining the orientation of the principal axes and serves as a guide to the interpretation of each axis. The next step is to determine the quality of the representation of each variable in the display: the "relative contribution to inertia". The various decompositions of total inertia, in conjunction with the principal co-ordinate values of the variables, make possible a complete interpretation of the results of correspondence analysis.

A last advantage of this factor analysis is that it provides the means for fitting external information (i.e., supplementary variables) into its graphic display. A supplementary variable makes no contribution to the axis, but its relative contribution to each principal axis can be examined. The fitting of these supplementary points can, for example, serve as a validity check (Lebart et al., 1984).

Like principal component analysis, correspondence analysis is a method of data reduction which produces a small number of uncorrelated composite scores (i.e., factors) which can then be used in place of the larger number of original variables in the subsequent analyses of data such as cluster analysis. We chose agglomerative hierarchical clustering, a minimum variance cluster analysis, which is processed using euclidian distance to determine cluster membership. This minimum variance method is designed to generate clusters in such a way to minimise within cluster variance. The use of hierarchical clustering enables one to take advantage of a valuable property of this algorithm which allows interpretation of several cluster solutions in terms of their reliability, on statistical criteria, and interpretability, on bioclinical criteria.

An example applied to behavioural and electrophysiological data

I present an example of multivariate descriptive statistical analysis applied to large populations of developmentally-disordered children in hospital. The aim of this study was to describe behavioural profiles (study I) on the one hand, and behavioural and electrophysiological profiles (study II) on the other. For this purpose, the parameters studied were first factor analysed using correspondence analysis. Then, the main factors identified by this analysis were entered into a hierarchical cluster analysis which subtypes children according to the similarity of their profiles. ADDAD software version 89.1 was used.

Behavioural assessment was carried out on 13 items extracted from the revised behaviour summarised evaluation scale (BSE-R). This consists of 29 initial items rated from 1 to 5 according to the severity of the disturbance: 1 if the disorder is never observed, to 5 if it is always observed. It has been validated (Barthélémy et al., 1997) and its content validity study using principal component analysis with Varimax rotation allowed identification of a first main factor (38 % of total variance) which comprises 13 items (Table 1). These items of behaviour, which describe the degree of severity of the autistic syndrome, were retained for further analysis.

Table 1
The 12 items of the BSE-R scale which describe the degree of autistic behaviour

1. Aloneness	ALO
2. Ignores people	IGN*
3. Poor social interaction	SOC
4. Abnormal eye contact	GAZ
5. Does not make an effort to communicate using voice and/or words	VOI*
6. Lack of appropriate facial expression and gestures	GES
7. Lack of initiative, poor activity	ACT
8. Inappropriate relating to inanimate objects or to doll	OBJ
9. Stereotyped sensorimotor activity	STE*
10. Unstable attention, easily distracted	ATT*
11. Bizarre responses to auditory stimuli	AUD*
12. Does not imitate the gestures or voices of others	IMI*
13. Does not share emotion	EMO

* items retained in study II

Electrocortical activity was assessed with an electrophysiological method using averaged evoked potentials in response to auditory stimulation (AEP). This procedure has been described fully elsewhere (Bruneau et al., 1985, 1987). Seven relevant parameters were extracted from the published results to assess electrophysiological patterns (Table 2a). They assess N1 amplitude of AEP recorded from Cz, Fz, T3, T4 and Pz sites at 80dB SPL intensity level (750 Hz tone bursts of 200 ms duration). The Cz/Fz and CzFz/T3T4 amplitude ratios were also computed. A glossary for each parameter, rated from 1 to 3, is given in Table 2b.

Table 2a
The 7 parameters which describe AEP recorded from 5 electrode sites at 80dB intensity level

1. Cz AEP amplitude (80 dB)	A8C
2. Fz AEP amplitude (80 dB)	A8F
3. T4 AEP amplitude (80 dB)	A8R
4. T3 AEP amplitude (80 dB)	A8L
5. Pz AEP amplitude (80 dB)	A8P
6. Cz/Fz amplitude ratio	CF8
7. CzFz/T3T4 amplitude ratio	CRL8

Study I

This concerned 186 developmentally-disordered children (129 boys, 57 girls), between 20 and 139 months of age (mean 65, SEM 1.9 months). The intelligence quotient (IQ), determined with standardised tests (Brunet and Lézine, 1976), ranged from 10 to 85 (mean 42, SEM 1.3). The children were diagnosed according to DSM-III R criteria (APA, 1987): autistic disorder (AD) 98 children, mental retardation (MR) 54 children, pervasive developmental disorders not otherwise specified (PDDNOS) 34 children.

Table 2b
Glossary of the 7 electrophysiological parameters

A8C, A8F, A8R, A8L, A8P parameters	1: AEP amplitude > 15 μV 2: AEP amplitude between 10 and 15 μV 3: AEP amplitude < 10 μV
CF8 parameter	1: Cz > Fz AEP amplitude 2: Cz =* Fz AEP amplitude 3: Cz < Fz AEP amplitude
CRL8 parameter	1: frontocentral > temporal AEP amplitude 2: frontocentral =* temporal AEP amplitude 3: frontocentral < temporal AEP amplitude

* AEP were considered equal when amplitude difference was less than 2 μV.

Correspondence analysis carried out on the 13 items of the BSE-R scale produced five interpretable factors which accounted for 66.9 % of total variance. Factor I (17.4 %) mainly opposed relationship (item IGN) and attention disturbances (item ATT). Factor II (15.9 %) revealed the association of perceptive disturbances (item AUD) and stereotyped behaviours (item STE). Factor III (12.8 %) was essentially a perception factor (item AUD). Factor IV (11.4 %) opposed attention disturbances (item ATT) and stereotyped behaviours (item STE). Finally, Factor V (9.4 %) opposed verbal communication disorders (item VOI) and imitation problems (item IMI).

The first three main factors, produced by correspondence analysis, served as the input of the cluster analysis in place of the 13 original variables. We retained two solutions on the basis of statistical criteria: a four cluster solution and a seven cluster solution. The proportion of variance accounted for by the four cluster solution was 49.7 % and by the seven cluster solution 65.9 %. The behavioural profiles of the four groups of children (G1, G2, G3 and G4) are illustrated in Figure 1a and those of the seven groups of children (g1, g2, g3, g4, g5, g6 and g7) in Figure 1b.

Group G1 (67 children, age 63 months, IQ 35) was distinguished on all 13 items by the severity of the

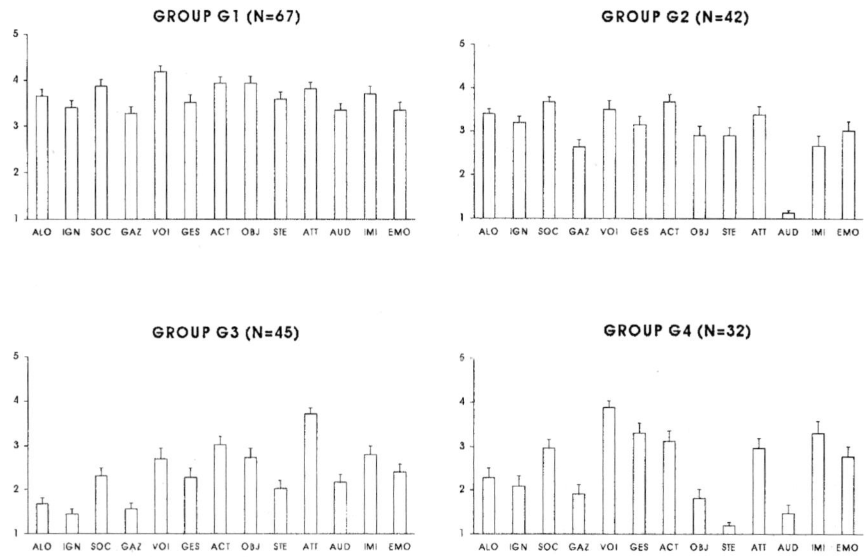

Fig. 1a
Graphic representation of the behavioural profiles which emerged from the four cluster solution via the mean (and SEM) of the initial 13 behaviour items.

disorders. Group G2 (42 children, age 75 months, IQ 47) was differentiated from group G1 primarily by the absence of auditory disorders (item AUD). Groups G3 (45 children, age 60 months, IQ 47) and G4 (32 children, age 62 months, IQ 44) had fewer behavioural disorders than the other groups, involving primarily relationship disorders (items IGN, ALO), but their profiles were very different. Group G3 was characterised by greater attention disturbances (item ATT). On the other hand, group G4 had mainly verbal communication problems (item VOI), but showed neither stereotyped behaviours (item STE) nor auditory disorders (item AUD). There was no significant age difference between the four groups. Groups G2 and G3, however, had a significantly higher IQ than group G1.

The study of the seven cluster solution made it possible to interpret how the clustering algorithm was produced. First, group G1 (homogeneous disorders) was composed of only group g2 (67 children). Group G2 (no auditory disorders) was composed of group g3 (27 children) and group g4 (15 children); these groups were different for items OBJ, ATT and IMI. Group G3 (marked attention disturbances) was composed of group g1 (31 children) and group g7 (14 children); these groups were identical only for items STE and ATT. Group G4 (main verbal communication disorders) was composed of group g5 (21 children) and group g6 (11 children); these groups were different for item AUD.

Study II

This involved 145 developmentally-disordered children (106 boys, 39 girls), between 25 and 146 months of age (mean 65, SEM 1.9 months). The intelligence quotient (IQ), determined with standardised tests (Brunet and Lézine, 1976), ranged from 15 to 85 (mean 48, SEM 1.5). The children were diagnosed according to DSM-III R criteria (APA, 1987): autistic disorder (AD) 73 children, mental retardation (MR) 38 children, pervasive developmental disorders not otherwise specified (PDDNOS) 34 children. The children included in this study had mild neurological signs but no EEG abnormalities.

Correspondence analysis was carried out on 13 variables: 6 of the 13 items of the BSE-R scale, i.e., the 6 behavioural items which described the first five main factors extracted in study I (Table 1, items: IGN, VOI, STE, ATT, AUD and IMI), and 7 electrophysiological parameters. It produced three interpretable factors which accounted for 54.3 % of total variance. Factor I (26.3 %) revealed the association of the intensity of the disorders (items IGN, AUD, IMI, STE) and frontocentroparietal electrophysiological reactivity (parameters A8C, A8F, A8P). Factor II (16.0 %) was essentially an electrophysiological factor. Factor III (12.0 %) revealed the association of attention disturbances (item ATT) and frontal electrophysiological reactivity (parameters CF8, A8F).

These three main factors produced by correspondence analysis served as the input of the cluster analysis in place of the 13 original variables. We retained a four cluster solution; the proportion of variance accounted for by this solution was 53.9 %. The behavioural and electrophysiological profiles of the four groups of children, C1, C2, C3 and C4, are illustrated in Figure 2.

Group C1 (30 children, age 55 months, IQ 39) was distinguished on all items of the BSE-R by the severity of the disorders. It had high AEP amplitudes at all electrode sites. Group C2 (49 children, age 66 months, IQ 44) also had high scores for all 6 behavioural items but was differentiated from group C1 primarily by fewer auditory disturbances (item AUD) and attention problems (item ATT). This group had low AEP on frontocentroparietal electrode sites (Cz, Pz and Fz); on the other hand, it had medium AEP on temporal electrode sites (T3 and T4). Groups C1 and C2 were significantly different for all five electrophysiological parameters which quantify AEP amplitudes.

Group C3 (35 children, age 76 months, IQ 51) was essentially characterised by some problems concerning verbal communication, attention and imitation (items VOI, ATT, IMI). It had low AEP at all electrode sites. Group C4 (31 children, age 61 months, IQ 57) had fewer behaviour disorders than the other groups, and only attention disturbances (item ATT). This last group had high AEP; Fz AEP amplitude was greater than that at Cz. Groups C3 and C4 were differentiated mainly by communication disorders (item VOI). Electrophysiologically, both groups were significantly different for all parameters except Pz AEP amplitude.

Fig. 1b
Graphic representation of the behavioural profiles which emerged from the seven cluster solution via the mean (and SEM) of the initial 13 behaviour items.

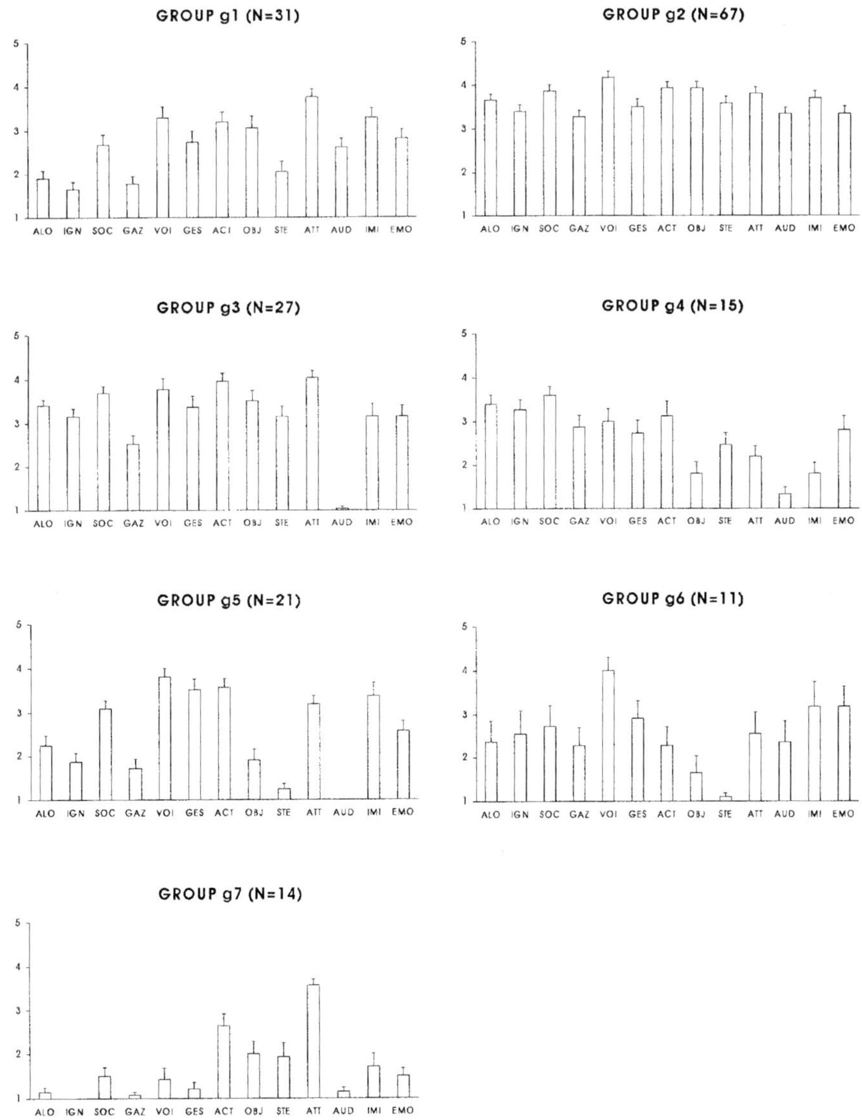

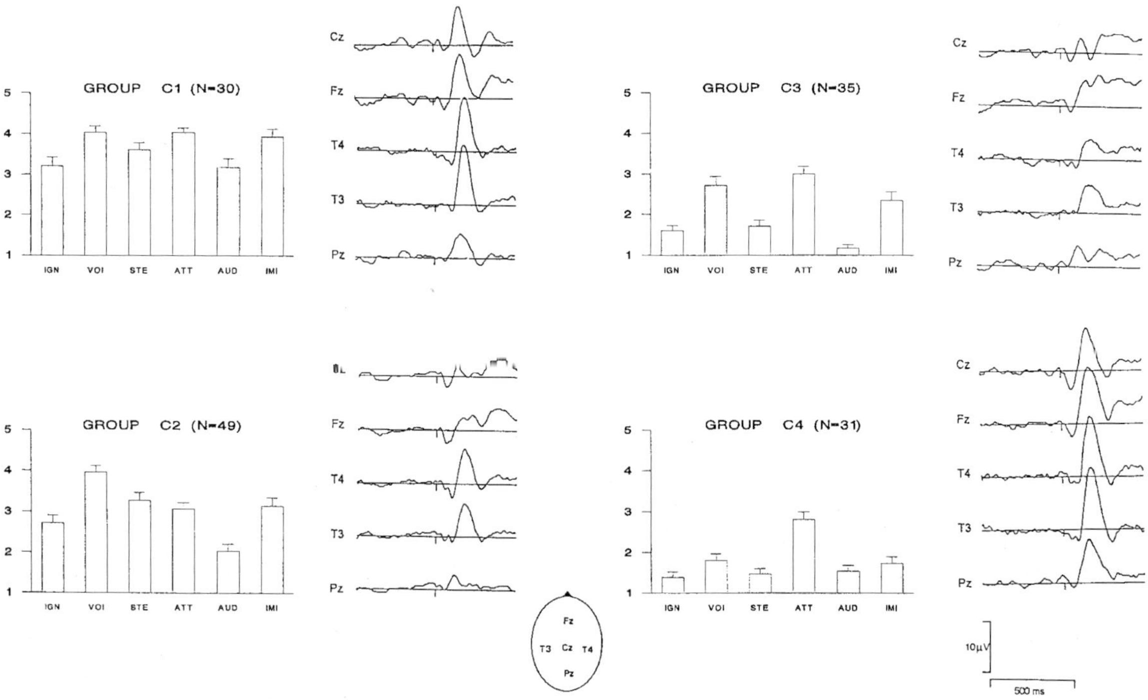

Fig. 2. Graphic representation of the behavioural and electrophysiological profiles which emerged from the four cluster solution via the mean (and SEM) of the 6 initial behaviour items on the one hand, and the grand mean AEP recorded from the 5 electrode sites on the other.

There was a significant difference between the four groups for age and IQ; group C3 was older than group C1 and groups C3 and C4 had a higher IQ than groups C1 and C2.

Thus, in the first study, correspondence analysis identified new main dimensions of behaviour, among 13 previously defined core autistic features previously extracted from the BSE-R scale (Barthélémy et al., 1997), i.e., contact (item IGN), attention (item ATT), auditory perception (item AUD), sensorimotility (item STE), imitation (item IMI) and verbal communication (item VOI). Cluster analysis following correspondence analysis, where the factor profiles serve as the input for the clustering procedure, identified several meaningful behaviour patterns. Two cluster solutions were reliable on statistical criteria and were also interpretable on clinical criteria. First, they revealed that the first main factor of correspondence analysis, which opposed relationship and attention disturbances, allowed autistic children (mainly in groups G1 and G2; 75.2%) to be dissociated from nonautistic children (mainly in groups G3 and G4; 79.2%). Factor I can thus be interpreted as an "autism factor". The subgroups were then separated, first on the basis of stereotyped behaviours and auditory disorders (Factor II, group G3 from group G4), and secondly mainly on auditory disorders (Factor III, group G1 from group G2). Finally, the study of the seven cluster solution, which was more difficult to interpret than the four cluster solution, allowed the four behaviour patterns to be refined and consequently to characterise smaller and more homogeneous subgroups of children. This approach allows the degree of homogeneity of the subgroups to be selected on the basis of statistical criteria, retaining different amounts of information extracted by factor analysis. The value of these methods was also discussed previously in relation to a subpopulation of 98 autistic children (Roux et al., 1995, 1997a). The factor structure of the data in this subpopulation was different from that in a larger population of developmentally-disordered children; the perceptive dimension predominated in autism (Roux et al., 1995).

Using objective statistical methods, it has thus been possible to identify data on disorder function which agree with clinical observations. These results suggest new working directions by drawing the attention of clinicians and neurophysiologists to phenomena which classical clinical investigation has overlooked. For example, the results concerning auditory perception, considered to be fundamentally involved in the autistic syndrome for many years (Ornitz and Ritvo, 1968; James and Barry, 1980; Ornitz, 1971, 1974, 1985; Grandin, 1994), have shown the necessity of developing specific assessment scales (Lenoir, 1994). Moreover, they allow more homogeneous subgroups of children to be identified objectively for further bioclinical studies, for example using neurophysiological, biochemical, genetic and/or neuroimaging information. In a parallel direction with research studies, the definition of subgroups independently of those described in the current diagnostic categories is an essential step towards the identification of early diagnosis and treatment strategies.

In the second study, relationships were identified between types of behaviour and certain patterns of electrocortical reactivity. Although these relationships were not strong, they reflect the association of the intensity of the disorders (items IGN, AUD, STE and IMI) and frontocentroparietal electrophysiological reactivity on the one hand (factor I), and attention disturbances (item ATT) and frontal electrophysiological reactivity on the other (factor III). These results were very similar to those in a subpopulation of 73 autistic children (Roux et al., 1997a). Thus, there is no real specificity of electroclinical relationships in autism, since they exist almost in the same way in a wider population of developmental disorders. Recently, we conducted another study on the same 145 developmentally-disordered children (Roux et al., 1997b) which also showed that correspondence analysis is well suited to the correlation of clinical and biological data. In this paper, the seven electrophysiological parameters previously studied were conjointly analysed with three clinical parameters which assess autistic behaviour, intellectual impairment and language and communication disorders (Hameury et al., 1995). This procedure identified two main bioclinical dimensions which reflect the association of intellectual impairment and centroparietal electrophysiological reactivity on the one hand, and autistic behaviour and temporal electrophysiological reactivity on the other. These studies, performed on large populations, provide a validation for numerous multidisciplinary studies of small samples of children. Descriptive analyses do not compete with other traditional statistical techniques; they have to be applied as techniques supplementary to other forms of analyses. These preliminary bioclinical analyses also show the interest of complementing the classical studies of clinical profiles, reviewed previously, with other relevant parameters in the biological field.

Multivariate descriptive statistical methods are first of all objective techniques which allow a more precise approach to the phenomena studied. They can do much to assist researchers and clinicians in detecting and explaining relationships among a complicated set of data. They have the advantage of deriving the classification of groups from the data set itself, without any initial working hypothesis. Owing to the fact that in the field of developmental disorders the bioclinical information to be analysed is often complex, factor analysis has proved to be an indispensable tool for extracting the main relevant tendencies from an array of data, providing a possible reduction of variables. This data reduction is helpful in aiding understanding of the structure or pattern which may be present in these complex multivariate data. Moreover, unlike principal component analysis, correspondence analysis has highly flexible data requirements. It is thus possible to gather suitable data quickly and easily, such as those obtained from rating scales. The value of such an analysis was also emphasized by Buitelaar (1991) who used it in pharmacological studies, and by Hamon et al. (1995) who applied it to clinical and electroencephalographic data. Principal component and correspondence analysis must be interpreted as complementary, rather than antagonist methods. The main limitation of multivariate statistical analysis is the number of subjects required, which can be a constraint on their use in the area of autism; clinical samples containing large numbers of autistic children are often difficult to obtain. We underline again that these techniques are too rigid, fixed or predetermined to be used as aids in the diagnostic process; more flexible techniques, such as expert systems or neural networks, should be more suitable for forming diagnostic categories.

Various handicaps or impairments, such as mental retardation, language disorders and neurological deficits, were previously considered to be involved in the heterogeneity of autism (Schopler, 1978; Wing and Gould, 1979; Rutter and Schopler, 1992). Furthermore, clinical research suggested an autistic continuum rather than a sharp boundary between core autism and noncore autistic-like groups (Wing, 1988, Waterhouse et al., 1996). Thus, the overlapping of the different diagnostic subgroups suggests that descriptive statistical methods, which do not require a initial selection of individuals such as by diagnostic category, are techniques suited to the study of populations of developmentally-disordered children. No initial hypothesis is required; on the contrary, descriptive methods can induce new hypotheses which can then be used in future analyses. The identification of more homogeneous subgroups of children would increase the deductive power of classical bioclinical studies. Such a multidimensional approach to developmental disorders thus opens new and interesting perspectives for further pathophysiological, bioclinical and therapeutic studies.

References

American Psychiatric Association (1987) Diagnostic and statistical manual of mental disorders 3rd edn revised. American Psychiatric Association, Washington, DC

Barthélémy C, Bruneau N, Adrien JL, Roux S, Lelord G (1990) Clinical, biological and therapeutic applications of the functional analysis of autistic disorders. Brain Dysfunct 3: 271-284

Barthélémy C, Lelord G (1991) Les échelles d'évaluation clinique en psychiatrie de l'enfant. Expansion Scientifique Française, Paris

Barthélémy C, Roux S, Adrien JL, Hameury L, Guérin P, Garreau B, Lelord G (1997) Validation of the revised Behaviour Summarized Evaluation scale (BSE-R). J Autism Dev Disord 27: 137-151

Benzécri JP (1969) Statistical analysis as a tool to make patterns emerge from data. In: Watanabe S (ed) Methodologies of pattern recognition. New York Academic Press, p 35-74

Benzécri JP (1973) L'analyse des données, Tome I: La Taxinomie, Tome II: L'analyse des correspondances. Dunod, Paris

Bruneau N, Roux S, Garreau B, Lelord G (1985) Frontal auditory evoked potentials and augmenting-reducing. Electroencephalogr Clin Neurophysiol 62: 364-371

Bruneau N, Garreau B, Roux S, Lelord G (1987) Modulation of auditory evoked potentials with increasing stimulus intensity in autistic children. In: Johnson RJ, Parasuraman R, Rohrbaugh JW (eds) Current trends in event-related potential research (EEG suppl 40). Elsevier, Amsterdam, p 584-589

Bruneau N, Barthélémy C, Martineau J, Adrien JL, Garreau B, Muh JP, Lelord G (1990) Clinical, electrophysiological, and biochemical markers and monoaminergic hypotheses in autism. In: Rothenberger A (ed) Brain and behavior in child psychiatry. Springer International, Berlin, p 217-234

Brunet O, Lézine I (1976) Echelle de développement psychomoteur de le première enfance. Le développement psychologique de la première enfance, 2nd edn. PUF, Paris

Buitelaar JK (1991) Psychopharmacology of autism. Utrecht, Nederland

Campbell M, Overall JE (1989) Diagnostic criteria and behavior patterns in infantile autism. Psychopharmacol Bull 25: 194-197

Dahl EK, Cohen DJ, Provence S (1986) Atypical development: DSMIII and the pervasive developmental disorders of early onset. J Am Acad Child Psychiat 26: 170-180

Eaves LC, Ho HH, Eaves DM (1994) Subtypes of autism by cluster analysis. J Autism Dev Disord 24: 3-22

Everitt BS (1989) Statistical methods for medical investigations. Oxford University Press, New York

Farmer EF, McGuffin P, Spitznagel EL (1983) Heterogeneity in schizophrenia: a cluster analytic approach. Psychiat Res 8: 1-12

Fein D, Waterhouse L, Lucci D, Snyder D (1985) Cognitive subtypes in developmentally disabled children: a pilot study. J Autism Dev Disord 15: 77-95

Frankel F, Hanna GL, Cantwell DP, Shekim W, Ornitz E (1992) Cluster analysis of child behavior checklists of 6 to 11 year old males with varying degrees of behavior disorders. Child Psychiat Human Dev 23: 69-85

Grandin T (1994) Ma vie d'autiste. Odile Jacob, Paris

Hameury L, Roux S, Barthélémy C, Desombre H, Sauvage D, Garreau B, Lelord G (1995) Quantified multidimensional assessment of autism and other pervasive developmental disorders. Apllication for bioclinical research. Eur Child Adolesc Psychiat 4: 123-135

Hamon JF, Juan de Mendoza JL, Camara PA (1995) Trypanosomiase: Détermination de groupes de patients à partir de données cliniques et électroencéphalographiques. Neurophysiol Clin 25:196-202

Hoffman DL, Franke GR (1986) Correspondence analysis: graphical representation of categorical data in marketing research. J Marketing Res 23: 213-227

James AL, Barry RJ (1980) A review of psychophysiology in early onset psychosis. Schizophrenia Bull 6: 506-525

Lebart L, Morineau A, Fénelon JP (1979) Traitement des données statistiques. Méthodes et programmes. Dunod, Paris

Lebart L, Morineau A, Warwick KM (1984) Multivariate descriptive statistical analysis: correspondence analysis and related techniques for large matrices. John Wiley, New York

Lelord G, Barthélémy C, Martineau J, Bruneau N, Garreau B, Hameury L (1991) Free acquisition, free imitation, physiological curiosity and exchange and development therapies in autistic children. Brain Dysfunct 4: 335-347

Lenoir P (1994) L'audition chez l'enfant autiste. Etude clinique et électrophysiologique des fonctions de perception et d'association transmodale. Thèse Université Paris VI

Ornitz EM (1971) Childhood autism: A disorder of sensorimotor integration. In Rutter M (ed) Infantile autism: concepts, characteristics and treatment. Churchill Livingstone, London, p 50-68

Ornitz EM (1974) The modulation of sensory input and motor output in autistic children. J Autism Child Schiz 4: 197-215

Ornitz EM (1985) Neurophysiology of infantile autism. J Am Acad Child Psychiat 24: 251-262

Ornitz EM, Ritvo ER (1968) Perceptual inconstancy in early infantile autism. Arch Gen Psychiat 18: 76-98

Overall JE, Gibson JM, Novy DM (1993) Population recovery capabilities of 35 cluster analysis methods. J Clin Psychol 49: 459-470

Prior MR, Boulton D, Gajzago C, Perry D (1975) The classification of childhood psychoses by numerical taxonomy. J Child Psychol Psychiat 16: 321-330

Rescola L (1988) Cluster analytic identification of autistic preschoolers. J Autism Dev Disord 18: 475-492

Rimland B (1971) The differenciation of childhood psychosis: an analysis of checklist for 2218 psychotic children. J Autism Child Schiz 1: 161-174

Roux S, Malvy J, Bruneau N, Garreau B, Guérin P, Sauvage D, Barthélémy C (1995) Identification of behaviour profiles within a population of autistic children using multivariate statistical methods. Eur Child Adolesc Psychiat 4: 249-258

Roux S, Adrien JL, Bruneau N, Garreau B, Couturier G, Gomot M, Barthélémy C (1997a) Classification of autistic syndrome using behavioural and electrophysiological assessment. Dev Brain Dysfunct 10: 28-39

Roux S, Bruneau N, Garreau B, Guérin P, Adrien JL, Dansart P, Gomot M, Barthélémy C (1997b) Bioclinical profiles of autism and other developmental disorders using a multivariate statistical approach. Biol Psychiat in press

Rutter M, Schopler E (1987) Autism and pervasive developmental disorders: concepts and diagnostic issues. J Autism Dev Disord 17: 159-186

Rutter M, Schopler E (1992) Classification of pervasive developmental disorders: some concepts and practical considerations. J Autism Dev Disord 22: 459-482

Salstone R, Fraboni M (1990) An empirical demonstration of the problem of cluster dissimilarity from different clustering methods in a single sample. J Clin Psychol 46: 930-933

Schopler E (1978) On confusion in the diagnosis of autism. J Autism Dev Disord 8: 137-138

Sevin JA, Matson JL, Coe D, Love SR, Matese MJ, Benavidez DA (1995) Empirically derived subtypes of pervasive developmental disorders: a cluster analytic study. J Autism Dev Disord 25: 561-578

Sherman M, Shapiro T, Glassman M (1983) Play and language in developmentally disorded preschoolers: a new approach to classification. J Am Acad Child Psychiat 22: 511-524

Siegel B, Anders TF, Ciaranello RD, Bienenstock B, Kraemer HC (1986) Empirically derived subclassification of the autistic syndrome. J Autism Dev Disord 16: 275-293

Skinner HA, Blashfield RK (1982): Increasing the impact of cluster analysis research: the case of psychiatric classification. J Consult Clin Psychol 50:727-735.

Szatmari P, Bartolucci G, Bremmer R (1989) Asperger's syndrome and autism: comparison of early history and outcome. Dev Med Child Neurol 31: 709-720

Waterhouse L, Morris R, Allen D, Dunn M, Fein D, Feinstein C, Rapin I, Wing L (1996) Diagnosis and classification in autism. J Autism Dev Disord 26: 59-86

Wing L, Gould J (1979) Severe impairments of social interaction and association abnormalities in children: epidemiology and classification. J Autism Dev Disord 9: 11-29

Wing L (1988) The continuum of autistic characteristics. In: Schopler E, Mesibov G. (eds) Diagnosis and assessment in Autism. Plenum Press, New York, p 91-110

Perspectives

B. GARREAU

At the end of this book, one might have the impression of a gap between the current technical possibilities of investigation in child psychiatry and the actual findings. Most studies have been done on groups and benefit to individuals does not yet appear evident. At least four factors may explain this breach between the progress in neuroimaging and its clinical consequence.

1. The various methods described in this book are being applied to children. Regardless of the procedure adopted, their use may create human problems, in addition to the ethical questions obviously raised. These examinations are currently being carried out on ever younger children, where parents are often in the process of coping with a serious diagnosis and its consequences for their personal and family lives. Accepting to undergo testing which may confirm a dread diagnosis and thereby increase their moral suffering can be very difficult at this time.

Moreover, as explained in the first chapters of this book, interpretation of the findings is intimately linked to the age of the patient, i.e. the stage of cerebral development. Although psychologists have described in great detail the main steps of normal development, relatively few brain imaging or neurophysiological studies have been devoted to the developmental process. This is particularly the case in pathology, where the functional consequences of abnormal development of the central nervous system are difficult to interpret. This may explain the caution of many authors.

2. Psychiatrists are not yet aware of the clinical utility of these methods. Morphological and functional imaging of the central nervous system has yielded considerable advances in physiology and pathology, especially in neurology. Electroencephalography, computed tomography and magnetic resonance imaging have proved their worth in the study of epilepsy, in vascular, neoplastic and degenerative pathology, in both adults and in children. In spite of this, the prevalent school of thought and, to a lesser extent, of knowledge among psychiatrists, and especially among those working with children and teenagers, does not yet incline them to use these methods which could nevertheless open up a considerable field of investigation in pathophysiology, diagnosis and treatment. Today many psychiatrists still hesitate to carry out examinations they consider useless for diagnosis and management of the specific patient.

3. The development of tools for clinical assessment is relatively slow. The small number of significant, reproducible and comparable results obtained by neuroimaging and neurophysiological techniques in developmental psychiatry is often due to the imprecise boundaries of diagnosic categories. It was not until the publication of the third edition of the Diagnostic Statistical Manual (DSM III) by the American Psychiatric Association (APA)in 1984, and the ninth edition of the International Classification of Disease (ICD IX) by the World Health Organization (WHO) that the scientific community had at is disposal unanimously recognised diagnostic criteria for the major childhood psychiatric syndromes. These criteria were broadened in the revised edition of the DSM III (DSM III R) in 1987 and further defined by the APA in the fourth edition (DSM IV) of 1994 and in the ICD X by the WHO. Thus it has been possible to compare neuroimaging and developmental neurophysiological findings obtained by various research groups for only a few years. In addition to these diagnostic criteria defined by international classifications, a certain number of specific assessment instruments have been developed for each syndrome.

4. Comparative studies are also difficult to conduct because of rapid changes in methodology and this is even more true of longitudinal studies. Position emission tomography has been widely employed for scarcely ten years and functional MRI

may be supplanting it. At the same time, existing machines have been constantly improved. With the latest generation of cameras we are able to detect and assess phenomena not measurable with the earlier ones. This is also true for quantitative EEG recording and processing methods.

In spite of these restrictions and limitations, imaging methods are of great value for the study of morphological, functional and neurophysiological development. There is no doubt about their value and the need for their widespread use in developmental psychiatry.

Progress in neuroimaging and in clinical observation methods, and co-operation between these two fields should enable them to benefit mutually from improved sensitivity and new possibilities. In clinical practice a morphological or functional imaging method is not an end in itself, but an essential tool to be used to prove or disprove a hypothesis. It is clear that "typical images" of childhood autism or hyperkinetic syndromes do not exist. But different images or neurophysiological features may be observed in children of the same age showing similar clinical pictures. Changes in the images or other features of the same child may also be detected in the course of development. This is why clinical data should not be limited to a nosological diagnosis, but should also include the results of assessment and testing of functions related to the imaging protocol. Ideally, these tests and neuroimaging should be carried out during the learning process. The aim could be to study a function or a strategy in a control group as compared to children with a given disorder regardless of their clinical picture, or the definition of subgroups with different features within a single syndrome.

Concurrently, methodological progress is under way in the field of cerebral investigations. The need for guidelines for choosing the appropriate imaging or developmental physiological exploration method is evident. On one hand, we should keep in mind the excellent results obtained using electrophysiological methods in the study of the temporal progression of a single task. And on the other, the fine analysis made possible by functional MRI and the remarkable anatomical-functional resolution of PET are essential for the definition of homogeneous clinical groups. Moreover, an increasing number of research groups is using complementary morphological and functional methods, for example, containing MRI with PET, SPECT or cerebral electrophysiology. For example we know the value of coupling of MRI and recordings of evoked potentials, to determine the origin of their components. Finally, we should not overlook the future contribution of methods yet to be used in developmental psychiatry such as functional MRI or magnetoencephalography.

The implementation, development and use of all these methods require collaborative programmes at two levels. First, close contact between clinicians, radiologists, neuropsychologists, physiologists, engineers, technicians, etc, is essential. Considering the cost of most current methods, this cross disciplinary approach should be implemented in specialised centres so as to carry out methodological studies and to define clinical applications. The work done in these centres should optimise the use of expensive equipment and avoid the unnecessary cost of numerous anarchic poorly-adapted sites. Second, national and international networks could enable complementary groups specialised in major pathologies to share and standardise examination protocols.

Morphological and functional imaging and developmental neurophysiology methods should potentially have repercussions in three fields: diagnosis, pathophysiology and treatment.

The most immediate contribution is to aid early diagnosis, particularly in child psychiatry, since most of these methods can be used with very young children. At this age the symptoms and signs are often subtle and mild. As a result, it is often difficult to differentiate between major, long lasting pathology and simple developmental delay. Functional imaging and development neurophysiological methods are now considered sufficiently sensitive and precise to confirm a differential diagnosis. This should lead to early intervention and appropriate treatment.

These methods will unquestionably make a considerable contribution to the neurophysiological approach to developmental psychiatry. The simultaneous use of functional tests and imaging methods is necessary to detect defects in functional anatomical systems. As mentioned in the introduction to this book, neuroimaging is at the interface between behavioural studies and basic biology. In this context, it can orientate genetic studies seeking candidate genes in certain developmental disorders. Subsequently, studies involving functional imaging and digital video will be very well suited to the study of psychomotor pathology, for example, postural defect, stereotyped and behaviour motor tics, etc.

The therapeutic utility of functional imaging and neurophysiologal methods is clear at two levels. First, for example, detecting a nonfunctional region of the cortex could have consequencies for a child's management. Should we implement only speech therapy for a child lacking language if he also shows cortical hypometabolism, or should teaching other means of communication also be recommended? Second, all child psychiatrists know the random nature of response to psychotropic drugs. Children with the same clinical picture may or may not respond to a particuliar medication, but why? Labelling receptors of the major neurochemical systems may answer this major question with immediate and concrete results for the children.

In conclusion, our intention in this book is to underline the sensitivity of various methods which may be applied during the course of cerebral development and to describe several current applications through the experience of representative research teams. In spite of the high initial cost of state of the art technical equipment, long-term benefits in term of diagnostic aid, screening, and therapeutic orientation are such that they should limit the consequences of handicapping conditions and lead in the long run to savings on health expenditures. During the next few years the applications and repercussions of each of these exploratory methods will become more clearly defined. The advances that we hope for and expect will be the fruit of our active collaboration with clinicians.

Index

D

E

G

H

I

J

K

L

N

O

P

X

COLOUR ILLUSTRATIONS APPENDIX

Part One

1. Cerebral development and neurophysiological investigations

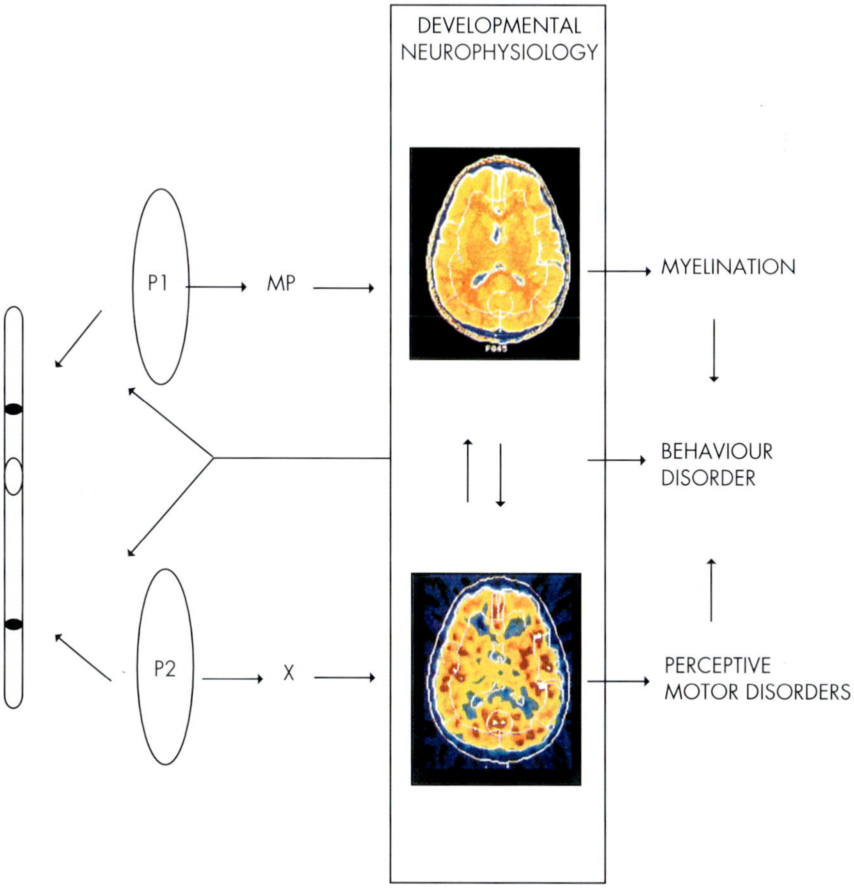

Fig. 7
Morphological and functional explorations are at the croossroads between clinical expression and more basic cell and molecular disorder.

Part One

8. Auditory evoked potentials (n1 wave) as indices of cortical development

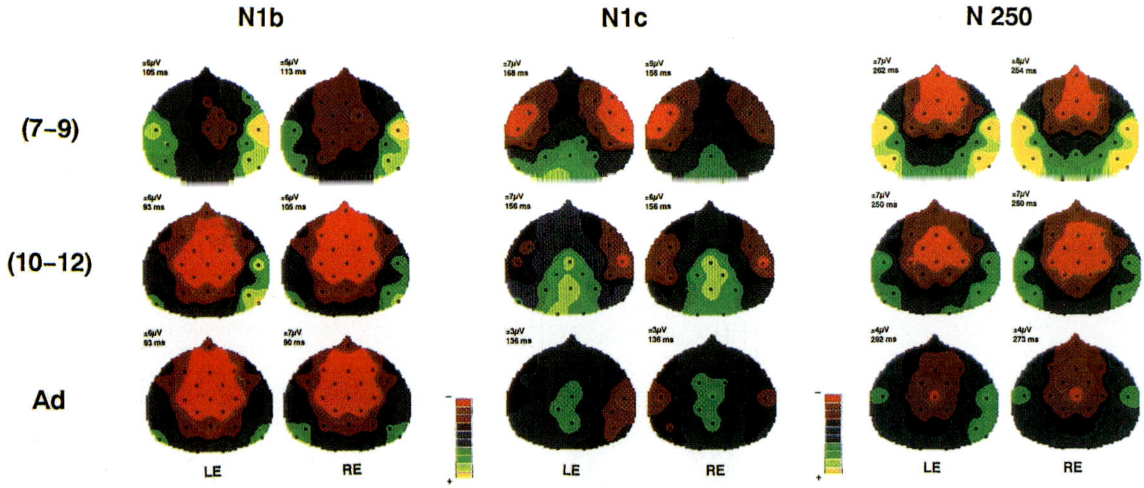

Fig. 2. Mean scalp potential distribution of N1b, N1c and N 250 to left ear (LE) and right ear (RE) tone stimuli in 8 children aged 7- 9-years, 8 children aged 10- 12 years and 8 adults.
Maps are plotted at the peak latency at the vertex for N1b and at the peak latency at the temporal site (T3, T4) contralateral to the ear stimulated for N1c.
For N 250, maps are plotted at the peak latency at Fz in children aged 7-9 and at the peak latency at Cz in children aged 10-12 and in adults.

Part Two

2. SPECT studies in subjects with Tourette's Syndrome

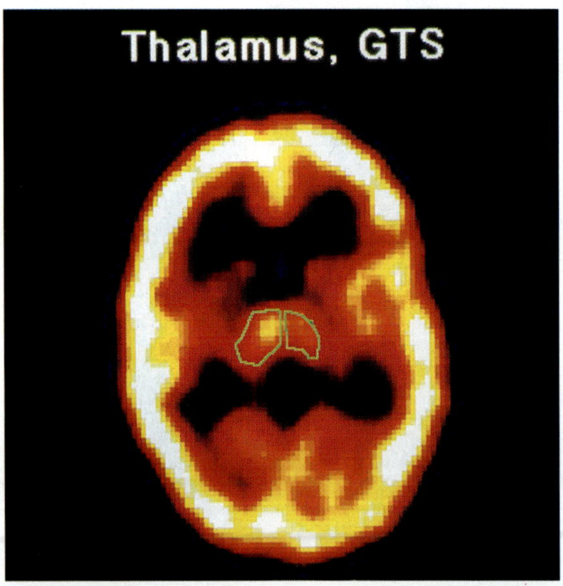

Fig. 2. SPECT of 13-year old boy with TS and ADHD and decreased number of pixels in left thalamus.

Part Two

3. Electrical brain activity and motor control in Tourette's syndrome and attention deficit hyperactivity disorder

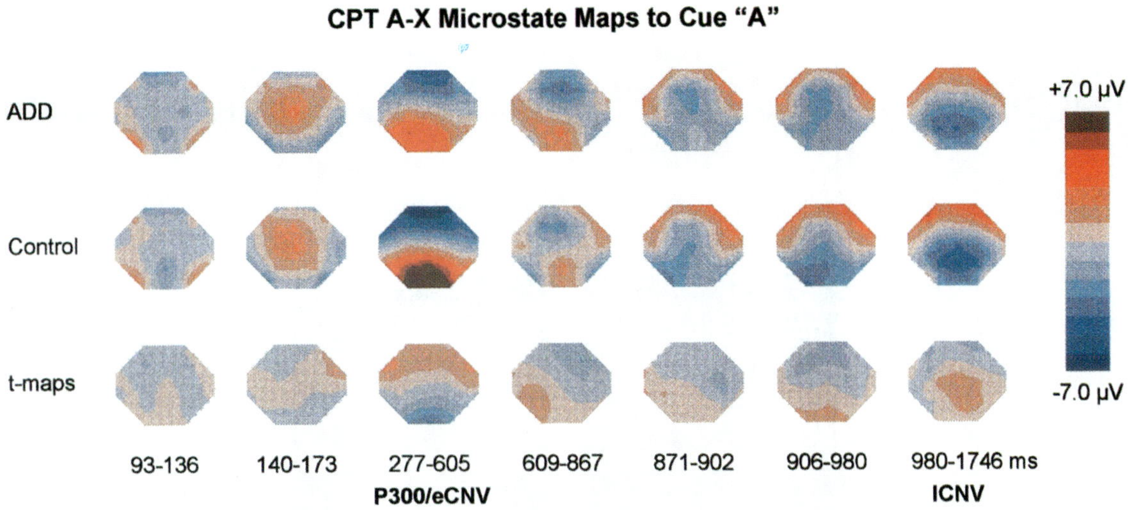

Fig. 3. Sequence of microstates and t-maps evoked by warning cue letter. Upper row shows the microstates for ADD (n = 11), middle row those for the control children (n = 9), lower row the t-maps for ADD minus control children.
Note: Inversion of positivity/negativity from early CNV to late CNV. Significant differences between groups at occipital area for early CNV.

Part Two

6. Functional brain imaging studies in childhood autism

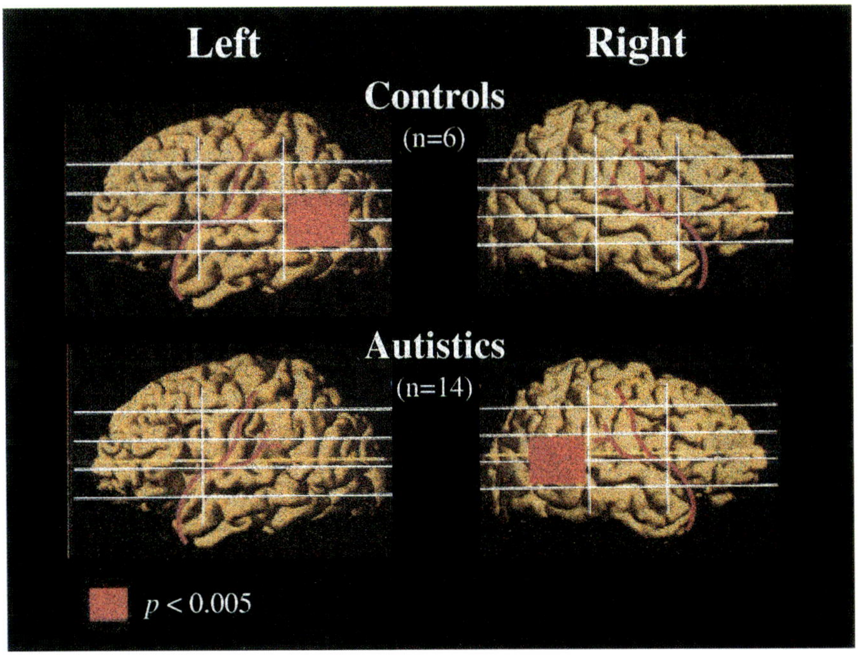

Fig. 1
A simple nonverbal auditory stimulus induced a significant rCBF increase in the left temporo-occipital cortex in control children (top) and in the right temporo-occipital cortex in autistic children (bottom).

Part Two

6. Functional brain imaging studies in childhood autism

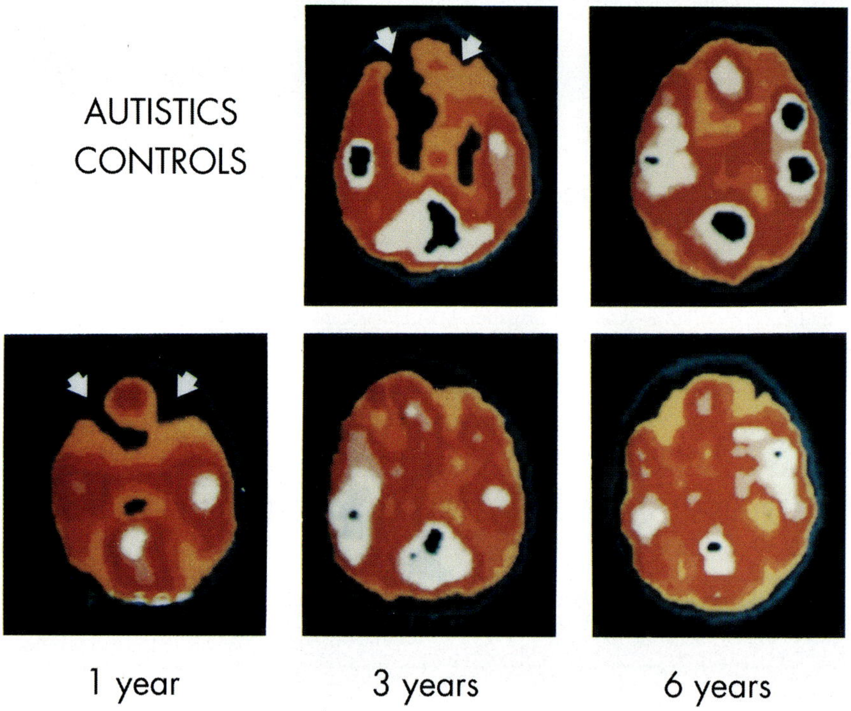

Fig. 2
SPECT rCBF images illustrating transient frontal hypoperfusion observed in autistic children.
(Top): An autistic child examined at 3 years and at 6 years. At the first examination we observed clear-cut bilateral frontal hypoperfusion (white arrows), while the later examination was a normal.
(Bottom): Three normal children's SPECT images obtained at different stages of development, indicating that frontal hypoperfusion is present at the age of one year (white arrows) but that the frontal lobes show a normal perfusion pattern by the age of three years.

Part Two

8. EEG investigations in autistic children

Fig. 1
Grand averages of topographical mapping of spectral power of EEG bands for 17 normal (left) and 17 autistic children (right). Significant differences between the two groups in spectral power in the alpha band are observed for all leads (from Garreau, 1994).

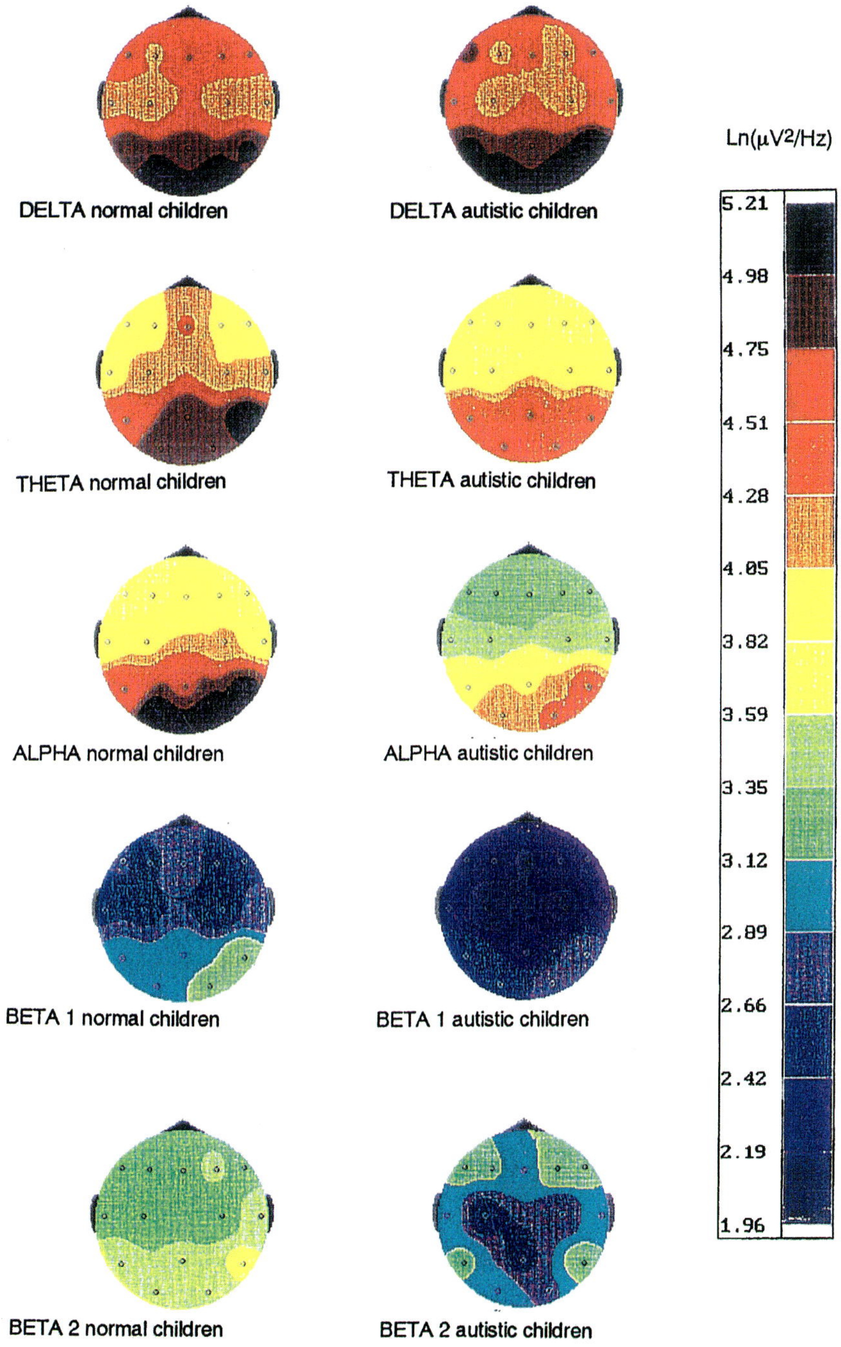

Part Two

8. EEG investigations in autistic children

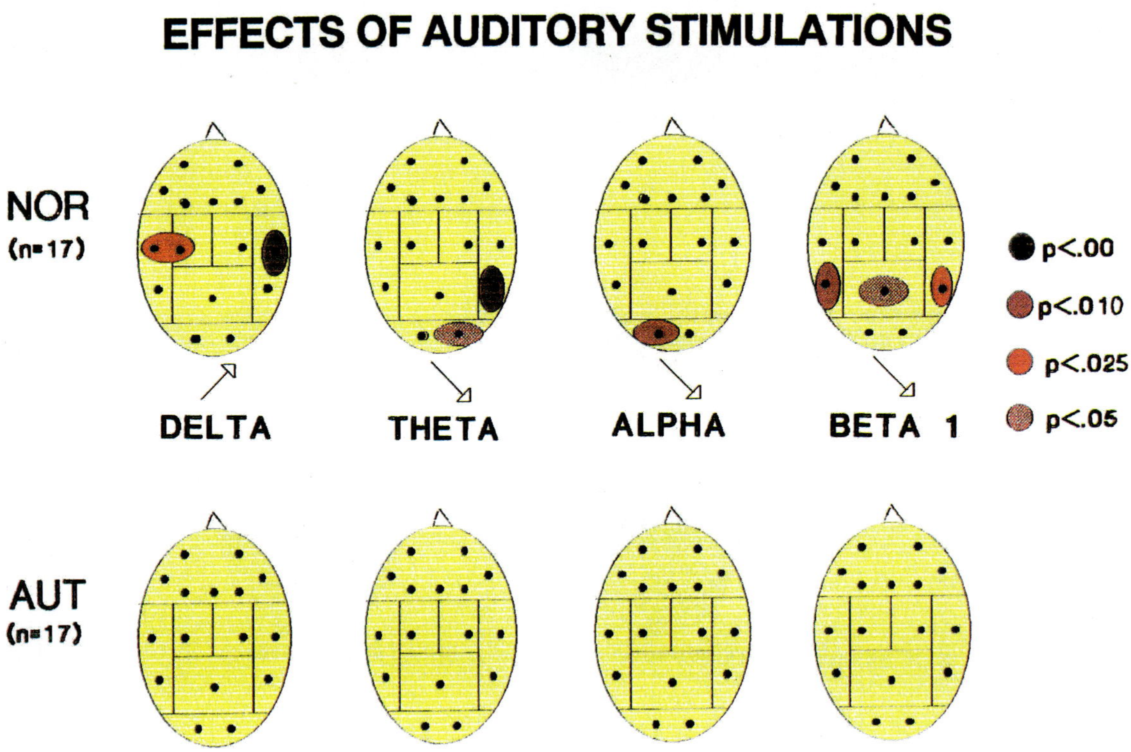

Fig. 2. Effects of auditory stimulation on the qEEG. In normal children, auditory stimulation increased spectral power in the delta band and decreased it in the theta, alpha and beta bands in both hemispheres. No such change was observed in autistic children (from Garreau, 1994).

Part Two

9. Neuroimaging in eating disorders in young people

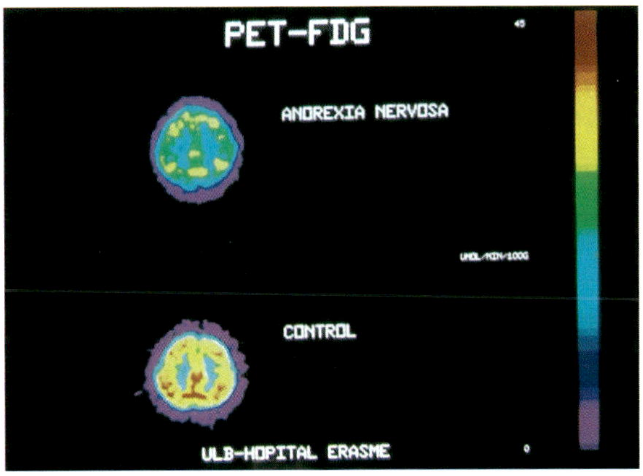

Fig. 1. Superior horizontal tomographic slice passing through the frontal and parietal cortices from an anorectic patient (upper slice) and a control subject (lower slice).
Absolute global and regional glucose cerebral hypometabolism was observed in anorectic patient.